EDGEWISE ORTHODONTICS

RAYMOND C. THURSOW, B.S., D.D.S., F.A.C.D.

Madison, Wisconsin

FOURTH EDITION

With **379** illustrations

The C. V. Mosby Company

ST. LOUIS • TORONTO • LONDON 1982

MOSBY

A TRADITION OF PUBLISHING EXCELLENCE

Editor: Samuel E. Harshberger
Design: Susan Trail
Production: Debbie Wedemeier

FOURTH EDITION

Printed in the United States of America

The C.V. Mosby Company
11830 Westline Industrial Drive, St. Louis, Missouri 63141

Library of Congress Cataloging in Publication Data

Thurow, Raymond C.
Edgewise orthodontics.

Bibliography: p.
Includes index.
1. Orthodontic appliances. I. Title. [DNLM:
1. Orthodontics. WU 400 T542t]
RK528.M4T48 1981 617.6′43 81-11216
ISBN 0-8016-4947-1 AACR2

C/CB/B 9 8 7 6 5 4 3 2 03/D/303

Preface

The human face is complex by any criterion. It encompasses all of the primary interfaces between the individual and the outside world. It houses the entryways for biological energy input as well as the sensory receptors for light, smell, and taste. Sound reception is accomplished at the dorsal boundary, and the face is also provided with an exceptional concentration of touch and temperature receptors.

Outgoing communication is also centered in the face, with speech and facial expression accounting for an overwhelming share of the average individual's communication to others.

All of these functions are interrelated with facial form in an intricate choreography that begins with our genetic heritage and goes on continuously throughout our lives. The teeth lie in a major adaptation area that links torso to face, interacts with head posture, and plays an important role in the breathing function. At the same time they are directly involved in the functions of taste, speech, and reception and preparation of food.

The teeth are maintained at the center of all this action by a uniquely adaptable mechanism that reacts to the slightest change in environmental forces. The root of a tooth is the most direct mechanical pathway from the outside world to the bony skeleton to be found anywhere in the body, and dentally applied forces can elicit responses throughout the surrounding skeleton.

With the dental supporting and attachment structure so exquisitely responsive to mechanical stimuli, lying in the midst of the most variable force field in the body, the teeth are subject to an endless array of malfunctions and malpositions.

Orthodontics is the art and science of applying orthopedic stimuli to resolve those malfunctions and malpositions. The clinician superimposes carefully controlled forces designed to warp the existing force field in a manner that will stimulate a favorable response in the underlying bony support.

The Edgewise appliance is the seminal mechanism of modern orthodontic therapy, the first to provide the capability of full control in all three axes and planes of space. The principles underlying the application of the Edgewise appliance pertain not only to the countless variations of the Edgewise but also to many other appliance mechanisms of different lineage insofar as they may be used to accomplish comparable effects.

The following chapters explore the various parameters that are involved in that therapeutic process for the serious student of dentofacial orthopedic therapy, whether in school or in active practice. This is definitely *not* a cookbook for another routine treatment protocol. It *is* an analytical review of basic information that is essential to the safe and effective selection and application of any dentofacial orthopedic therapeutic modality for a particular patient.

Raymond C. Thurow

Contents

PART **I**

Engineering in dentofacial orthopedics

■ Dentofacial orthopedics is the art and science of inducing changes in the bone structure of the face, primarily by means of corrective forces introduced through the dentition. As such, it is intimately concerned with the bewildering array of forces that play continuously on the teeth and bones from the earliest stages of embryonic development and continue throughout life.

All active bone surfaces respond to the forces of their immediate environment. Sutural interfaces, including those between tooth roots and bone, are especially responsive. These provide great opportunities for improvement in the development of the face as well as the dentition during the growing years. Alveolar bone never loses its capacity to respond to environmental forces, including those which may be imposed by therapeutic appliances. This ability makes effective therapy a very real possibility at any stage of life.

With the position of each tooth from minute to minute and day to day determined entirely by the combined effects of environmental forces, it becomes obvious that a knowledge of how forces behave is essential to an adequate understanding of tooth position and its modification.

The language of forces is the language of engineering, a field usually considered to be far removed from the healing arts; but arbitrary academic barriers cannot alter the fact that biological systems enjoy no special exemption from basic physical laws.

The orthodontist is an engineering layman, and that status will not be changed by this book; but the next nine chapters will provide an orthodontically oriented review of the essential mechanical "facts of life," with the concepts and the vocabulary that are essential to a full understanding of clinical orthopedics of the face.

1

Therapeutic energy management in the dentofacial complex

Orthodontic therapy is a dentofacial orthopedic process that is accomplished by modification of the complex matrix of mechanical energy that is a part of the very life of the facial structures.

Mechanical forces influence the growth, development, shape, and function of the dentofacial complex throughout life. The multifunctional nature of this area is unique in its diversity, and all of these functions combine with the genetic program to produce and maintain a spectacular variety of human facial forms.

The objective of dentofacial orthopedic therapy for a growing child is to optimize the attainment of full genetic potential. Countless environmental influences can intervene in the progression of growth and development, often with disastrous results from the viewpoint of oral and facial health and well-being. Redirection of those processes, with timely guidance toward the most beneficial form and functional capabilities attainable within the genetic program, can do much to minimize the effects of unfavorable genetic and environmental influences.

Adult therapy can no longer influence growth; the facial structures have already achieved their full size. These structures are the foundation on which any corrective effort must be built, and treatment can still provide great benefits in optimizing form and function, even within those narrower confines.

Details of the functional and facial orthopedic aspects of therapy cover broad areas that often go well beyond the scope of this book, which is directed primarily at active therapeutic mechanisms. Physiologic considerations are the basis for all such mechanical therapy, so they are covered in considerable detail as they relate to corrective therapy.

THE THERAPEUTIC ARENA

The dentition provides unique direct mechanical access to the bony skeleton of the face. In no other part of the body is it possible to apply outside forces so directly or precisely to a bony structure. Therapeutic manipulation of the teeth is accomplished at the tissue level by the orthopedic changes that are stimulated in the underlying bone, and some of these changes can extend far beyond the dental area. Conversely, seemingly remote structures and functions can be responsible for important effects on dental relationships.

Therapeutic changes are effected by superimposing extrinsic appliances on existing structures to alter the natural energy fields by either addition or redirection of forces. Functional appliances redirect natural forces. Active appliances introduce outside forces that interact with the natural forces to stimulate the planned desirable tissue response.

The basic flow of active therapy begins with the introduction of outside forces into the appliances, which in turn store, distribute, and apply those forces to the appropriate teeth and tissues. This pattern can be represented by a simple flowchart (Fig. 1-1).

Outside forces are introduced to the appliance and processed there through the intermediate stages. In the appliance the forces are stored, distributed, and finally applied to the teeth and tissues to ultimately produce the physiologic responses to therapy.

The appliance functions as a "black box" in this scheme, with energy flowing within it in often inscrutable ways. The point of entry of a force into the system may be a long way from its often widely dispersed areas of action.

Orthodontics has always had its full measure of searchers for the "Holy Grail" of a black box that could be plugged into this system without the need for examining or understanding its inner workings. There has also been an endless succession of false prophets with claims that they have found the secret. As with all nostrums, these claims can usually demonstrate some measure of success in limited circumstances, and this provides the basis for inappropriate extrapolation.

The appeal of such standardized black boxes can be irresistible in the absence of a high level of diagnostic skill and critical analysis of their real value for a partic-

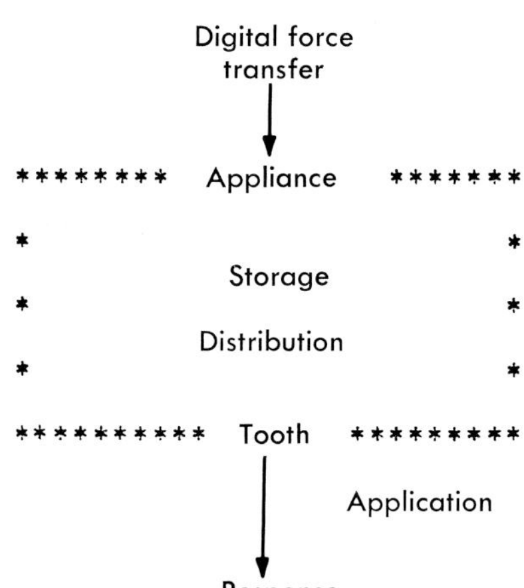

Fig. 1-1. The flow of forces in an orthodontic appliance system. Note that the tooth becomes a part of the appliance force distribution mechanism; it is the component that actually applies therapeutic forces to the responsive tissue structures.

ular patient. Most run a relatively brief cycle of several years of popularity within any given population, but may recur repeatedly in other areas that lack information on earlier experiences elsewhere.

This book is based on the thesis that a professional in the healing arts has a responsibility to know and to understand the therapy that is being used. Rather than a cookbook for pushing the buttons on a black box, it is essentially a detailed dissection—a design, engineering, and service manual—of those black boxes, intended to provide a rational basis for skilled dentofacial orthopedic therapy.

One of the greatest sources of confusion in understanding the contents of the orthodontic black box is that it is filled with components that are outwardly similar in appearance and/or function. But these components are actually so versatile that they may, by design or indirection, serve completely different functions in the operational process scheme for different situations.

The following brief descriptions of the key stages of the therapeutic process provide the basis for all later discussions. Note that the stages represent processes, not hardware. Each of these processes can be accomplished by many different mechanical means, and most appliance components are capable of performing more than one process.

Outside force: the motive power for all therapy

The term *outside* as used here means outside the immediate area of action; it may originate in nearby or remote structures.

Human muscle provides all of the motive power for dentofacial orthopedic changes in bone, including the movement of teeth. This muscle force can be classified by source into the following major categories:

1. Patient
   a. Functional forces: This is the functional environment that will be a part of the patient throughout life. It consists of the perioral musculature and all of the more remote musculature that interacts with it. These muscles produce a full-time fluid force field that may have both positive and negative effects on therapeutic efforts.
      (1) Tongue
      (2) Lips and the muscles of facial expression
      (3) Muscles of mastication and related musculature of the head and neck
   b. Extrinsic forces: More remote parts of the body may also interact mechanically with the facial area. These are primarily digital forces, applied either directly or through other objects.
      (1) Habits such as sucking, holding, and biting
      (2) Placement and activation of therapeutic appliance components
2. Therapist: The digital forces that are applied by another person account for most of the action of fixed orthodontic appliances. Each adjustment visit is an occasion for the critical selective recharging of the energy storage components of the appliance. The ultimate success of treatment is totally dependent on the skill with which this transfer of energy is accomplished.

Transfer. Transfer is the critical insertion of energy into the appliance, which converts it from a passive device to an active component of the dentofacial energy complex.

Energy transfer from its source into the appliance is usually a brief episode. With functional appliances and oral habits it may be an ongoing process, but with fixed appliances such as edgewise it is a conscious manual act. The patient places elastic components, stretching them as they are applied. The therapist activates the various components as they are placed and secured. In every situation a manual force is applied directly to one or more appliance components to accomplish the storage of energy in the appliance.

Storage. Elastic storage of applied forces is essential to the operation of all orthodontic appliances that apply corrective forces directly to the teeth. This includes all except functional appliances that are limited to deflection or redirection of perioral muscle forces.

External forces are applied episodically to recharge the mechanism. This is done every few weeks by the orthodontist or perhaps daily by the patient. It is elastic storage that keeps energy available for gradual release to stimulate the desired therapeutic changes over the period between outside applications.

Selection and design of the elastic storage components establish the key factors of *force level* and *duration,* which in turn affect patient comfort, treatment time, and adjustment intervals.

Storage components may be classified by material into two broad groups.

Elastomers. Rubber bands, other elastomeric modules, and elastic thread are typical examples.

Metals. Coil springs, free-end finger springs, archwires, and auxiliaries in endless variety are examples of metallic storage components.

Storage components may also be more specifically identified in the following classification based on configuration:

1. Rubber elastic components (applied by patient)
   a. Rubber bands are used for primary energy storage over a broad range of force levels in both intraoral and extraoral appliances.
   b. Woven elastic straps provide an alternative form of storage module in the higher force ranges required for extraoral appliances.
2. Coil springs
   a. Intraoral forces can be stored between appliance components in both compression and tension coil springs of many different physical characteristics.
   b. Heavier coil springs are also available for use instead of rubber elastics as the storage components for both intermaxillary and extraoral traction.
3. Ligatures
   a. Elastic ligatures (standard modules or tied elastic thread) may be used to store force between tooth and archwire or between teeth.
   b. Wire ligatures have negligible elasticity and storage capacity. The limited elasticity that may appear to be derived from a wire ligature is actually an effect of the elasticity of archwire or periodontal membrane that is merely transmitted by the wire ligature.
4. Archwires: Archwire elasticity covers a broad range. The lighter wires may be used as the primary energy storage module of an appliance, but the heavier wires are so stiff that they function only as distribution units while required energy storage is accomplished with other appliance components.

5. Finger springs: A wire spring with a single free end engaging a tooth is called a finger spring. These are typically used as dual-function energy storage and application components on rigid removable appliances, but they may also be used in conjunction with fixed appliances.
6. Auxiliary components: Most auxiliary appliance components are specifically designed to function as energy storage units. These are commonly formed into special-purpose springs of endless variety.
7. Patient tissues: The tissues surrounding teeth moved by outside forces store some of this force elastically.

The periodontal membrane is the major tissue component in the energy storage complex, and it is also the most important. The forces stored in the periodontal membrane are those which are gradually dispersed to the reactive subcomponents of the periodontium to induce the actual tissue changes of tooth movement.

Gingival tissues also store orthodontic forces elastically, often over an extended period of time. These stored forces are usually unwanted and frequently tend to induce rebound movements that require long-term control with retaining appliances.

Distribution. All elastic storage is accomplished by restraining the two ends of the storage unit between other appliance components. This sets up the initial stage of the distribution system. One underlying law of mechanics is inescapable: The forces at the two ends of an elastic storage unit are equal and opposite.

Either or both of these ends may be a point of initial application of force for storage, or the force may have been introduced at some remote point. Either or both ends may be a point of application of force to a specific tooth, or they may be remote from the points or areas of intended application.

Regardless of the points of input or the points of application, it is the function of the orthodontic appliance to distribute the resultant forces from all sources and storage units to either points of intended movement or over broad "anchorage" bases of teeth and tissue. Appliance components attached to storage units distribute the resultant forces to the teeth, often through other components that in turn store at least part of the force in the process.

The archwire is a primary force distribution component in most fixed appliances, even in those where it may also serve in a storage mode. Removable appliances and auxiliaries may serve either or both functions. The sometimes bizarre configurations and multifunctional applications required to achieve desired force parameters in a structure that will fit into the oral environment make identification and control of specific functions and ultimate force levels and applications a most challenging undertaking.

Application. Force application is the process that transfers the force from the black box appliance through the tooth to the supporting tissues. The tooth/appliance interface where the initial transfer occurs may take many forms. Any positive contact between tooth and appliance will result in a transfer of force that will continue until the contact force diminishes to zero. The contact then becomes functionally nonexistent. Negative force application may also be accomplished by some appliances that disengage the natural contact between tongue or labiobuccal tissues and teeth.

Fixed attachments, such as those used in the edgewise appliance, modify the contours of the teeth to provide discrete precise points for the transfer of force from the elastic appliance components to the teeth. These precise interfaces facilitate the force transfer and provide essential directional control for this critical transfer process.

Response. The ultimate response of changes in the form of facial structures is the objective of the entire therapeutic process. Those changes may be local alterations in alveolar walls or more remote responses in sutures and other related tissues, but all are the result of physiologic responses within the structure of the dentofacial complex to the forces that are injected into the supporting bone by the roots of the teeth.

INTEGRATING THE OVERALL PROCESS

The preceding is the essence of dentofacial orthopedic therapy. Integrating these processes to produce a beneficial effect for the individual patient is what orthodontics is all about. That can only be accomplished with a full understanding of the interplay of mechanics and physiology, the mechanism and the patient.

No one component of the overall process can be singled out as most important because none can stand alone and all are important. That includes, above all, an understanding of the black box that is the orthodontic appliance, and its interaction with the living tissues of the dentofacial complex. No patient's welfare should ever be abandoned to the uncontrolled or unsupervised myriad forces unleashed by these devices, regardless of their apparent simplicity or sophistication.

2

Ever-balanced forces

Orthodontics, like all of dentistry, is continually involved in the subject of *balance.* Balanced occlusion is a most familiar term to all dentists, but it has a much broader meaning for the natural dentition than the rigid mechanical syntheses of prosthetics. Living teeth maintain a dynamic balance with their ever-changing environment that goes far beyond a simple cusp/condyle/fossa relationship.

Balance is a part of all of life. Chemical balance, fluid balance, and mechanical balance are in continuous operation at all levels from the subcellular unit to the total organism and its environment. The awakening interest in ecology is a recognition on a broader scale of these principles, which are so familiar to the orthodontist in the more circumscribed environment of the head and neck.

All of these influences are important to the dentition, but in orthodontics mechanical balance takes on a special significance. The dentition is essentially a mechanical device with mechanical functions, and dentistry is concerned directly with the maintenance, improvement, or restoration of that mechanism.

Orthodontics is mostly concerned with improvement, by repositioning the individual components for improved health, efficiency, and longevity. The accomplishment of this orthodontic improvement requires even deeper involvement in mechanics than most other dental procedures, because it depends heavily on *actively working* mechanical devices that bring movement and variable forces into the picture.

Restorative dentistry is primarily an exercise in structural engineering, building or rebuilding to provide static resistance to the forces of occlusion. Rigidity, strength, and durability are the prime considerations. Load distribution on teeth and tissues is an important consideration, but primarily in the very special situations that require optimum distribution of overloads on teeth carrying more than their normal load. Orthodontics uses working mechanisms that actually store and introduce supplementary forces, superimposing them on the natural forces already acting on the teeth. Resiliency rather than rigidity is the first consideration, with requirements for strength and durability greatly reduced.

But mechanics and its preoccupation with forces is only half the story. Orthodontic and functional dental forces operate in a reactive, living environment that is extremely sensitive to their influences. Forces *within* these tissues are just as important as those in the orthodontic mechanisms themselves, for it is at this tissue level that actual orthodontic response takes place.

Successful orthodontic therapy cannot be based on either physiology or mechanics alone; it is the end result of the *combined effects* of all of these internal and external actions and reactions, with the outcome finally expressed in the deceptively simple phenomenon of tooth movement.

BALANCE AND FREE-BODY ANALYSIS

All considerations of tooth position and positioning revolve around the element of *balance.* Supporting tissues adjust continuously to maintain balance with environmental forces. Environmental forces in turn are always in balance with each other and with the resisting stresses and strains within the tissues.

This predictable state of balance provides the basis for application of free-body analysis, a powerful analytical tool in the planning and execution of orthodontic treatment.

The basic idea of free-body analysis is that in a static system of forces, such as an orthodontic appliance and associated teeth, all forces must always be in balance. In this system there is no movement other than tooth movement or other slow physiologic changes, so that at any given time the entire complex can be considered to be in a state of static equilibrium. If there were any unbalanced force in a system such as this, something would move in response to it. The fact that nothing is moving proves that all forces are in balance, and this makes it possible to determine what forces are at work and in what direction they are operating. The basic requirement for static analysis is that *there must be no movement within the system.*

Balanced linear forces

All linear forces must be in balance. The principles necessary to an understanding of most orthodontic situations can be illustrated by the simple teeter-totter shown in Fig. 2-1. Here a 50-pound child at one end is balancing a 100-pound child at the other end in a very familiar situation. We know the weights of the children, and from this we can determine all the other operating forces. For simplicity, the weight of the board will be ignored, just as the weight of the appliance is ignored in the mouth.

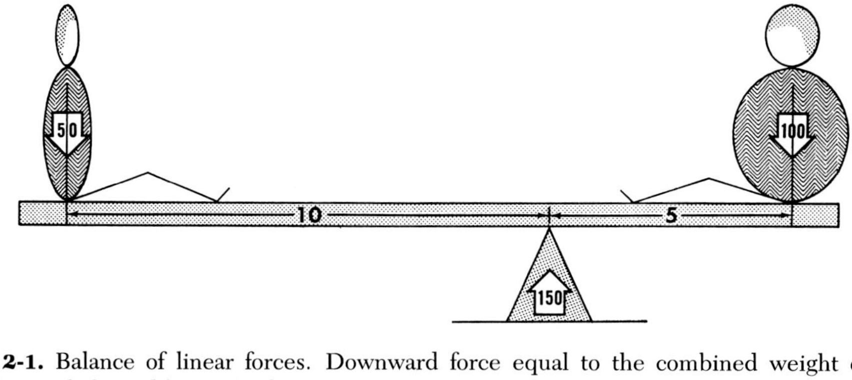

Fig. 2-1. Balance of linear forces. Downward force equal to the combined weight of the children is balanced by upward force at support.

The board is in balance as it is illustrated. Every force acting on it is balanced by an equal and opposite force. The most obvious forces, acting in a downward direction, are the weights of the two children. These are balanced by a less obvious upward resisting force under the fulcrum that exactly equals their combined weights. If this equal and opposite force did not exist, the entire board would move up or down accordingly. This illustrates the second requirement for static balance, that *all straight-line (linear) forces must be balanced by equal opposite forces.* In mathematical terms, the algebraic sum of linear forces must be zero.

There are no horizontal or angular forces in this illustration. If any did exist, they, too, would have to be in balance or the board would slide in one direction or another.

Balanced moments

In static analysis rotational forces are expressed in terms of moments, the units of measure for the rotating effect of leverage. *All moments around ANY point must be in balance.* The remaining forces in this illustration are rotational, the type of forces that would cause the board to tip if they were not in balance.

If the board were to tip, it would obviously rotate around the supporting fulcrum. Any such rotation is prevented by the children's positioning themselves so that the rotational moments around the fulcrum are equal in both directions. They balance each other.

Moments are measured by the product of force multiplied by its distance from the fulcrum. This distance is called the *moment arm.*

In the illustration the heavier child is seated 5 feet from the fulcrum, so the moment is determined by multiplying the 100-pound weight by 5 feet. This gives a moment of 500 pound-feet in a clockwise direction. The smaller child is seated 10 feet from the fulcrum, so the effect in terms of moments is 50 pounds times 10 feet, or 500 pound-feet. What is lacking in pounds is made up in feet. This moment is counterclockwise so that it balances the moment of the heavier child. The two moments are equal and opposite, so the board is in rotational equilibrium. These moments are shown on either side of the fulcrum in Fig. 2-2.

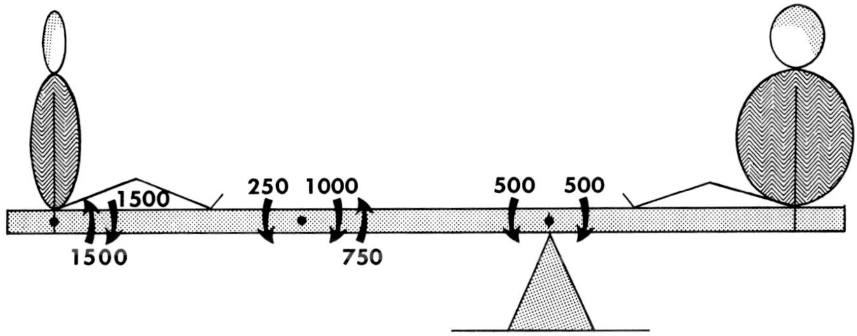

Fig. 2-2. Balance of moments in the same situation shown in Fig. 2-1. The algebraic sum of moments around *any* point is zero.

Units for measuring moments. Moments are identified by the units of force and distance used for measuring the components, as pound-feet in the preceding paragraph. The force unit is usually named first to avoid confusion with foot-pounds and similar units of work. Rotational moments have nothing to do with work units, in spite of the similarity in the names of the units with which they are measured. Other common units for measuring moments are ounce-inches, gram-centimeters, and kilogram-meters.

Selecting the center of moments. Up to this point the same results could have been determined by means of lever formulas, but the advantage of the more broadly applicable static analysis lies in simplifying more complex problems, such as those found in orthodontics. In the case of the children on the balanced board it was easy to identify the supporting fulcrum, but in the case of an archwire there are several brackets and other attachments in contact with the wire. Which of these is the fulcrum?

As long as the system is static, it makes no difference which point is selected as the fulcrum. Nothing is moving anyway. With this type of analysis we can ignore the fulcrum and choose any arbitrary point as a center of moments.

Convenience is the major consideration in selecting this reference point for moment analysis. Going back to Fig. 2-2, we could just as well select the point under the smaller child, who contributes nothing at all to the rotation of the board around that point. The larger child is seated 15 feet away, producing a moment of 100 pounds times 15 feet or 1500 pound-feet. This must be balanced in some way, and the only possible balancing force is the 150-pound upward thrust of the support, 10 feet away. This also contributes 1500 pound-feet, so the opposing moments are equal.

It is not necessary to use one of the points of force application for figuring moments; any point will do. Fig. 2-2 also shows the moments around the point midway between the smaller child and the fulcrum. Here the smaller child contributes a moment of 50 pounds times 5 feet, or 250 pound-feet, counterclockwise. This is augmented by the upward thrust at the fulcrum, which also produces a counterclockwise moment around this point: 150 pounds times 5 feet, or 750 pound-feet. These two combine to give a total counterclockwise moment of 1000 pound-feet. The heavier child is 10 feet away from this point, contributing a moment of 100 pounds times 10 feet, or 1000 pound-feet in the opposite (clockwise) direction.

The example used to illustrate balance of forces in Figs. 2-1 and 2-2 presents exactly the same force relationships found in the case of a tooth subjected to a lateral (tipping) force. Fig. 2-3 shows such a tooth with its supporting bone.

The alveolar crest occupies the position of the fulcrum, the external force on the tooth replaces the larger child, and the apical region of the alveolus replaces the smaller child. If the tooth is regarded as a free body, we observe that external forces are being applied at these three points, ignoring the fact that forces will be applied to the root over an *area* centered on these points rather than on a single point (a child sitting on a board also applies weight over an area).

The principle of equal and opposite forces tells us that the alveolus at each point of force application will also be subjected to an equal and opposite force. This

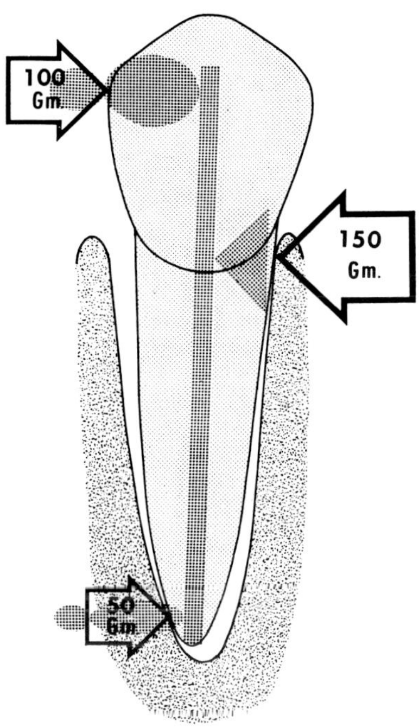

Fig. 2-3. The relationships of forces on a tipping tooth are identical to those on the boards in Figs. 2-1 and 2-2. Note that the force at the alveolar crest region equals the sum of the force on the crown *plus* the resisting force in the apical region.

concept holds true in all orthodontic situations where one object acts on another, whether they be teeth, bone, wires, brackets, or other objects. Forces at points of interaction are *always* reciprocal.

Measurement of the moment arm. In Fig. 2-2, all measurements from force to center of moments were made along the board. This bypassed one additional factor that must be considered in measuring moments: the way in which the distance from force to axis is measured. This distance cannot always be measured directly from the point of force application as it was in the illustration.

Distance from force to center of moments (axis) must be measured along a line perpendicular to the direction of the force. The board shown in Fig. 2-2 satisfies this condition. Fig. 2-4 shows the correct way to measure the moment arm in two other situations. The actual mechanical arms shown could be replaced by a solid arm in the position of the moment arm with no change in the rotational effect. Stated simply, the moment arm is always the *shortest distance* from the center of moments to the *line* of force orientation, regardless of the point of application.

Couples. When a body (such as a tooth) is subjected to two equal forces acting in opposite directions along parallel lines, these forces will produce the same net moment around *any point* in the plane in which they are acting. Such a pair of forces is called a *couple.* Fig. 2-5 illustrates a couple, showing the same moment around three different points. It would also be the same around any other point in that plane.

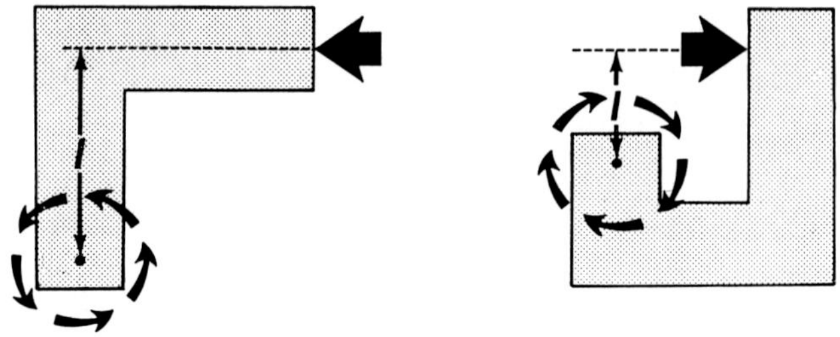

Fig. 2-4. Moment arm, l, is measured from the center of rotation to the line of the force, along a line perpendicular to the line of the force. The moment arm may or may not coincide with the mechanical arm.

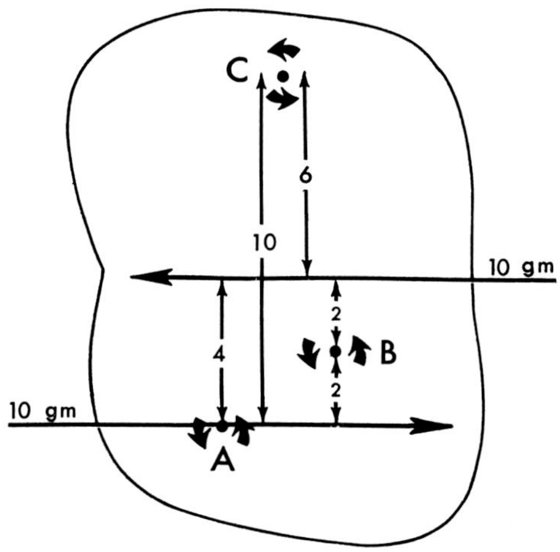

Fig. 2-5. The moment of a couple is the same around *any* point in the same plane. This illustration shows a pair of 10-gm forces 4 mm apart, operating to produce a counterclockwise moment of 40 gm-mm on a molar. Three typical reference points are shown. At *A*, the moment arm for the upper force is 4 mm, so this 10-gm force will produce a moment of 40 gm-mm. The lower force is directed through point *A*, so it will have no rotational effect. At *B*, both 10-gm forces are operating with 2-mm moment arms, so each produces a moment of 20 gm-mm. At *C*, the lower force is operating on a 10-mm moment arm to produce a counterclockwise moment of 100 gm-mm; this is partially balanced by the upper force, which is operating on a 6-mm moment arm to produce a clockwise moment of 60 gm-mm. The net operating moment is again 40 gm-mm counterclockwise.

The moment of a couple is most easily measured by multiplying *one* of the forces of the couple by the distance separating the lines of the forces (*A* in Fig. 2-5).

In describing a couple it is not necessary to identify either the actual forces or their points of application. Their moment is the same at all points, and the two opposite linear forces cancel each other out so there are no linear effects. It is enough merely to say that a couple is acting with a given moment. This moment can then be considered to be operating around any point in its plane. Actual rotation in response to the moment will depend on resisting forces.

APPLICATION OF FREE-BODY ANALYSIS

The laws of statics are universal in their application. They apply to any object or system, and to *any part* of an object or system. Using this concept, we may figuratively dissect and isolate any part of a mechanical system as a free body and consider the forces acting upon it. These forces must be in balance, or the part would not have been in a stable condition. This approach can greatly simplify the problem of understanding the forces on an individual tooth or other local area, for it helps to cut the total problem into pieces of manageable size. Teeth or small sections of an archwire can be separated easily from the overall problem and studied individually.

In free-body analysis all outside forces are considered to be acting at the "cut" surfaces where the section was figuratively removed from its surrounding parts. Of course, these must also balance. Internal forces can then be taken up from this point as they relate to the outside forces and to each other.

SUMMING UP

In static free-body analysis the following conditions must be satisfied:

1. The part under study must be clearly delineated. There are no limitations on the selection, size, or complexity of the free body, but it must be clearly identified.
2. All forces acting at the interfaces between the body and outside objects or forces must be identified. Force values must be assigned to enough of these forces to make it possible to determine the others.
3. There can be no movement of the free body in relation to the immediate environment. This is a static analysis and does not consider the effects of inertia, acceleration, or velocity that are associated with movement.
4. All linear forces acting on the free body must be in balance. This condition will be satisfied if the body is not in motion. Each force must be countered by an equal and opposite force or combination of forces. Mathematically stated, all linear forces must add algebraically to zero. The same condition also applies to forces within the free body.
5. All moments around *any* point must be balanced by equal and opposite moments or combinations of moments. This condition also applies to moments within the free body.

A *couple* is a general case involving conditions 4 and 5. Two equal and parallel forces operating in opposite directions cancel each other as linear forces, but produce a resultant moment. The couple can therefore be identified by its moment alone. This moment is the same around *any* axis perpendicular to the plane of the couple, and it can be balanced by any opposite moment or combination of moments.

3

Elastic properties

Elasticity is a characteristic of all the solid materials we find around us. Their elastic properties vary widely, from the conspicuously elastic to the apparently inelastic. These properties play a major role in structural integrity and functional effectiveness, which is why they are the primary considerations in the selection of material for any mechanical function.

Storing and delivering delicate forces in an oral environment place extreme demands on the materials that are used in orthodontic appliances. Their elastic performance is central to their design, application, and success.

Any application of force through an elastic component induces and uses some combination of force and displacement. The force distorts the elastic material by moving one part in relation to the rest; this is what places force in storage. The force is released as the material returns to its original form.

It is the relationships between force and distance and their effects on the material that determine the effectiveness of an individual component in any specific situation. Some applications require large deflections while others require small ones. Some require high force levels while others require low ones. Regardless of the requirements, the important parameters can be described precisely in terms of three basic elastic properties.

THE THREE BASIC ELASTIC PROPERTIES

Three characteristics must be measured if the forces in an elastic mechanism are to be fully described. These can be used to describe both the mechanism itself and the materials of which it is constructed. This is important for the orthodontic practitioner, who must select both the material and the design for the application, because any change in one characteristic will require a compensatory change in the others for comparable performance.

The three basic properties of elastic materials and devices follow:

1. *Stiffness* is a force/distance ratio that is a measure of *resistance to deformation.* It is a measure of the force required to bend or otherwise deform the material a definite distance, but it has no relationship to the maximum force or distance that can be sustained. Other things being equal, a stiffer wire can store proportionately more force, but other things are seldom equal.
2. *Strength* is a force value that is a measure of the *maximum possible load,* the greatest force that the wire or arch arrangement can sustain or deliver if it is

Stiffness	Strength	Range
	Material	
Modulus of elasticity (E)	Resiliency	Elastic limit Proportional limit
Slope of stress/strain curve	Area below stress/strain curve	Deflection at the proportional limit (or other arbitrary point on the stress/strain curve)
Spring constant Load/deflection rate Stress/strain rate		Working range
	Effects of length	
	Bending	
$\frac{1}{(\text{Length})^3}$	$\frac{1}{\text{Length}}$	$(\text{Length})^2$
	Torsion	
$\frac{1}{\text{Length}}$	Not dependent on length	Length
	Effects of cross-section	
	All wires	
Moment of inertia (I) for bending	Section modulus (Z) for bending	$\frac{1}{c}$
Polar moment of inertia (J) for torsion	Polar section modulus (Z) for torsion	For bending or torsion
	Round wires in bending and torsion	
$(\text{Diameter})^4$	$(\text{Diameter})^3$	$\frac{1}{\text{Diameter}}$
	Rectangular wires in bending	
$(\text{Thickness})^3$	$(\text{Thickness})^2$	$\frac{1}{\text{Thickness}}$
Width	Width	Not dependent on width
	Helical spring in axial tension or compression	
$\frac{1}{(\text{Coil diameter})^3}$	$\frac{1}{\text{Coil diameter}}$	$(\text{Coil diameter})^2$
$\frac{1}{\text{Number of coils}}$	Not dependent on number of coils	Number of coils
	Effects of cross-section of wire in helical springs are the same as in torsion	

Fig. 3-1. Some factors related to the three basic elastic properties of wires under various loading conditions. Most of these are discussed in detail in later chapters and defined in the glossary.

loaded to the limit of the material. When this term is applied to a material, it indicates its total capacity for storing force, usually in comparison to some other material. *Resiliency* and *toughness* are other terms sometimes used to describe this force storage capacity.

3. *Working range,* or simply *range,* is a linear value that is a measure of *how far* a wire or material can be deformed without exceeding the limits of the material. This tells how far a tooth can be moved with a single adjustment.

These properties can be expressed in absolute terms, but they can be very useful in orthodontics on a simple comparative basis without direct measurement of unit values. The orthodontist is concerned primarily with the *change* in response that might be expected with a change in material, wire size, or bracket arrangement. The knowledge that force or movement will be doubled under certain circumstances can be useful even without precise measurement.

Information concerning these properties will be presented here in both absolute and relative terms, depending on which are most directly applicable to the clinical situation.

Stiffness, strength, and working range do *not* vary in direct proportion to one another in most cases, so we must be continually aware of all three. Often a gain in one must be paid for by a loss in another.

Comparing the three properties further we find that *stiffness* indicates the rate of force delivery but gives no indication of how much force can be applied or how much distance can be covered. It is equally important under all loading conditions. *Strength* and *range* are both measures of the maximum capacity of the material. Strength measures the load or force that can be carried at this maximum capacity, and range measures the amount of movement (displacement) that is attained under maximum load.

Factors that influence stiffness, strength, and range

One factor that affects the properties of stiffness, strength, and range in orthodontics is the mechanical arrangement by which force is applied to the teeth. This includes bracket width, length of archwire, span, and loops. A second factor is the form of the wire itself—the size and shape of the cross-section. A third factor is the material, including the alloy formula, its hardness, and the state of heat treatment. These will be discussed in the chapters that follow. Fig. 3-1 shows many of the interrelationships of these factors in tabular form.

4

Archwires and beams

The board shown in Figs. 2-1 and 2-2 can be easily recognized as a beam, but one might have to take a second look at an archwire to recognize that it is also a beam. To an engineer any long, slender structure that is subjected to lateral (bending) loads is a beam, and under this definition an archwire qualifies with flying colors. This is a big advantage in our study of the behavior of archwires, for the subject of beams has been well explored in the engineering field. Beam behavior can be predicted precisely, and with just a moderate understanding of the principles of beam behavior an orthodontist can predict the function of an archwire in the mouth without resorting to mathematical calculations.

Engineers are very practical in approaching a subject such as this; they go directly to the heart of a problem without wasting effort on unnecessary details. The same approach will be used here; only the essential facts of beam theory will be discussed, without concern for details that have no direct clinical application.

Beams function by bending whether they are supporting a building or moving a tooth. The important information for design purposes in either of these applications is the amount of bending involved under anticipated force loads. A beam in a building must bend very little, and it is designed accordingly. In orthodontics we are more often looking for the exact opposite: an archwire with the greatest possible flexibility. This flexibility must be planned in the design, and when considered together with capacity for force storage it will deliver the forces required for tooth movement.

BEAM LOADING

Beams can be loaded in several different ways, but only the simplest is applicable in most orthodontic situations. This is point loading, in which each load is applied at one point. A typical example is an archwire engaged by a ligature wire or the edge of a bracket. In engineering practice many beams must support loads distributed over their entire length (such as beams supporting floors and roofs), but the only comparable situation in orthodontics is that in which a bolus of food is forced against an arch during mastication.

CANTILEVER BEAMS

The simplest type of beam is the cantilever, which most orthodontists encountered in their earlier study of restorative dentistry. This beam is rigidly supported

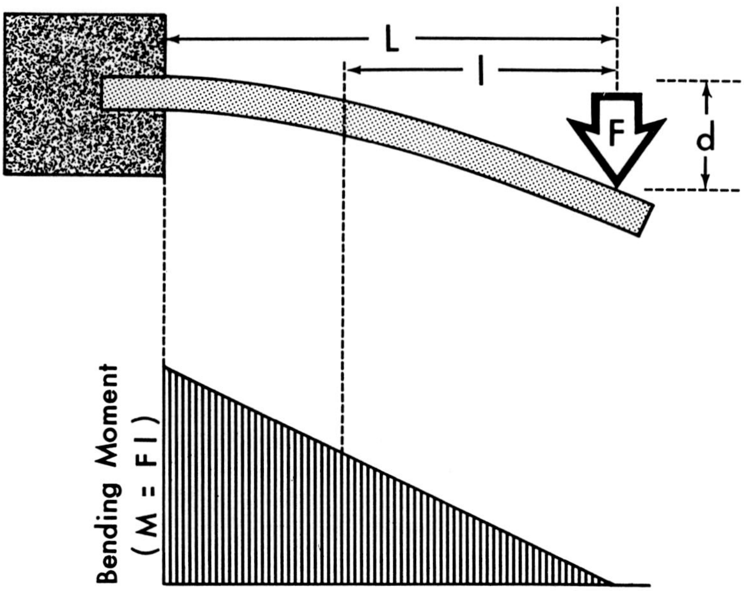

Fig. 4-1. A cantilever beam. *F,* Force or load; *d,* deflection; *L,* working length of beam; *l,* length of moment arm for any point on the beam. The bending moment at any point is *Fl;* these moments for all points along the beam are shown in the bending moment diagram below the beam. This diagram shows that the bending moment is zero under the point of force application, increasing uniformly to a maximum at the support.

at one end and carries a load on the extended arm (Fig. 4-1). A cantilever bridge is expected to be rigid, but a cantilever archwire can be very flexible. The same laws of bending apply to both. From the discussion of moments in Chapter 1, it is obvious that the load on this beam produces a moment at the supported end equal to the load multiplied by its distance from the support (the moment arm). When a free end of the beam extends beyond the load as shown, the outer end has no effect.

Bending moments

Moments such as those present at the supported end of the cantilever are called *bending moments,* since they are responsible for the bending of the beam. The moment actually puts a rotating force at every point along the beam. There are no hinges so the beam cannot pivot; however, it does the next best thing by pivoting on itself (bending). The stiffness of the material resists this bending, so the amount of bending is inversely proportional to the stiffness.

Bending moments are imposed on the entire length of a beam between the support and the load. These bending moments are highest at the supported end, diminishing uniformly to zero at the point of application of the force. The graph below the beam in Fig. 4-1 shows how the moments decrease from a maximum at the support to zero under the load and beyond.

The support contributes an equal countermoment, maintaining the balance of moments. As in all static force situations this same force picture can be reversed,

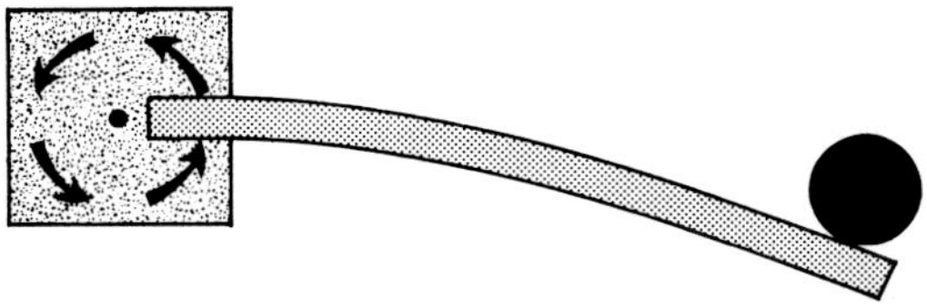

Fig. 4-2. Forces on the beam shown in Fig. 4-1 will be exactly the same if the "force" is replaced by a fixed stop and force is applied as a moment at the "support" end.

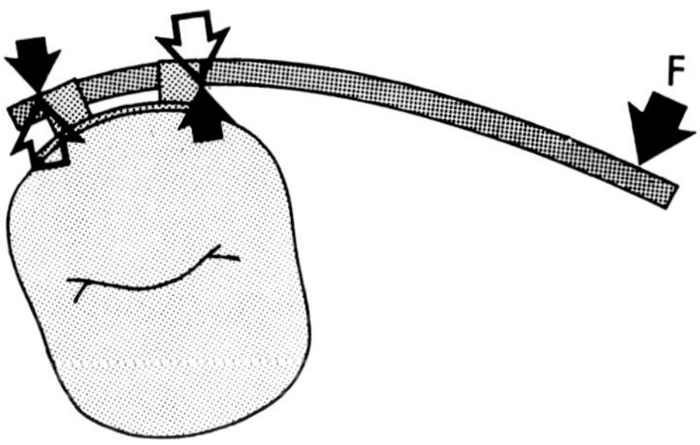

Fig. 4-3. An archwire in a bracket presents the same force relationships as in Figs. 4-1 and 4-2. Solid arrows show forces acting on the wire; open arrows show forces acting on the tooth. The paired forces on the brackets produce a couple with a moment comparable to that shown in Fig. 4-2.

considering the applied force to be the rotating moment at the "support" end and the resisting force at the "force" end (Fig. 4-2).

A comparable orthodontic situation is shown in Fig. 4-3. If the archwire is inserted in the bracket and activated by bending it down at *F*, we think of the force picture shown in Fig. 4-1. If the wire is first engaged at *F* and then activated by bending it to engage the bracket, we think of the situation in Fig. 4-2. In either case, all forces and their effects are the same.

Critical (dangerous) section

The maximum bending moment in a cantilever is at the supported end. In beam terminology the location of this maximum bending moment is called the *critical* or *dangerous section*. This is the section of the beam that will be bent the most, and that will fail first under an overload. Knowing the location of critical sections in an orthodontic appliance is important for two reasons. Most obviously, this tells us where we can expect a permanent set and where preventive measures should be taken to reduce breakage. Less obviously, but just as importantly, it tells us where to place loops to most effectively increase the working range of the wire.

Maximum bending moment and working limits (strength and range)

Every beam or wire has a maximum bending moment beyond which it cannot function without excessive deformation or failure. The maximum allowable bending moment depends on the cross-section of the beam (large or small, round or rectangular), on the physical properties of the metal, and on the degree or incidence of deformation or failure that can be accepted in service. Even though such limits may not be sharp cutoff points, as will be shown later, they are still clinically useful.

The *force* required to produce the maximum bending moment depends on the *strength* of the beam.

Working range indicates the *deflection* (amount of bending) that is acceptable before the maximum moment is reached.

Stiffness determines the force required for a specific deflection in the range below the maximum limit. Stiffness indicates resistance to bending, but it has nothing at all to do with how far the beam can be bent. There is no relationship whatever between stiffness and the maximum allowable bending moment.

INTERRELATIONSHIPS BETWEEN STIFFNESS, STRENGTH, AND RANGE IN BEAMS

The three-way relationship between stiffness, strength, and range in beams is an unclosed triangle. Stiffness and range combine to establish the value of the

	Beam Type	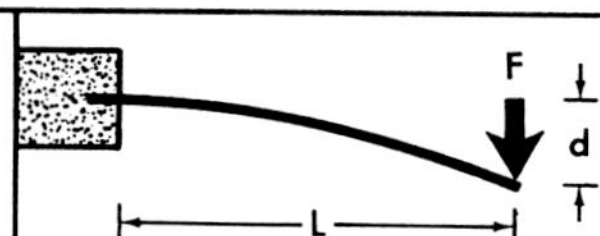	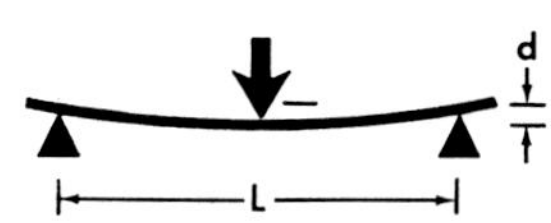
	Bending Moment Diagram	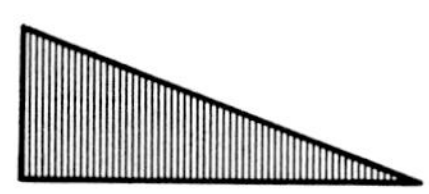	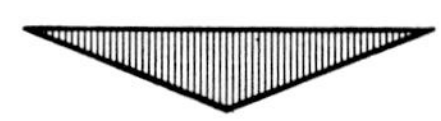
	Maximum Bending Moment	FL	$\frac{FL}{4}$
	Deflection (d)	$\frac{L^3F}{3EI}$	$\frac{L^3F}{48EI}$
	Dangerous Section	support	center
Relative	Stiffness	$\frac{1}{16}$	1
	Strength	$\frac{1}{4}$	1
	Range	4	1

Fig. 4-4. Bending properties of frequently encountered beam types. *F*, force or load; *L*, length; *d*, deflection; *E*, modulus of elasticity; *I*, moment of inertia of the cross-section.

working range but do not have any consistent direct relationship with each other.

Stiffness is a force/distance rate value defining the level of force required to accomplish a specific deflection. It has *no relation* to how far a beam can be bent. Equivalent measures include the bending rate, spring rate, or spring constant.

Range is the extreme acceptable bending deflection. It is a measure of distance alone, without regard for the force that may be required to accomplish the deflection.

Strength is a value derived from the combined effects of stiffness and range. It is the force required to produce a deflection to the limit of the working range.

OTHER BEAM TYPES

The cantilever is only one type of beam. Many other types are in use, classified according to the relationship between beam, load, and supports. Different beam types place different demands on the material through variations in the distribution of moments and in the location of the critical sections. Fig. 4-4 shows some of the most common beam types and their important characteristics.

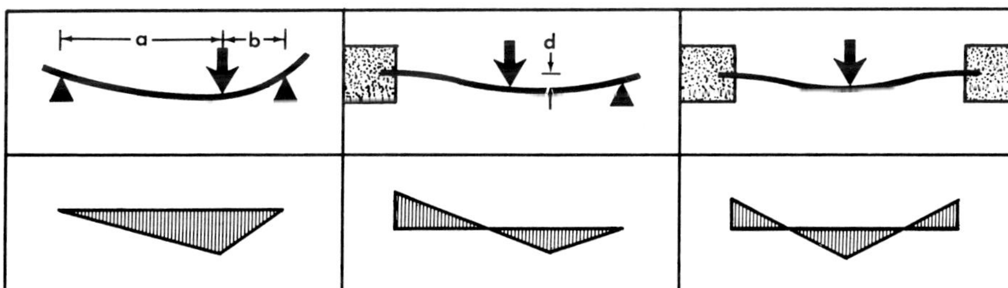

			Effect of Span (L)
$\frac{Fab}{L}$	$\frac{3FL}{16}$	$\frac{FL}{8}$	
$\frac{Fb}{3EIL}\left[\frac{a(b+L)}{3}\right]^{\frac{3}{2}}$	$\frac{7L^3F}{768\ EI}$	$\frac{L^3F}{192\ EI}$	
load	fixed support	supports and center	
> 1	1.9	4	$\frac{1}{L^3}$
> 1	$\frac{4}{3}$	2	$\frac{1}{L}$
< 1	.7	$\frac{1}{2}$	L^2

Fig. 4-4, cont'd. For legend see opposite page.

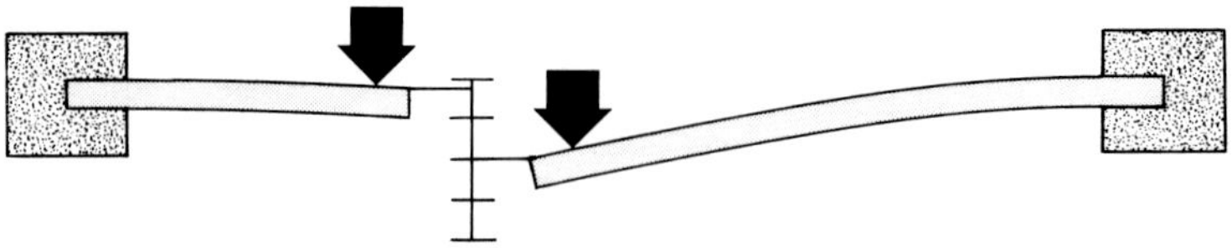

Fig. 4-5. *Stiffness* is *inversely proportional to the cube of length.* The beam on the right, twice as long as the beam on the left, is deflected eight times as far by the same load.

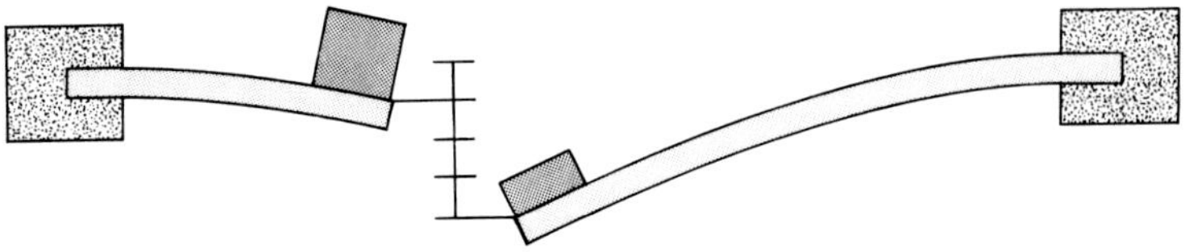

Fig. 4-6. *Working range* is proportional to the *square of the length.* When loaded to capacity, the beam on the right will be deflected four times as far as the beam half its length.

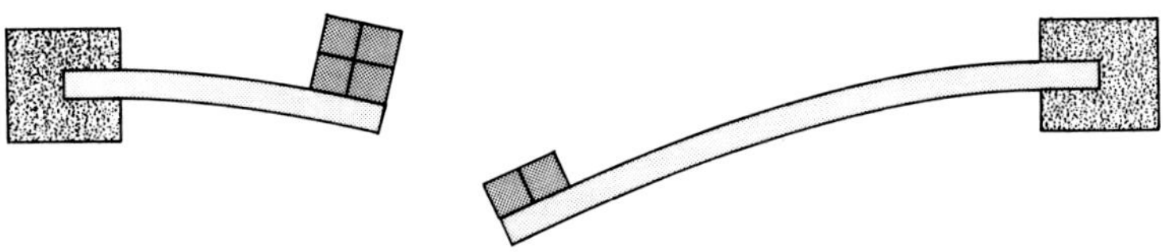

Fig. 4-7. *Strength* is *inversely proportional to length.* The beam on the right has a maximum load capacity only one-half as great as the beam half as long on the left.

The orthodontist does not always have a free hand to select the optimum mechanical arrangement, for the mechanism must be fitted to the teeth and the mouth of a patient. When the required arrangement has a marked effect on arch performance, other measures must be taken to compensate. This may require the selection of a different size of wire or the addition of loops. Bracket width and tube length can be very important here, and the dimensions recommended in Chapter 15 have been selected on the basis of these considerations.

It will be noted that the symbol 'L^3' appears in all of the formulas for deflection shown in Fig. 4-4. This indicates that deflection is always proportional to the *cube* of the length of the beam, which means that stiffness is inversely proportional to the cube of the length. Doubling the length of any beam, keeping the load and support arrangement unchanged, will produce *eight times* as much deflection (Fig. 4-5), or an eightfold reduction in stiffness.

The formulas for maximum moment show that it is *directly* proportional to length. Doubling the length of a beam doubles the bending moment, reducing the maximum load-carrying capacity by one-half. Lengthening the span, therefore, does not decrease load-carrying capacity as rapidly as it increases deflection. *Strength* is *inversely* proportional to length of span. The beam can be longer than the span (Fig. 4-6).

EFFECT OF LENGTH OF SPAN

Each type of beam has its own characteristic stiffness, strength, and range. These characteristics are affected by length in the same way for all beam types, so length can be considered an independent characteristic in addition to the basic beam configuration.

Doubling the length of a span and loading it with the new maximum load (one-half the original load) will still deflect it four times as far as the shorter beam. This means that working range has been increased four times by doubling length. *Working range* is always proportional to the *square* of the length (Fig. 4-7).

These effects of length are summarized in formula form in the last column of Fig. 4-4.

5

Effects of cross-section on force storage in bending

The cross-section of a wire may be round or rectangular in any of a broad range of dimensions. The size and shape of the cross-section have profound effects on the stiffness, strength, and working range of a wire in the mouth, making it the most potent single factor available for the control of orthodontic force application.

When a wire is bent, the metal is stretched along the outside curvature and compressed along the inside curvature (Fig. 5-1). It is this combination of tension and compression that resists the bending and actually accomplishes the energy storage in the spring action of the wire. The picture is simplified by the fact that metals usually behave identically under tension and compression, so that deformation is equal in the opposite sides of the wire. The metal midway between the two extremes, which is neither stretched nor compressed, is called the *neutral axis*. The neutral axis is like a flat ribbon through the center of the wire, midway between the outer and inner curved sides.

ROUND WIRES

Range

The parts of the wire farthest from the neutral axis take the brunt of any bending action. They are stretched and compressed the most, so they accomplish most force storage. These sections of the wire are called the *extreme fibers,* a term that is descriptive of the shape and action of this section of the wire and nothing more. The metal is not strictly fibrous, and the extreme fiber could never be dissected out of the wire as a separate piece.

The greater the distance between the extreme fiber and the neutral axis, the more it will be stretched or compressed in bending. This distance (usually abbreviated "c") is the index of the working range of a bending wire. Working range (or maximum acceptable bend) is inversely proportional to c. This dimension is half the thickness of the wire in the plane of the bend, which is the radius for round wires.

As an example of the variation in working range for round wires, a wire .010 inch (.25 mm) in diameter can be bent exactly twice as far as a wire .020 inch (.50 mm) in diameter without overloading the material (Figs. 5-2 and 5-3).

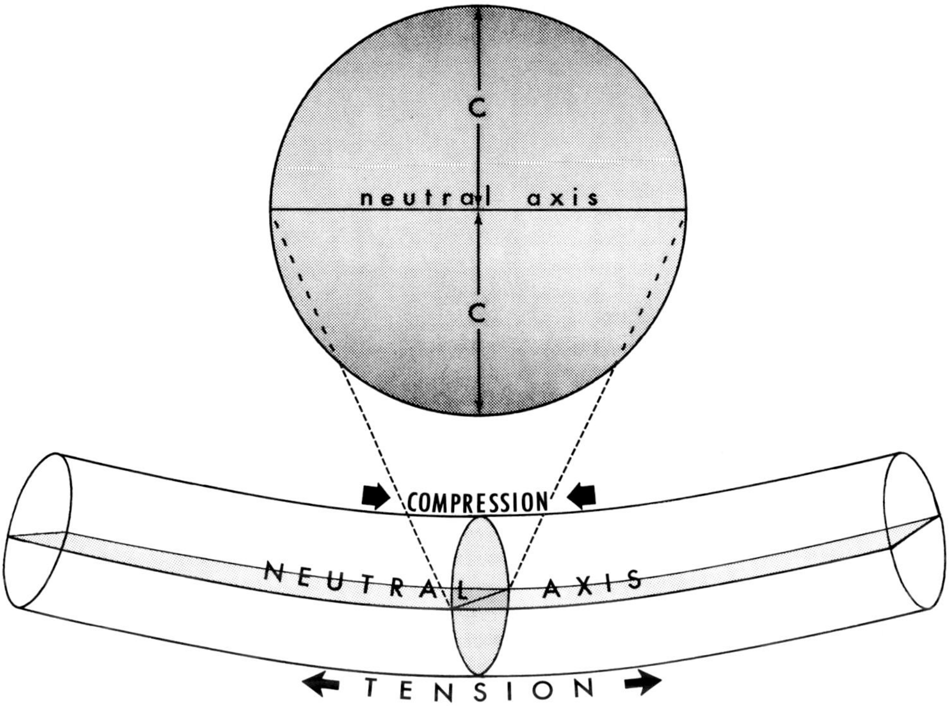

Fig. 5-1. One side of a bending beam is under tension; the other is under compression. The neutral axis is the plane that divides these two regions. At the neutral axis there is no tension, compression, change in length, or force storage.

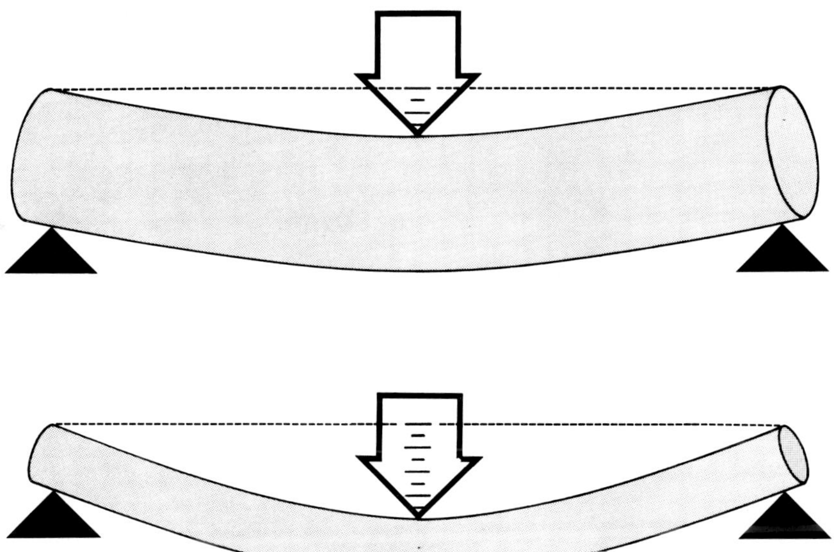

Fig. 5-2. *Range* is inversely proportional to diameter. A .010-inch (.25-mm) wire, loaded to its (smaller) capacity, can be deflected twice as far as a .020-inch (.50-mm) wire without exceeding its elastic limit.

A

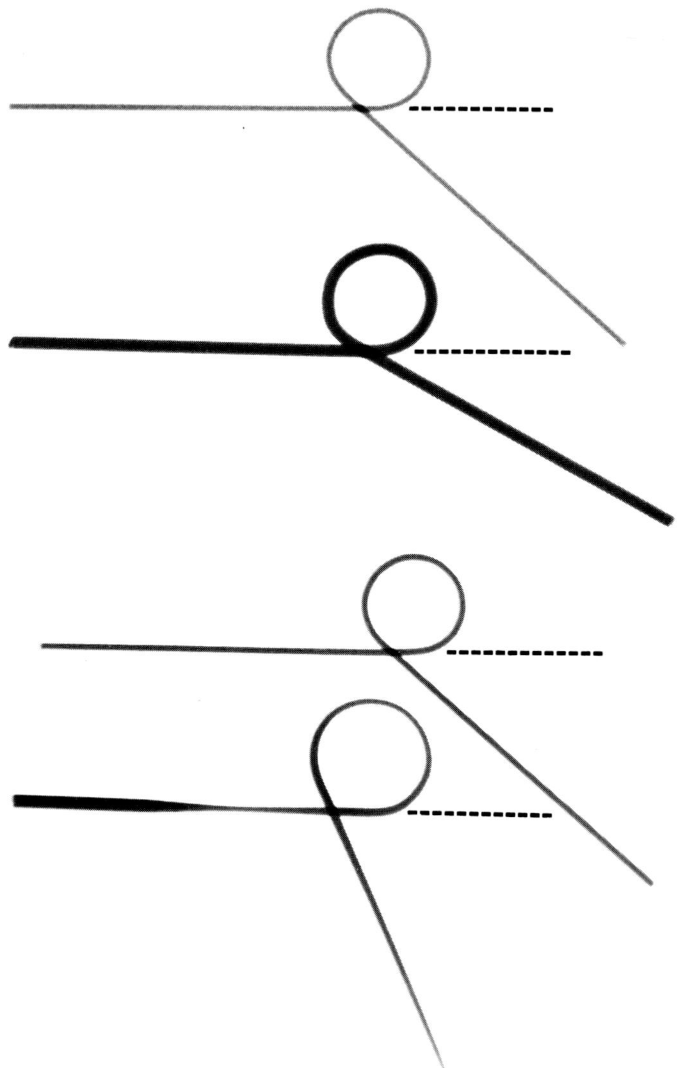

B

Fig. 5-3. Effect of diameter on bending range. Shadowgraphs of .011-inch (.275-mm) and .022-inch (.55-mm) wires, each bent 360 degrees around the same mandrel (dashed line) and released. Note in **A** that the heavier wire has undergone more plastic deformation (greater permanent set). In **B** the same two wires are shown, with the larger wire electrolytically reduced the diameter of the smaller one. Note that the heavier wire now shows less permanent set (more rebound) than the lighter wire, demonstrating that most of the original plastic deformation occurred in the outer part of the wire. The difference between the two wires is due primarily to the fact that the radius of the bend in the "core" of the heavier wire was increased by the added thickness of the wire; therefore the original bend was not quite as sharp as in the smaller wire.

Stiffness

Stiffness of wires depends on a value called the moment of inertia (usually abbreviated "I") of the cross-section. The mathematical basis for the moment of inertia may be found in Appendix A, but the moment of inertia can be easily visualized if one imagines a thin slice cut out of the wire and suspended on the neutral axis. For a round wire this would look something like a phonograph record balanced horizontally on two fingers at opposite edges. Spinning the slice around this axis will produce an inertial effect that resists the start of the spin and tends to keep the slice spinning once it has started. The strength of this effect is proportional to the moment of inertia of the section.

This may seem a far cry from bending wires, but the moment of inertia is exactly proportional to the stiffness of a wire. The extreme fibers lying farthest from the neutral axis are the major contributors to stiffness, just as mass in this part of the section is a major contributor to inertial effects. Ratios between moments of inertia are the same as ratios between measures of stiffness.

The moment of inertia varies with the *fourth power* of wire diameter, so changes of cross-section affect stiffness much more than they affect any other property. A wire .010 inch (.25 mm) in diameter is actually only one-sixteenth as stiff as a wire .020 inch (.50 mm) in diameter. Sixteen times as much force will be required to bend a .020-inch (.50-mm) wire the same distance as a .010-inch (.25-mm) wire, so doubling wire diameters (Fig. 5-4) will actually change the associated bending forces from ounces to pounds!

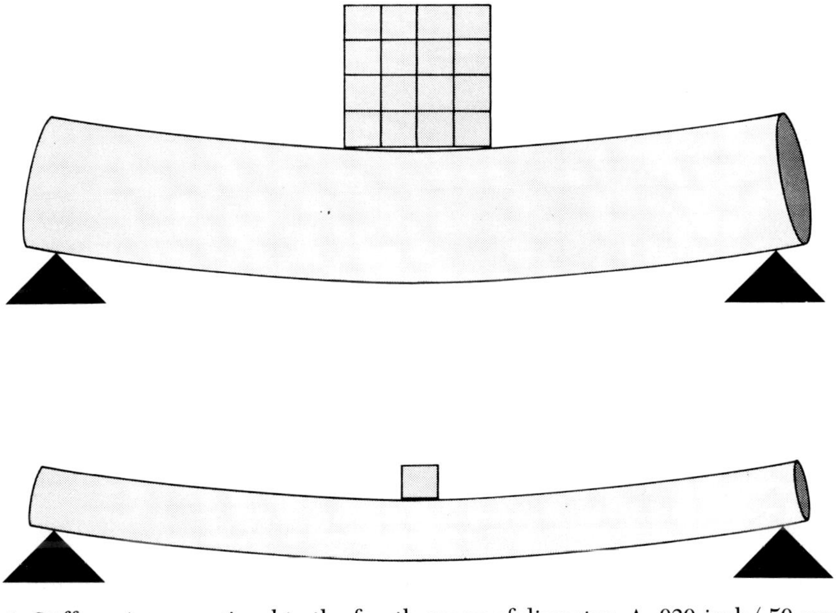

Fig. 5-4. *Stiffness* is proportional to the fourth power of diameter. A .020-inch (.50-mm) wire requires sixteen times as much force to deflect it the same distance as a .010-inch (.25-mm) wire.

Actual moments of inertia for wire sizes used in orthodontics will be found in Appendix A. These values provide a ready reference in comparing stiffness.

Strength

As the term is used here, strength is a measure of the total load-carrying capacity of a wire. Relative values depend on a combination of working range and stiffness. Working range limits the distance that a wire can bend, and stiffness determines how much force will be required to reach that point. The engineering term that defines strength in terms of the wire's cross-section is *section modulus,* usually represented by the letter "Z". The section modulus is derived by dividing the moment of inertia by c, expressed mathematically by the formula $Z = \frac{I}{c}$. This is the basic bending formula that relates stiffness, strength, and range. The same formula may be restated to define the other factors as $c = \frac{I}{Z}$ or $I = cZ$.

Section modulus and strength are important in orthodontics because they indicate the maximum force that the wire can store or deliver. This maximum force is reached clinically when a wire is tied or otherwise adjusted so tightly that it takes a significant permanent set.

Whether we are seeking high forces or low forces, these factors must be considered. In some situations a limitation on available force may serve as a safety factor to prevent excessive force application, while in others it may make sufficient force unattainable without redesign of the appliance. Strength is also important in resistance to bending by the forces of mastication.

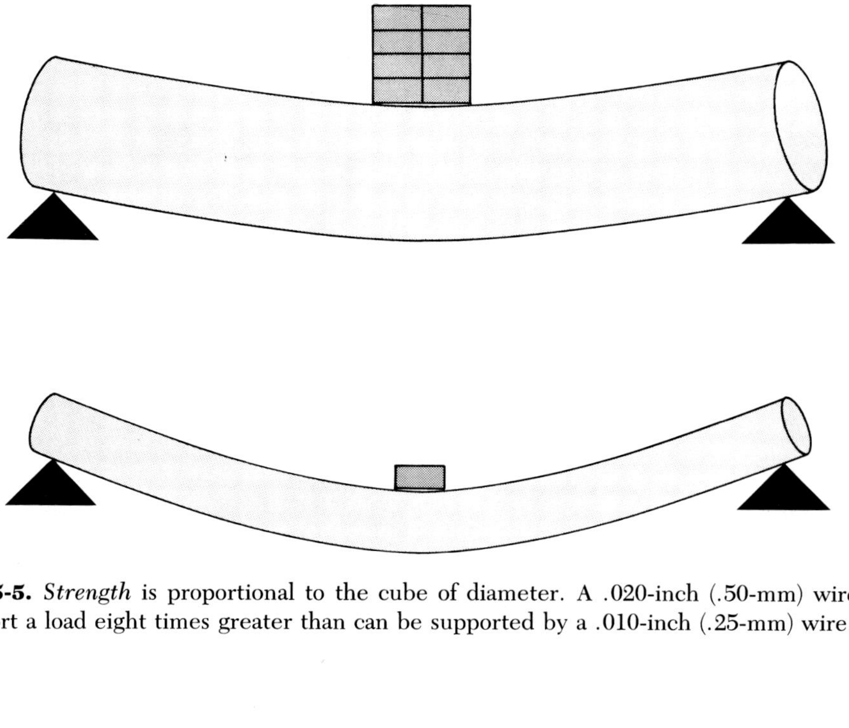

Fig. 5-5. *Strength* is proportional to the cube of diameter. A .020-inch (.50-mm) wire can support a load eight times greater than can be supported by a .010-inch (.25-mm) wire.

Section modulus and strength are proportional to the *cube* of the diameter of round wires; thus the .010-inch (.25-mm) wire can carry a total load one-eighth as great as the .020-inch (.50-mm) wire (Fig. 5-5).

RECTANGULAR WIRES

Width and thickness

In round wires width and thickness are always the same, so both are called the diameter and treated as a single dimension. Width and thickness can vary independently of one another in rectangular wires.

Width of a bending wire is used to describe the dimension perpendicular to the direction of bending in the plane of the neutral axis. Thickness is the dimension in the plane of the bend. These terms are applied strictly in relation to the direction of bending, regardless of which dimension may be larger.

Effect of width and thickness on range

Width has no effect on the bending range of a wire. Range is *inversely related to thickness* and is dependent on c as in round wires.

Effect of width on stiffness and strength

Width has a simple proportional relationship to the stiffness and strength of rectangular wires. Doubling the width will double both stiffness and strength (Fig. 5-6).

This effect of width is also present in round wires, but it is obscured by the fact that thickness and width must always be equal and so are not separately identified.

Effect of thickness on stiffness and strength

Separate identification of the effects of width and thickness in rectangular wires leaves less effect for thickness than was found for the diameter of round wires.

While the *stiffness* of round wires was proportional to the fourth power of diameter, for rectangular wires it is proportional only to the *third power* (cube) of the thickness. A .020- × .020-inch (.5- × .5-mm) wire is eight times as stiff as one .010 × .020 inch (.25 × .5 mm) when it is bent flatwise (Fig. 5-7).

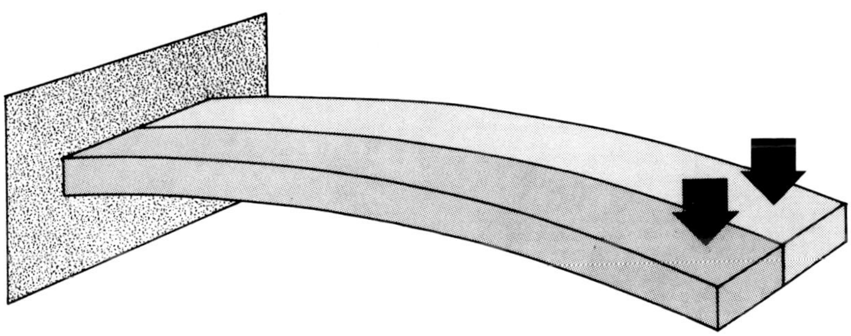

Fig. 5-6. *Strength* and *stiffness* are directly proportional to width in rectangular wires. Doubling width will double total load capacity as well as the force required for the same amount of bending deflection.

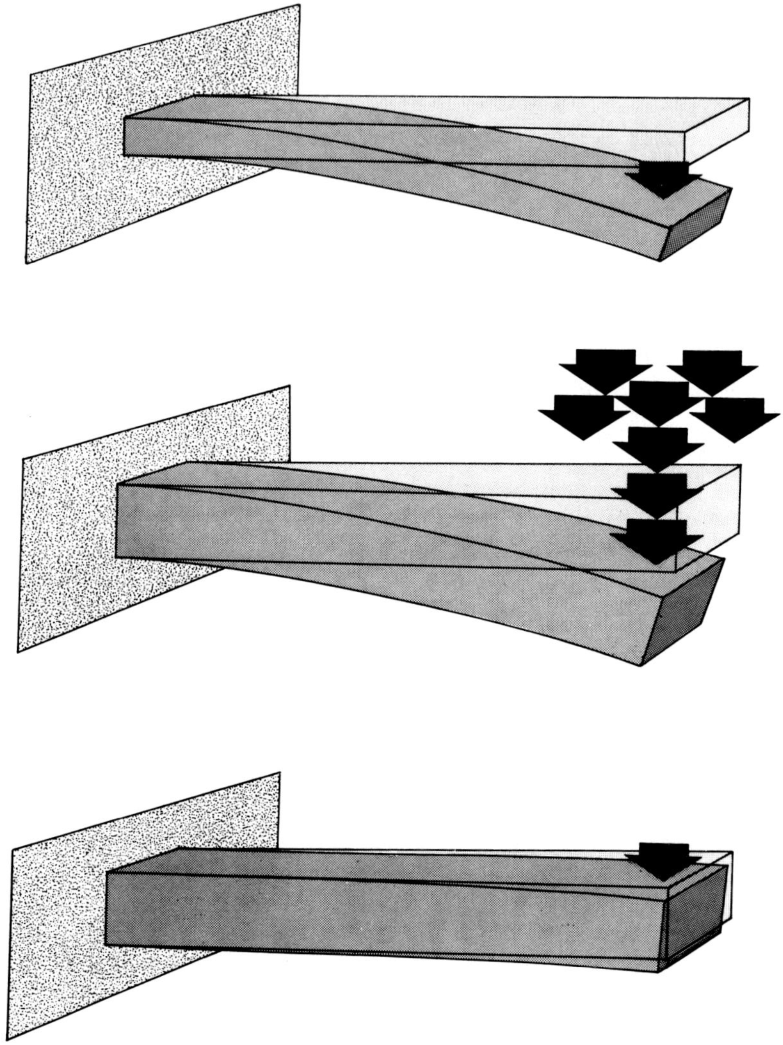

Fig. 5-7. *Stiffness* is proportional to the cube of thickness. Eight times as much force is required to deflect a .020- × .020-inch (.5- × .5-mm) wire the same distance as a .010- × .020-inch (.25- × .5-mm) wire; the same force will deflect the thicker wire only one-eighth as far as the thinner wire.

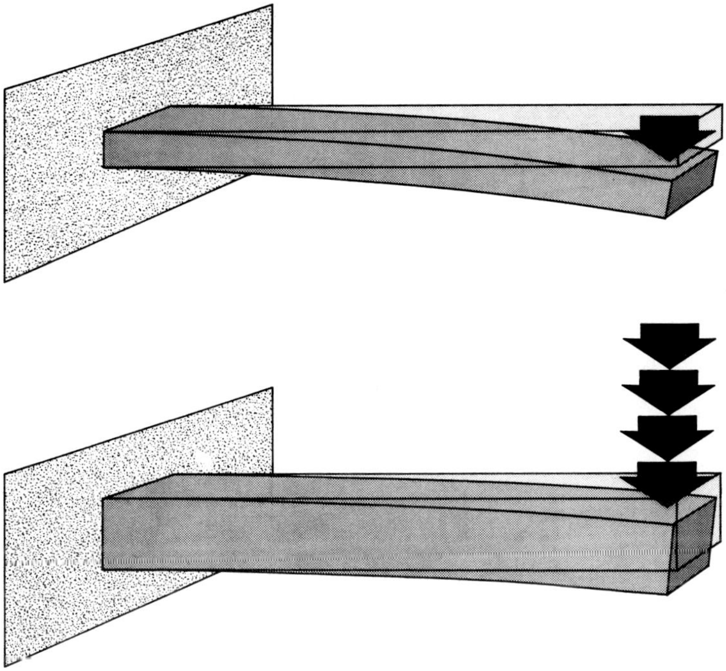

Fig. 5-8. *Strength* is proportional to the square of thickness. A .020- × .020-inch (.5- × .5-mm) wire can support a maximum load four times as great as a .010- × .020-inch (.25- × .5-mm) wire loaded flatwise.

Strength of round wires is proportional to the cube of the diameter, but in rectangular wires it is proportional only to the *square* of the thickness. Maximum load for a square wire is four times that which can be supported flatwise by one only half as thick (Fig. 5-8).

COMPARING WIRES FOR STIFFNESS, STRENGTH, AND RANGE

Appendix A shows the values of c, section modulus (Z), and moment of inertia (I), for all wires of orthodontic size.

These values are functions of wire dimensions alone and are the same for all materials. They provide a precise comparison of the elastic properties of different sized wires made of the same material.

Elastic properties can also vary widely between different materials. Properties of materials combine with the dimensional effects just discussed to determine the properties of a specific wire, so the material and the dimensions must be considered together for a complete picture.

The tables in Appendix A can be used to compare the elastic properties of any wires of the dimensions shown, as long as the wires being compared are made of the same material. To compare any two wires, find the values in the appropriate column and compare the two figures. The ratio of the two figures is the comparative range, strength, or stiffness, as the case may be.

Text continued on p. 38.

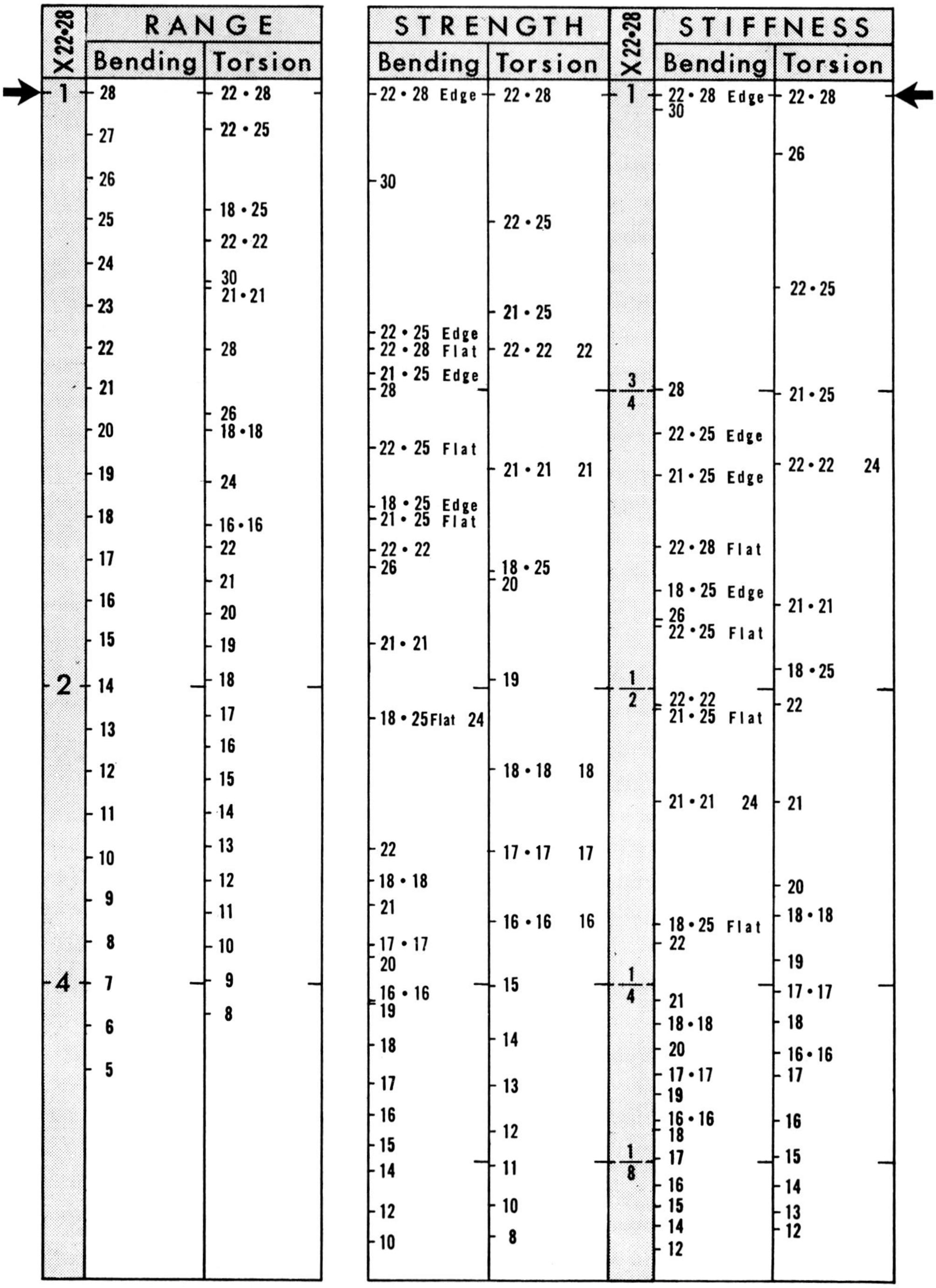

Fig. 5-9. Elastic properties of wires of different sizes compared to .022- × .028-inch (.55- × .70-mm) rectangular wire.

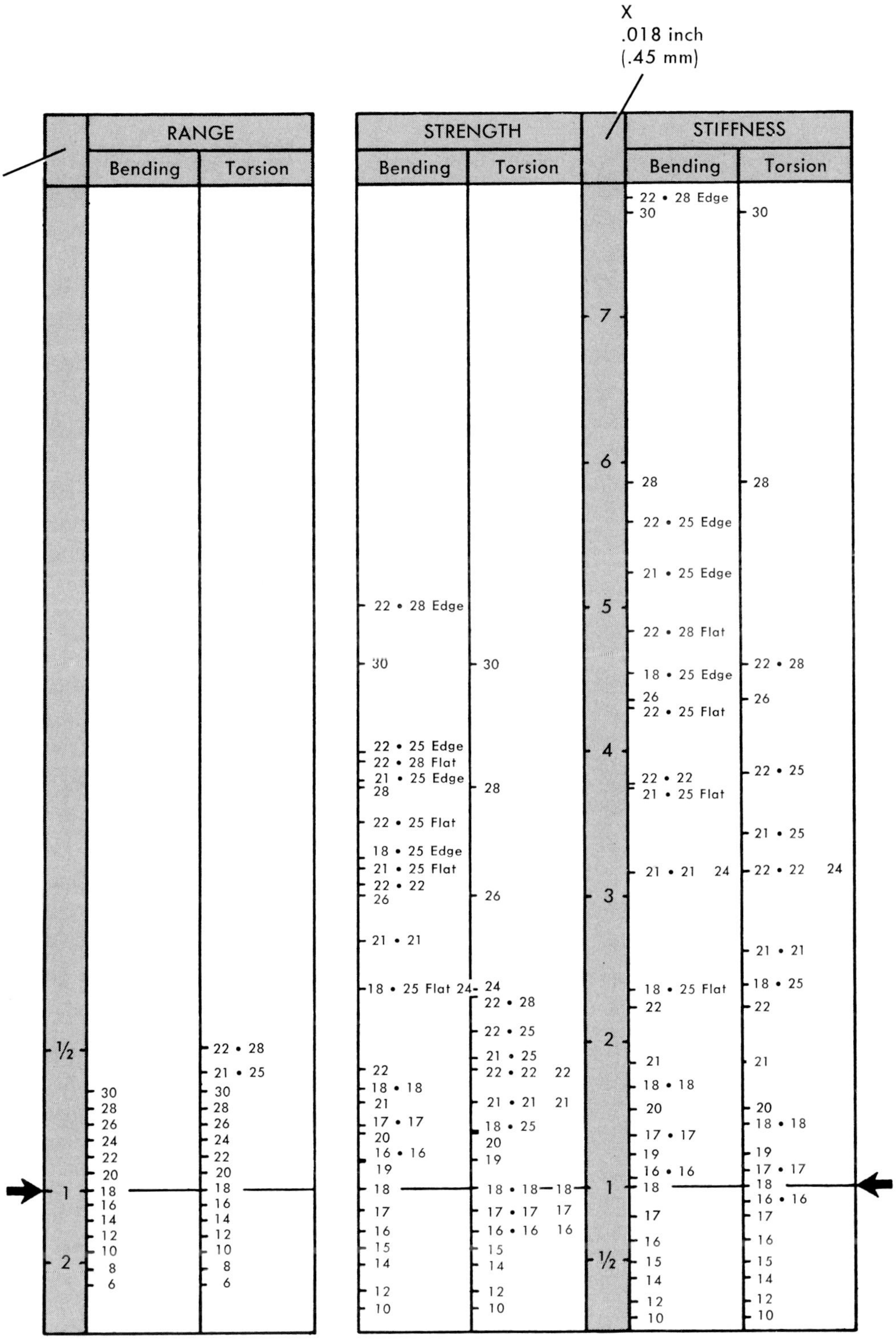

Fig. 5-10. Elastic properties of wires of different sizes compared to .018-inch (.45-mm) round wire.

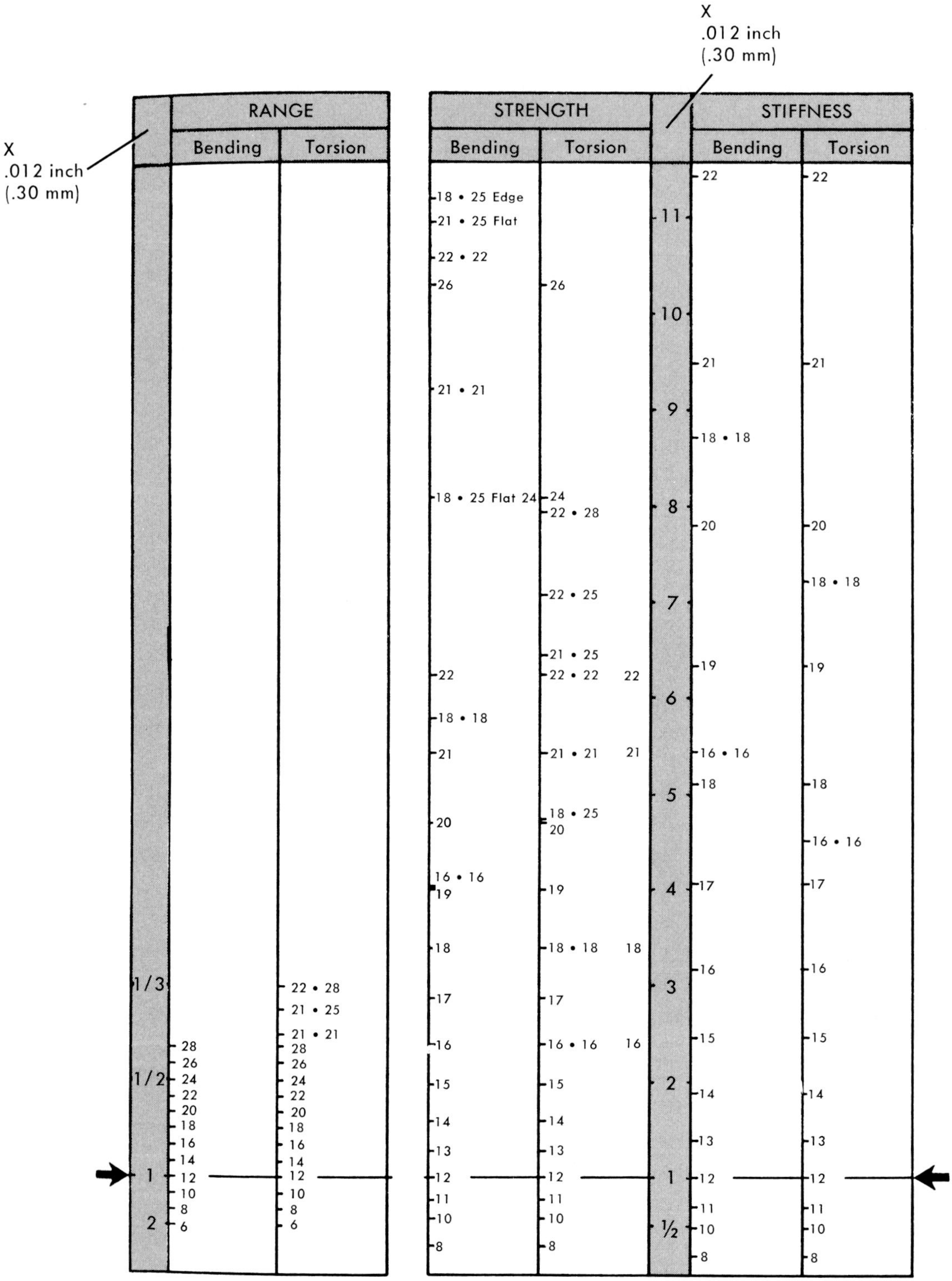

Fig. 5-11. Elastic properties of wires of different sizes compared to .012-inch (.30-mm) round wire.

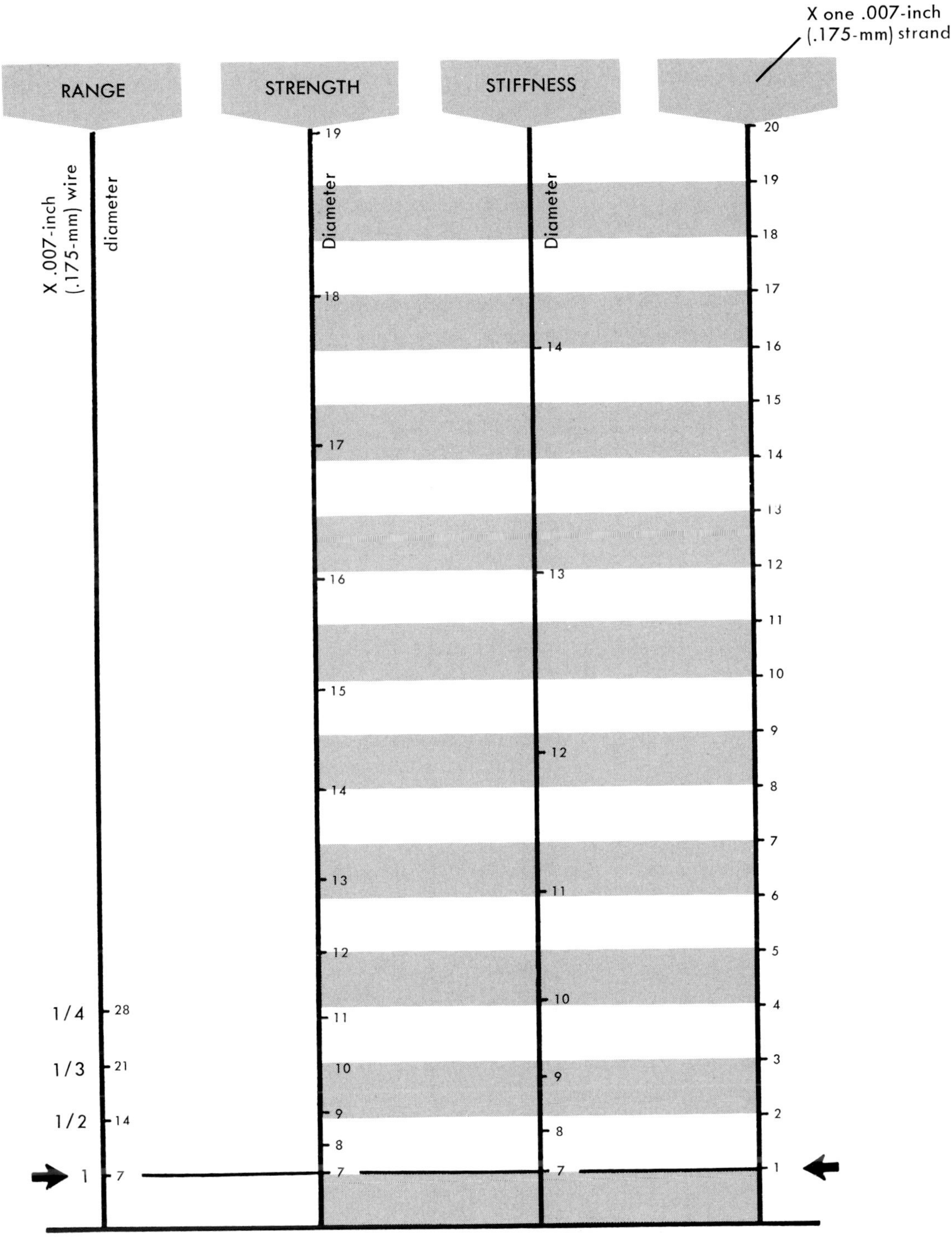

Fig. 5-12. Bending properties of wires compared to .007-inch (.18-mm) round wire. Multiple strands multiply stiffness and strength by the number of strands; thus the numbers at the right can be used to compare such multiple wires with single strands of larger dimensions. Example: twelve strands of .007-inch (.18-mm) wire will have the stiffness of a .013-inch (.33-mm) wire and the strength of a .016-inch (.40-mm) wire.

To reduce the need for such calculations, Figs. 5-9 to 5-12 compare wires of common dimensions on a graphic scale. In each case the scales have been adjusted to place a wire of one size at a common level for the three characteristics. This makes it possible to directly compare all properties of any other sized wire to a wire of the reference size.

Dimensions in the tables are shown in thousandths of an inch (mils). Metric conversion values may be found in Appendix B.

6

Torsion

Torque and *torsion* are similar words that describe the twisting of a beam or wire and its effects. Torque is the force (stress) that causes the twist. Torsion is the actual twisting (strain) that takes place in the material as a result of the torque.

The word *torque* has taken on an altered meaning in orthodontics, where it is used to describe the effect on a tooth of the force delivered by a twisted (torqued) archwire. To avoid confusion, the word *torque* will be reserved for this orthodontic application whenever possible, and *torsion* will be used to describe other twisting phenomena.

A round wire in torsion may be viewed as a string of flat disks that are rotated slightly on one another. Each section through the wire remains perfectly flat as the wire is twisted, so that a series of circles drawn around the wire will keep their flat circular form (Fig. 6-1).

The cross-sections of a rectangular wire under torsion undergo a deformation such as that shown in Fig. 6-2, and the actual changes become very complex. There is no need to consider these changes in full detail, because a relatively small limiting effect on the working range of a rectangular wire is their only pertinent effect.

EFFECTS OF CROSS-SECTION IN TORSION

Wires in torsion exhibit elastic properties similar to those seen in bending, and they can be described in the same basic terms. These values are also tabulated in Appendix A (Tables 1 and 3).

Range

The distance to the extreme fiber (c) is the governing factor in range under torsion, just as it was in bending. For round wires, c is one-half the diameter in both cases (Fig. 6-1). For rectangular wires in torsion, c is the distance from the center of the wire to an outer corner instead of to one of the sides. Range in torsion is proportional to the diameter of round wires and to the diagonal of rectangular wires.

Stiffness

Stiffness in torsion is proportional to the polar moment of inertia. This is similar to the moment of inertia in bending, except that the neutral axis is a line down the center instead of a broad ribbon. The moment is determined around the center of the section instead of the diameter (the slice of a round wire is spun like a phono-

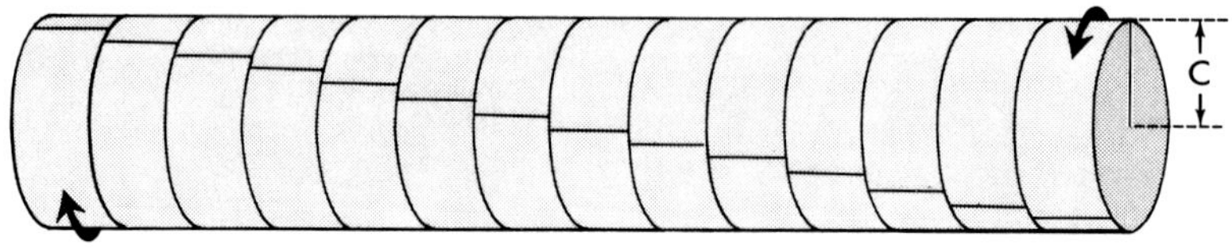

Fig. 6-1. The stress in torsion tends to slide one "slice" of the wire in relation to another. The effect is pure shear, with no tension or compression. There is no distortion of any of these individual circular sections; the wire retains its original outward shape.

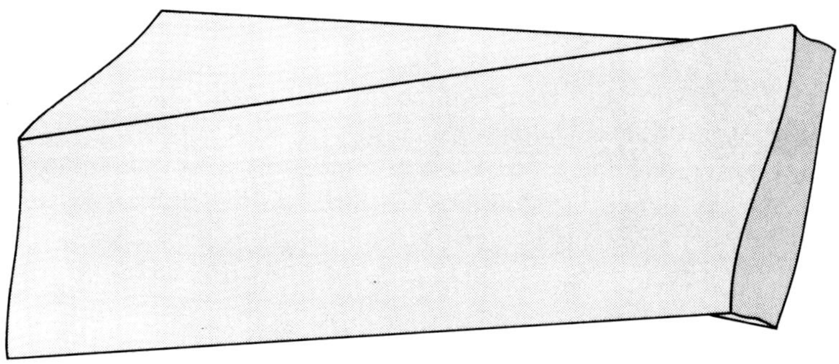

Fig. 6-2. When a rectangular wire is twisted, there is distortion of the surface and of the cross-section.

graph record on a turntable instead of crosswise). The polar moment of inertia is usually identified by the symbol "J" instead of "I," but it is used in the same way as the moment of inertia in bending. Thickness and width affect stiffness in direct proportion to their effect on the moment of inertia, so stiffness in torsion is also proportional to the fourth power of the diameter for round wires. For rectangular wires, there is no distinction between thickness and width in torsion. (See Appendix A, Table 3, for specific values.)

Strength

Strength of wires in torsion depends on the polar section modulus, which is based on the polar moment of inertia in the same way that the bending section modulus is based on *I*. These values can also be used and compared in the same way as for bending. The only difference is that there need be no differentiation between thickness and width for rectangular wires because these two factors work together in torsion. For round wires strength is proportional to the cube of the diameter as in bending. For rectangular wires comparisons are best made on the basis of values for the polar section modulus, which is shown in Appendix A, Table 3.

EFFECTS OF LENGTH IN TORSION

There are *no* exponential effects of length in torsion, so we have a markedly different response when compared to bending.

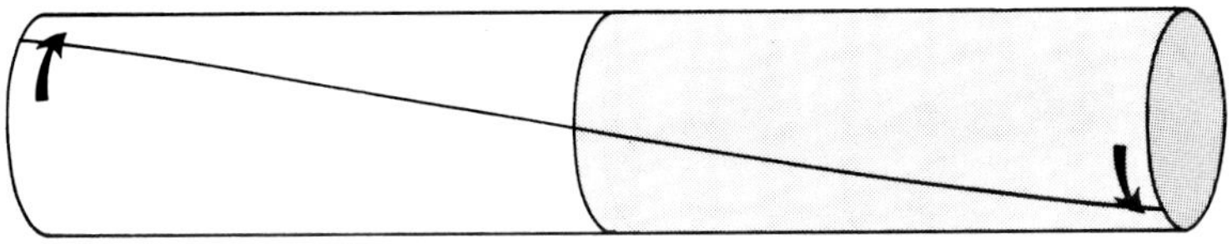

Fig. 6-3. Doubling the length of a wire will double its working range in torsion; the total twist that can be applied at full working load is directly proportional to length. Stiffness is inversely proportional to length. Strength is independent of length; each segment can sustain the same load whether there is additional wire at either end or not.

Strength

Length has absolutely *no effect* on strength. A given torqueing load will cause a definite twist over a certain length of wire, and strength is determined by the amount of such twist that this section can sustain. This section of wire will behave the same whether it is rigidly supported at the end or attached to an additional length of wire (Fig. 6-3). Its maximum permissible load is the same for any length.

Range

Range in torsion is directly proportional to length. Adding the shaded section shown in Fig. 6-3 to double the length will cause the ends to twist twice as far under the same load.

Stiffness

Stiffness in torsion is inversely proportional to length, essentially a mirror image of range. Fig. 6-3 also illustrates this parameter; doubling the length will increase the rotational deflection or proportionately reduce the force requirement for the same deflection. This is an entirely different relationship than exists in bending, and that difference can be very important. Changes in length are not the powerful modifiers that they are in bending.

SIGNIFICANCE OF DIFFERENCES BETWEEN BENDING AND TORSION

Cross-section affects the responses to bending and torsion in essentially the same way, but the substantial differences in the effect of length have very important clinical implications.

All three elastic properties are very limited in short lengths of wire, and the small influence of length in torsion makes it difficult to effect significant increases by increasing lengths.

This limits rectangular wires to very small torqueing adjustments on individual teeth and is one more advantage of a somewhat free fit in adjacent slots, as described on p. 171.

This same characteristic must be considered in arch bends and loop design as discussed on pp. 253-255, to avoid premature failure due to overloads in the segments subjected to torsion.

7

Orthodontic metals

Up to this point wire loading has been considered without regard to the structural material itself. These rules of structural design apply for any material, but differences in materials can shift the range of forces in which a specific design must operate.

Several different metals are used in orthodontic appliances, and their physical properties and mechanical behavior are the very lifeblood of orthodontic therapy. We take delicate wires, bend and twist them far beyond their usual working limits, and then place them in the mouth of a patient who pounds them unmercifully for weeks and months on end.

Through all this these wires are expected to be easily formed when we want to bend them, steadfast in their new form under oral stress, and gentle in their action on the teeth. Pushing materials to the limit in this way makes both the materials themselves and the design of the appliance of critical importance.

These demands are the exact opposite of what is usually expected of metals in most engineering applications. Industrial products are deliberately built heavy enough to provide a comfortable margin of safety to compensate for deficiencies in design and for the usual variations and minor flaws present in all materials. Where design calls for lightness and flexibility, as in a watch spring, precise engineering design limits loads to provide a similar margin of safety.

Orthodontists must burn the candle at both ends by applying heavy stresses to delicate structures, but this is as it should be. To do less would deprive patients of the optimum service to which they are entitled. The objective of this discussion is to help the orthodontist burn the candle at both ends without burning fingers. By not *unnecessarily* abusing materials, and by designing appliances to use the full potentials of the materials with maximum effect, it is possible to effect great gains in treatment efficiency.

Manufacture

Modern foundry techniques produce a consistent product by ordinary commercial standards, but the demands on orthodontic materials, especially wires, are such that the usual commercial test specifications are not adequate to ensure completely predictable behavior in clinical application. Suppliers work diligently to provide a product with consistently high properties. On the whole they succeed very well, but variations must inevitably appear from time to time.

A look at the processes and problems involved in wire manufacture leaves one with about the same impression as a look at the developing dentition; it is remarkable that the final result can be as dependably good as it actually is.

MAKING ORTHODONTIC WIRE

Sources

Stainless steel orthodontic wires are procured by suppliers from commercial sources of stainless steel. These alloys are usually standard formulas based on specifications of the American Iron and Steel Institute but often processed especially for orthodontic use. Even after the most careful manufacture, most orthodontic wires are further selected to provide a product that far surpasses basic commercial standards.

The quantities used in orthodontics, even on a national scale, are so small that the orthodontic specialty is among the smallest of customers. When one of the smallest of customers is also one of the most demanding, it becomes clear that those in orthodontics owe a collective vote of thanks to the suppliers who have often worked out of all proportion to this small volume of production to give the excellent wires that we are privileged to use today.

Most special-formula alloys are actually different stainless steels, but there are some notable exceptions such as chrome-cobalt (Elgiloy) and titanium alloys such as Nitinol.

Gold materials are usually manufactured by the suppliers, each to their own specifications. This has led to a much wider variation in gold products than in steel wires. Some gold alloys are still occasionally used in orthodontic treatment, although they have been largely replaced by other metals.

Melting

The physical properties of metals are influenced at every step in production beginning with the selection and melting of the alloying metals. This composition, which fixes the general properties of the metal, is more variable than might be expected. Fig. 7-1 shows the specifications for some standard stainless steel alloys, with permissible variations in the component materials.

The ingot

Dentists are so accustomed to differentiating between cast and wrought metals that it is easy to forget that a wire is actually a processed casting. One of the critical operations in wire making is pouring the molten alloy into a mold to produce an ingot. An ingot is far from being a uniform chunk of metal; like any casting, it will have varying degrees of porosity and inclusions of slag in different parts.

A magnified view of the inside of an ingot would show it to be made up of crystals of the component metals. In metallurigical terminology these crystals are usually called *grains*, and it is this granular structure that controls many of the ultimate mechanical properties.

Type	Chemical composition (%)						
	Cr	Ni	C (max.)	Mn (max.)	Si (max.)	P (max.)	S (max.)
302	17.00–19.00	8.00–10.00	0.15	2.00	1.00	0.045	0.030
304	18.00–20.00	8.00–12.00	0.08	2.00	1.00	0.045	0.030
416	12.00–14.00	None	0.15	1.25	1.00	0.06	0.15 min.

Fig. 7-1. Chemical composition for typical stainless steels.

Grains in a casting are formed in definite patterns typical of the individual metals, but they are far from perfect because of the conditions under which they must form. When the ingot is cooling and solidifying, many different grains are forming at once. These growing crystals crowd and even surround one another, so that the ingot becomes a conglomeration of many irregularly shaped grains of different materials. The size and distribution of the grains depend on the rate of cooling and the size of the ingot.

The pouring and cooling processes also affect porosity. Porosity in the ingot comes from two sources. Gases that are either dissolved in the metal or produced by chemical reactions within the molten mass form bubbles that are trapped in the metal. In addition, as the ingot cools and shrinks, the late-cooling interior section must shrink inside an already hardened shell. This shell does not permit the volume to adjust completely to the shrinkage, so additional vacuum voids result. Before further processing is begun, or very early in processing, the ingot is trimmed to remove the undesirable parts.

The microstructure of a metal is the very basis of its physical properties and mechanical performance, and every step in production is directed at getting the most out of the original grain structure of the ingot.

Rolling

The first mechanical step is rolling the ingot into a long bar. This is done by a series of rollers that gradually reduce the ingot to a relatively small diameter. Through all this rolling and the later processing into the final wire, the different parts of the original ingot never completely lose their identity. The metal that was on the outside of the ingot is on the outside of the finest wire. Likewise, the ends of the ingot will be at the ends of the wire, even though it may be miles long. Wire is actually a grossly distorted ingot, so it is easy to see that different pieces of wire from the same batch may differ depending on which part of the ingot they came from.

The individual grains of the ingot also keep their identity through the rolling process, at least until certain heat treatments are applied. Each grain is elongated in the same proportion as the ingot. The squeezing, massaging action of rolling the ingot has a very important effect on the grain structure, actually increasing the strength of the metal. Where the original crystals fitted together rather indifferently, with gaps and voids scattered among them, the mechanical action of rolling forces them into long, fingerlike shapes that are closely meshed with one another. This causes an increase in the hardness or brittleness of the metal as the grains are forced to interlock ever more tightly with one another in a form of work hardening. Even the atoms that make up the crystal structure are forced into new positions, filling in gaps and irregularities that may have been left in the original crystal.

Each pass through the rollers increases the work hardening, until finally the structure becomes so "locked up" that it can no longer adjust enough to adapt to the squeezing of the rollers.

If rolling is continued beyond this point, the surface will start to show many small cracks and begin to crumble. Before this happens the rolling process is interrupted and the metal is annealed by heating to a suitably high temperature. At annealing temperature the atoms become mobile enough to move about within the mass, breaking up the tight crystalline structure and relieving some of the internal stresses brought about by the rolling. When the metal has cooled again, the annealed structure more nearly resembles that of the original casting, but it is more uniform. Grain size can be controlled in annealing by adjustment of the time and temperature of annealing and the rate of cooling.

Drawing

After the ingot has been reduced to a fairly small diameter by rolling, it is further reduced to its final size by drawing. This is a more precise process in which the wire is pulled through a small hole in a die. The hole is slightly smaller than the starting diameter of the wire, so that the walls of the die squeeze it uniformly from all sides as it passes through, reducing the wire to the diameter of the die. Drawing subjects the entire surface of the wire to the same pressures instead of squeezing from only two opposite sides as in rolling.

The effect on grain structure in drawing is much the same as in rolling. Before it is reduced to orthodontic size, a wire is drawn through many series of dies and annealed several times along the way to relieve work hardening.

These intermediate annealings are very important to strength, and especially to resistance to breakage. The task of heating and cooling a large coil of wire so that all parts are treated alike is not as easy as it may seem. It must be done slowly to prevent the outer coils from being heated more than those on the inside, and temperatures must be carefully controlled. Even with the most careful procedures situations can arise in which one part of a coil will be affected differently. Such variations can create many problems in sampling for quality control.

The actual number of drafts through the dies, as well as the frequency of annealing, depends on the alloy being drawn. Gold is extremely ductile and can be reduced considerably with each draft. Ordinary carbon steel requires many more steps than gold, and stainless steel requires many more than carbon steel. Gold work hardens slowly, so that it also needs less frequent annealing than the more rapidly work-hardening steels.

Spring properties of wire

Hardness and spring properties of most orthodontic wires depend almost entirely on the effects of work hardening during manufacture. This means that the entire drawing and annealing schedule must be planned carefully with the final size and properties in mind. If the metal is almost in need of another annealing at its final size, it will have maximum work-hardening and spring properties. If drawing is carried too far, the wire will be brittle and will break easily. If drawing is not carried far enough after the last annealing, there will be too much residual softness and very low working range and strength.

Wires can be reduced through much of the range of orthodontic sizes without an intermediate annealing. When wire is annealed in processing at one size and different parts of the batch are then drawn to different final sizes, the smaller of the wires will be subjected to additional work hardening. This effect is rather small for small size differences and because of the different drawing schedules that are used, it is not consistent. Such differences can make the smaller wire proportionately harder, which is desirable so long as brittleness does not become excessive. This increased hardness in wire of small diameters was clearly noted in some bending tests, such as those reported in Chapter 17.

Rectangular wires

Rectangular wires can be made by drawing the material through a rectangular die or by rolling round wires to a rectangular shape. There appears to be little significant difference in the wires formed by the two processes, but this is difficult to evaluate because of other variables. Round wires made by drawing vary as much in physical properties as most rectangular wires; therefore it would be unrealistic to attribute specific differences to the rolling or drawing process. Drawing can, however, produce sharper corners on rectangular wire, and the engagement of these edges in a rectangular slot can be an advantage in the application of torque.

Hardening and heat treatment

The properties of metals can be altered after fabrication by heat treatment either before or after delivery to the orthodontist. Annealing is one form of heat treatment that was discussed in connection with manufacture, but there are many other processes. Each metal behaves differently under the application of heat, so these processes must be considered separately for each major class of metals.

CARBON STEEL

Carbon steel is not an orthodontic metal because of corrosion problems, but its behavior is so basic to the subject of heat treatment that it provides a basis for discussion of other metals as well.

Composition of carbon steel

Carbon steel is mostly iron, but the small amount of carbon that is added to the alloy makes a tremendous difference in its response to heat. These steels are actually a mixture of pure iron, called *ferrite,* and iron carbide (Fe_3C). In metallurgy, iron carbide is called *cementite,* because it sometimes gives the appearance of cementing the ferrite grains together. Because carbon is so light in relation to iron, pure cementite is only 6.69% carbon. It is easy to see from this how even very small percentages of carbon can cause a large change in the crystalline structure of steel.

Ferrite, the pure iron, is a soft, ductile material without much structural strength. Cementite is hard enough to scratch glass and is comparably brittle; therefore, used by itself, it would also be a poor structural material.

Steel is a mixture in which these two mediocre materials support and reinforce one another, much like glass fibers and plastic. The physical properties of steel depend almost entirely on the proportions of ferrite and cementite and on the way in which they are intermixed with one another. Various alloying materials contribute to the properties of steel, but most of them work indirectly by modification of the ferrite-cementite structure.

Heat treatment of carbon steel

Heat treatment is the key to controlling the important internal structure of steel, making it soft when it must be worked and hard or tough when those qualities are needed.

High temperatures. At the high end of the temperature scale (over 1400° to 1500° F or 750° to 800° C), steel is a homogenous material with all of the carbon in solid solution in the iron. The iron carbide is completely decomposed at this temperature. Steel in this form is called *austenite,* a name that should be remembered for future reference with respect to stainless steel. In carbon steel, austenite is stable only at these high temperatures where it becomes a starting point for later changes that take place during cooling.

Low temperatures. At the low end of the temperature scale (below 450° F or 225° C) an entirely different material known to metallurgists as *martensite* is formed. This is almost pure cementite, the hardest and most brittle form of the iron-carbon combination. Martensite will begin to form as the mass of cooling metal reaches the 450° F (225° C) range, and the transformation is complete at about 200° F (90° C).

Intermediate temperatures. Between these high and low extremes of temperature, many intermediate phases are formed. These are various mixtures of ferrite and cementite, with crystal structures tending toward hardness in the low-temperature ranges and toward softness and ductility at higher temperatures. Many of these other forms have names of their own and play important parts in steel production, but they are not of concern in orthodontics.

The properties of the metal when it reaches room temperature depend on the amount of time that it spends in the different intermediate temperature ranges as it cools. If it is cooled rapidly, by quenching, it will go past all the intermediate stages and into the martensite range so fast that the product will be almost pure martensite—hard and brittle (if there is enough carbon present for all of the iron). If it is cooled more slowly, other crystal structures will be formed, and some of these will also be stable at room temperature. If these forms are allowed to develop, the amount of martensite will be correspondingly reduced and the product will be more workable. By various special manipulations, such as quenching in baths of molten salt, temperatures can be changed very rapidly from one range to another. These treatments bypass certain temperatures and give ample time for full development of desired crystalline structures at others.

Tempering. When steel is quenched in water, the resulting martensite is so brittle that the steel is unsuitable for most mechanical applications. This is remedied by reheating to intermediate temperature ranges (usually below 1000° F [525° C]) under carefully controlled conditions to permit a partial transformation into softer forms. This reheating is called tempering. Quenching and tempering are commonly used in this sequence to bring carbon steel into the most favorable condition for machining and other applications.

Effect of alloying on heat treatment

Other metals are added to steel alloys for many reasons, but one of the most important is to control the rates and temperatures of the heat transformations just discussed. Some alloying metals make certain otherwise unstable phases stable at room temperature and may modify the physical properties of the final product in other ways. A few alloying metals, such as the chromium in stainless steel, contribute physical properties of their own to the final alloy.

STAINLESS STEEL

The stainless steel alloys include a wide range of compositions and physical properties. Only a few of these are suitable for orthodontic use. All standard stainless steels are classified and numbered for identification according to a standardized system set up for all steels by the American Iron and Steel Institute. This system uses type numbers from 300 to 502 for stainless steel. Fig. 7-1 shows the composition of typical stainless steel alloys in the 300 and 400 series.

Types 501 and 502 are low-chromium (4% to 6%) steels not used for orthodontic appliances.

Martensitic stainless steels (400 series)

Alloys in the 400 series contain little or no nickel; they are primarily alloys of iron and chromium. These alloys can be heat treated much the same as carbon steel, forming martensite at room temperature. For this reason they are known as the martensitic stainless steels.

The heat hardenability of these alloys would seem to make them ideal for orthodontic appliances, but they have another property that rules out their use for most of the severe service we demand. The martensitic alloys are brittle and fracture much too easily under a sharp blow to endure in the mouth or to withstand the bending to which we must subject them. However, they are very useful for the construction of many orthodontic instruments.

Austenitic stainless steels (300 series)

Types numbered in the 300 range make up the most widely used group of stainless steels, and this group includes those usually used in orthodontic appliances. These alloys contain iron and chromium, but they also contain significant quantities of nickel. The nickel content has a stabilizing effect on austenite, which is stable in carbon steel only at high temperatures. In these chrome-nickel stainless steels the austenite is stable even at room temperature, so these alloys are called austenitic stainless steel. Austenite alone would be excessively soft at room temperature, but the large proportion of chromium in these alloys gives them the necessary strength. This chromium also gives them their high resistance to corrosion.

Types 302 and 304 are commonly used in orthodontic appliances. These and many other alloys that contain about 18% chromium and 8% nickel make up the 18-8 group of stainless steels.

Hardening of austenitic steels. Because of the stability of the austenite in these steels, they cannot be hardened like carbon steel by quenching or similar heat treatment. The only way in which these steels can be hardened is by cold working. Austenitic steels harden rapidly with the usual realignment of the crystalline structure under cold working.

Work hardening also brings about some transformation of part of the austenite into martensite, which adds to the hardening effect. The austenite in these metals is stable at room temperature, but just barely so; even disturbing the crystalline structure by cold working is enough to permit transformation of some of the material to the harder martensite.

Annealing austenitic steels. Stainless steel requires a higher temperature for annealing (1800° to 2000° F or 1000° to 1100° C) than does carbon steel. At this temperature all of the effects of cold working are eliminated, and the metal returns to its softest, most workable state. Orthodontic bands and ligature wires are usually supplied fully annealed. Rapid cooling is not an essential part of the annealing process, but in air it is important for corrosion control, as will be described later. These materials are ordinarily either quenched or treated in an inert atmosphere to maintain their stainless properties.

Stress relief of stainless steel

A most important heat treatment process for orthodontic stainless steel is the relatively low-temperature process of stress relieving, which is used both in manufacturing and at the time of clinical application. This is a level of heat treatment at which internal stresses are relieved by minute slippages and readjustments in intergranular relations, without the loss of hardening that accompanies the higher-temperature process of annealing.

Work hardening is the result of forced interlocking of grains and atoms of the metal. Many of these grains are locked in situations in which the material is under stress, even when the piece as a whole is not stressed. These microscopic regions are under pressure or tension, more or less working against one another.

When a wire with such internal stress is bent to store energy for an orthodontic application, the previously stressed areas cannot do their full share. Force applied to these stressed regions will bring them to their load limit sooner than usual because some of their reserve has already been used up by the prestressed condition. If the new load is in the same direction as the internal stress, the two loads actually augment one another. In either case action of the wire is weakened by the internal stress (Fig. 7-2).

Stress relief eliminates such prestressed areas within the wire and puts it into

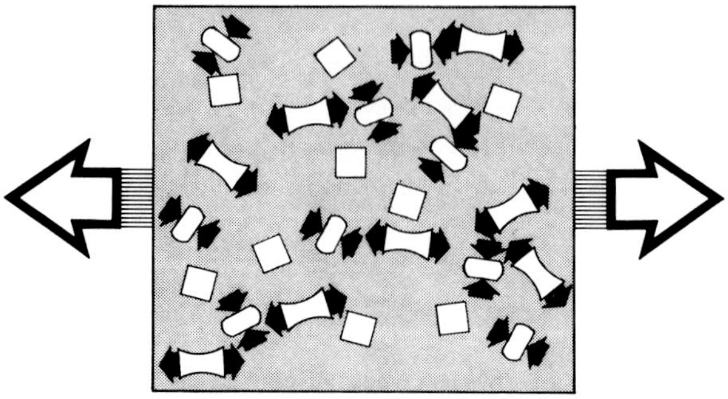

Fig. 7-2. A pictorial representation of the random tension and compression stresses present in a metal after mechanical manipulation. Residual tension areas are already under stress of the same nature as that being imposed by the outside load, so they reach their limit of strength before the unstressed areas do; residual regions of compression are relieved by the outside load, actually working with it instead of resisting its action.

condition to work more effectively. Tests described in Chapter 17 clearly show these effects.

As internal stresses are relieved, there may also be some change in the shape of the wire. This is the second reason for stress relieving in orthodontics. A wire that is bent to form an arch is full of residual stresses that tend to slowly return it toward its original form. This goes on gradually at ordinary temperatures, causing a progressive change in arch form called *elastic memory.* A stress-relieving heat treatment accelerates those changes in shape so that the wire will become more stable. When this treatment is applied to an archwire, the form should always be checked and the arch reshaped as required after the heat treatment.

Stress-relieving effects depend on both time and temperature, and they can be controlled by the adjustment of either of these factors. In general, low-temperature treatment (400° to 700° F or 200° to 350° C) over a long period of time is most desirable, but this is feasible only in the manufacturing process. The arch formed for a patient in the chair cannot be treated for hours or even for too many minutes. Fortunately, however, most of the benefits of heat treatment can be produced in a few minutes or less at temperatures of 800° F (425° C), especially if the wires have been treated previously to eliminate the stresses of the wiremaking process.

Commercial specifications usually call for a long period of time for all heat-treating processes, including stress relieving. This is as much for the practical considerations of commercial production as for purely metallurgical reasons.

In commercial production long treatment periods are not only practical, they can actually be more precisely controlled than short periods. When these treatments are applied to large, bulky coils or bundles, a long time is required to reach a uniform temperature. After hours in a furnace, a heavy coil of wire may still show a difference of more than 100° between inside and outside layers. It takes a long time for even a small bundle of orthodontic wires to reach a uniform temperature throughout. Under such circumstances uniform results are best achieved by prolonged low-temperature treatment.

In the orthodontist's office the entire problem is different. One small wire is treated at a time, and as it is placed in an oven it will reach maximum temperature almost instantly. In less than one minute such a wire will undergo most of the possible stress-relieving changes. The small remaining changes will take place much more slowly and add little to the wire properties.

An oven is the most reliable medium for heat treatment because of its relatively uniform temperature. Much of the deterioration of such ovens is due to expansion and contraction as they are heated and cooled. This, together with long warm-up times, makes it most practical to keep a heat-treating oven in continuous operation day and night.

Rapid treatment can also be carried out by heating the wire directly with an electric current from a welder or special heat-treating power source, but this is not appreciably faster than oven treatment. Most electrical techniques use a rapid rise to a somewhat higher temperature, stopping the heat application as soon as that temperature is reached.

A major problem with electrical heat treatment is lack of uniform temperature, especially in loops bent into the wire. Heated wires radiate heat in all directions. When loops bring wires close together, some of this heat goes to the adjacent wire, so the temperature rises much more rapidly there than in the rest of the wire. This is dramatically illustrated by slowly raising the temperature of a small-diameter wire containing loops until it glows. The loops will always reach incandescence first.

Intergranular corrosion of stainless steel

Carbon is an undesirable impurity in austenitic stainless steel, but it is difficult to eliminate it completely. Carbon does not enter into the physical structure of these steels, except in the formation of a small amount of martensite in cold working, but at temperatures between 800° and 1200° F (425° and 650° C) it starts a chain of corrosion that can result in actual physical failure of the metal. At these temperatures carbon reacts with chromium to form chromium carbide (CCr_4). This reaction is called *sensitization*. At temperatures above the 1200° F (650° C) range, chromium carbide breaks up into the component elements. Below sensitizing temperatures, the reaction between carbon and chromium cannot take place; thus at either higher or lower temperatures the metal is safe from sensitization.

Chromium carbide is harmless in itself, but chromium tied up as the carbide cannot contribute to the corrosion resistance of the metal. Minute amounts of carbon can have a devastating effect, because most of the carbon in these metals is precipitated between the grains. Here it inactivates the chromium at the grain boundaries, opening them to corrosion. Since only the surfaces of the grains are involved, inactivation of even a very small part of the total chromium will have a great effect on the material. The grain boundaries are already the weak points in the structure, so corrosive attack on these surfaces can actually cause the metal to disintegrate; the grains literally fall apart.

Prevention of intergranular corrosion is one of the most important problems in manipulating stainless steel at high temperature. Two means of prevention are available: (1) keeping out of the sensitizing temperature range (800° to 1200° F or 425° to 650° C) and (2) controlling the carbon.

Controlling temperatures to prevent intergranular corrosion. The chromium carbide reaction takes time. Speed in handling the metal in the sensitizing temperature range, as during soldering, can be a very effective means of minimizing sensitization. Stainless steel should always be quenched immediately after soldering, to bring it down to a safe temperature as rapidly as possible. This is also the reason for quenching after annealing. At annealing temperatures the chromium and carbon exist as separate elements; if the metal is cooled rapidly from annealing to room temperature, there is no opportunity for them to combine to form chromium carbide.

Both low-temperature and high-temperature solders can be used to advantage to control intergranular corrosion if they are used properly. With low-temperature solders (silver solders that melt below 1100° F, or 590° C), the objective is to heat to soldering temperature, solder, and then quench as quickly as possible. This is the most commonly used procedure in soldering stainless steel.

Higher-temperature solders (gold solders that melt well above 1200° F, or 650° C) also can be used, but only if the entire piece of steel can be heated to this high temperature. The metal is then above the sensitizing range while it is being soldered, so it is safe. It must still be quenched immediately after soldering. If only part of the steel is heated to this high soldering temperature, there will be a zone outside the soldering area that is in the sensitizing temperature range; therefore this method is useful only for small pieces. Soldering at these temperatures may also cause some annealing, which may or may not be desirable.

Stabilization to prevent intergranular corrosion. The second possibility for control of intergranular corrosion is to make carbon unavailable for the sensitizing reaction. This is done at the time that the alloy is manufactured, either by keeping the carbon content exceptionally low (below 1.08%) or by adding other metals that tie it up in different compounds. Columbium and titanium are commonly used for this purpose. These metals form carbides at higher temperatures than chromium, so the cooling steel is held at these temperatures long enough to allow the formation of other carbides before the chromium carbide reaction can take place.

Steel that has been treated in any of the foregoing ways to reduce the available carbon is called *stabilized steel.* The method of stabilization is usually chosen on the basis of cost, availability, or technical requirements; the final effect of each is about the same.

Stabilized steel is less susceptible to intergranular corrosion, but it is still not 100% safe. Improper handling by the user can easily nullify the advantage. These steels are stabilized as they are delivered, but there is no compensation for carbon introduced later. In orthodontics a plentiful supply of carbon is always available in the organic debris present in the mouth. Leaving these deposits on a piece of steel as it is welded or soldered will immediately carbonize them and infuse the surface of the steel with carbon. Extreme care should be taken to avoid this and any other carbon contamination of stainless steel that is to be heated.

GOLD ALLOYS

Precious metals behave much the same as austenitic stainless steel under heat treatment, but at lower temperatures. Most gold alloys can be annealed by heating to 1200° F (650° C), and quenching. This simplifies the process of annealing but makes it almost impossible to solder gold without annealing it.

Some special alloys, such as those which are high in platinum, can be hardened materially by temperature manipulation, usually by heating to about 800° to 1000° F (425° to 550° C) and cooling slowly. The slow cooling permits optimum grain growth (crystal formation) for the production of a hard material.

Many different gold alloys are available, each with its own peculiarities, so it is important to carefully follow the manufacturer's instructions for heat treatment. Differences between these alloys are too great to permit further generalization.

Work hardening

Gold alloys work harden much more slowly and to a lesser degree than steel. This can be a great advantage. To the manufacturer, low work hardening means that drawing is much easier, with fewer intermediate anneals required. To the orthodontist, it means that these materials are less brittle and will take much more manipulation before they have hardened enough to become brittle and break.

CHROME-COBALT (ELGILOY)

Chrome-cobalt (Elgiloy) is a unique alloy that has been available for orthodontic use for some time. Its elastic properties are enough like stainless steel that it requires no changes in appliance design, and the usual adjustment procedures can easily keep force parameters within the same range as with steel.

The significant differences are in workability and heat treatment potential. The softer tempers offer formability unparalleled by any but the gold alloys, with the added advantage of the availability of heat treatment to bring elastic properties of the formed wire into the longer working range of stainless steel.

This alloy work hardens rapidly. It is available in several "tempers," all with the same stiffness. The higher tempered materials have a higher working range achieved through a combination of work hardening and heat treatment in manufacture. These can be heat treated to further increase their working range, but the selector should consider formability first. The additional work hardening imposed in forming can increase the brittleness that is associated with all high-tempered materials. When heat treatment is to be used, even the softest temper will have a very adequate working range for most applications, while providing the greatest ease of initial forming with negligible brittleness.

TITANIUM ALLOYS

The most widely used titanium alloy is Nitinol, a nickel-titanium alloy, but some other forms show similar mechanical properties. The elastic properties of these materials differ significantly from those of other orthodontic alloys.

Stiffness is much lower and working range much higher, producing spectacular flexibility. This requires complete redesign and redesignation of component functions. These are special-purpose materials that should not be used as simple replacements for conventional wires in conventional techniques.

The negative aspects of these alloys revolve around their more difficult formability and increased brittleness that are always the other side of the coin of increased working range.

8

Elastic behavior of metals

Metals fill a major role in the storage and distribution of mechanical energy in an orthodontic system. The design of any specific mechanical device such as an orthodontic appliance is a matter of juggling the requirements for force management with the available space and the properties of the material for desired results. With the wide range of possibilities often available with all three of these variables, it is obvious that many very different solutions may be possible.

The orthodontic mechanism offers a wide range of options even with the frequently limited working range that we find available to us. Working within close limits of space, applying forces to highly responsive delicate tissues, and using materials to the very limits of their capacity, the orthodontist must continually balance all of these factors against one another. Neither space, materials, nor the patient's response allows any comfortable margin or freedom to "overdesign," which is a choice that is available with most mechanical devices. Any significant change in one factor is almost certain to impose significant limitations on another.

This chapter will describe the behavior of forces within a wire, those properties at the very heart of the orthodontic appliance that govern the transfer of force from the orthodontist's fingers to the appliance for storage, and the later distribution and delivery to the teeth.

STRESS

When force is applied to a mechanical part, that force is called a *stress*. Most stresses come from outside the material itself, but under some conditions, such as cold working or uneven cooling, one part of the material may impose a stress on another part of the same piece. These are the internal stresses that were discussed previously in connection with stress relieving.

A *stress is a force*, whether it is internal or external. Stress is measured in units of force, such as ounces or grams.

Types of stress

Stresses are usually classified into three types depending on their action on the material. All stresses can be resolved into one or more of these three basic stresses, as illustrated in Fig. 8-1.

A *tension* stress tends to pull the material apart. The two forces that must work against one another to apply this stress pull directly away from one another.

A *compression* stress is the direct opposite of tension in every way.

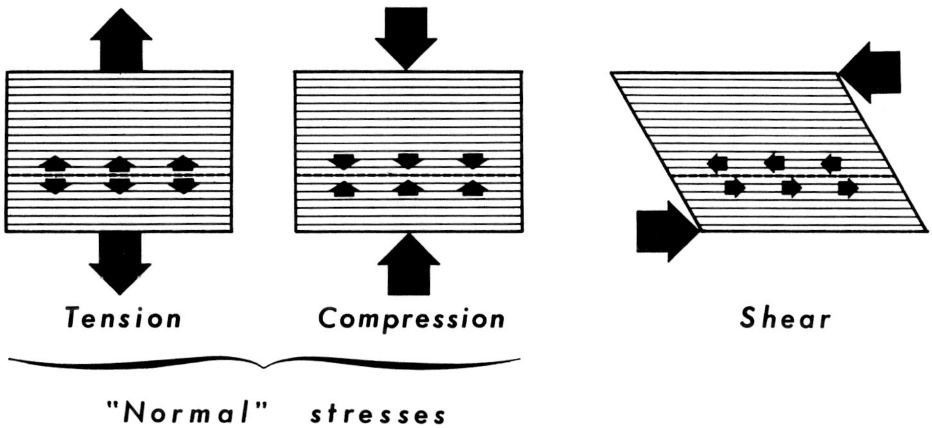

Fig. 8-1. The three basic types of stress.

Tension and compression stresses, taken together, are called *normal* stresses because the force is normal in the geometric sense (at right angles) to the affected planes of the material.

A *shear* stress is applied by two forces acting in opposite directions but *not* in the same line. These stresses tend to slide one part of the material past another along planes parallel to the applied forces. This is the familiar couple, which will rotate the piece unless a counter-couple is applied elsewhere.

All three of these stresses are present in most working mechanical parts, but they are usually not of equal magnitude or importance. Tension and compression account for most of the effects in bending, while shear is the only one of the three involved in torsion or torque.

STRAIN

When a material is subjected to stress, it is changed in shape. The change may be difficult to detect in heavy, rigid structures, but nevertheless it is there. No material is completely rigid. This forced change in shape is called a *strain*. Strain is measured in units of length such as inches or millimeters.

This internal distortion produces the internal stresses that balance (resist) the externally applied stress.

ELASTICITY

Stress and strain go together; it is impossible to have one without the other. The relationship between the two depends on the material that is stressed. A light stress can produce a large strain in a dish of gelatin, but even a heavy stress will produce only a microscopic change in a granite rock.

In deforming under stress, a material absorbs and stores energy from the force. This stored force is ready for instant release as the stress is removed and the material is freed to return to its original form. This tendency of a stressed material to return to its original form is called elasticity.

In orthodontics the relationship between stress and strain tells us how much our materials will bend and how much force they can store for later application to the teeth. Careful measurements over the complete working range of the material also tell which material or which size of wire will be most effective in storing and applying orthodontic forces.

Measuring stress and strain; the stress-strain diagram

Measuring stress and strain can be readily accomplished with a high degree of accuracy. Each metal has its own typical response, which varies within certain limits depending on processing, so the results of these tests are frequently used for quality control in manufacturing.

The old standby workhorse of materials testing is the stress-strain tensile test. Most other tests are variations of this one or are related to it in some way. The tensile test is the essence of simplicity, and machines for carrying it out are available in all force ranges from grams to hundreds of tons.

In a tensile test a piece of the test material is stretched, usually until it breaks. It is stretched gradually, with the force steadily increased while the force (stress) and the amount of stretch (strain) are measured at regular intervals. These measurements show exactly how much strain is produced by each level of stress. Plotting the entire series of measurements for a single test piece on a graph will show exactly how the material responded through the entire test. This graph is called the *stress-strain diagram* (Fig. 8-2). This same graph may also be called the *tensile curve* or the *elastic curve.*

The general form of the elastic curve is similar for most metals. It always begins at the origin of the graph, the lower left-hand corner where both stress and strain are zero. As stress is applied, strain is produced, and both increase simultaneously. This is indicated by the line of the graph rising upward and to the right. The line is usually straight in this first part of the curve, indicating that stress and strain are proportional to one another. Doubling the stress will double the strain.

This proportionality is the basis for Hooke's law of springs, which is usually encountered in early science courses. According to Hooke's law, a spring will stretch in proportion to the applied force. Actually, this law holds true only in the lower, straight portion of the elastic curve, but springs are normally designed to function only within this range where response is proportional.

The slope, or steepness, of the elastic curve is an indication of how much the material has resisted being stretched. If the line is almost vertical, it shows that a large force was required to produce a small amount of stretch; if the line is nearly horizontal, it indicates that a small force stretched the test piece a great distance. Of course, the apparent steepness of the line depends on the selection of the scales on the graph, so comparisons between materials must be based on the actual ratio between stress and strain rather than on the appearance of the graph alone.

Modulus of elasticity. This brings us to the modulus of elasticity (Young's modulus), a figure in millions of pounds per square inch that is found in most tables of physical properties. The modulus of elasticity is an expression of the steepness of the elastic curve in absolute terms, thus it is actually an index of stiffness or resistance to stretching. It is useful primarily as a basis for comparing different materials

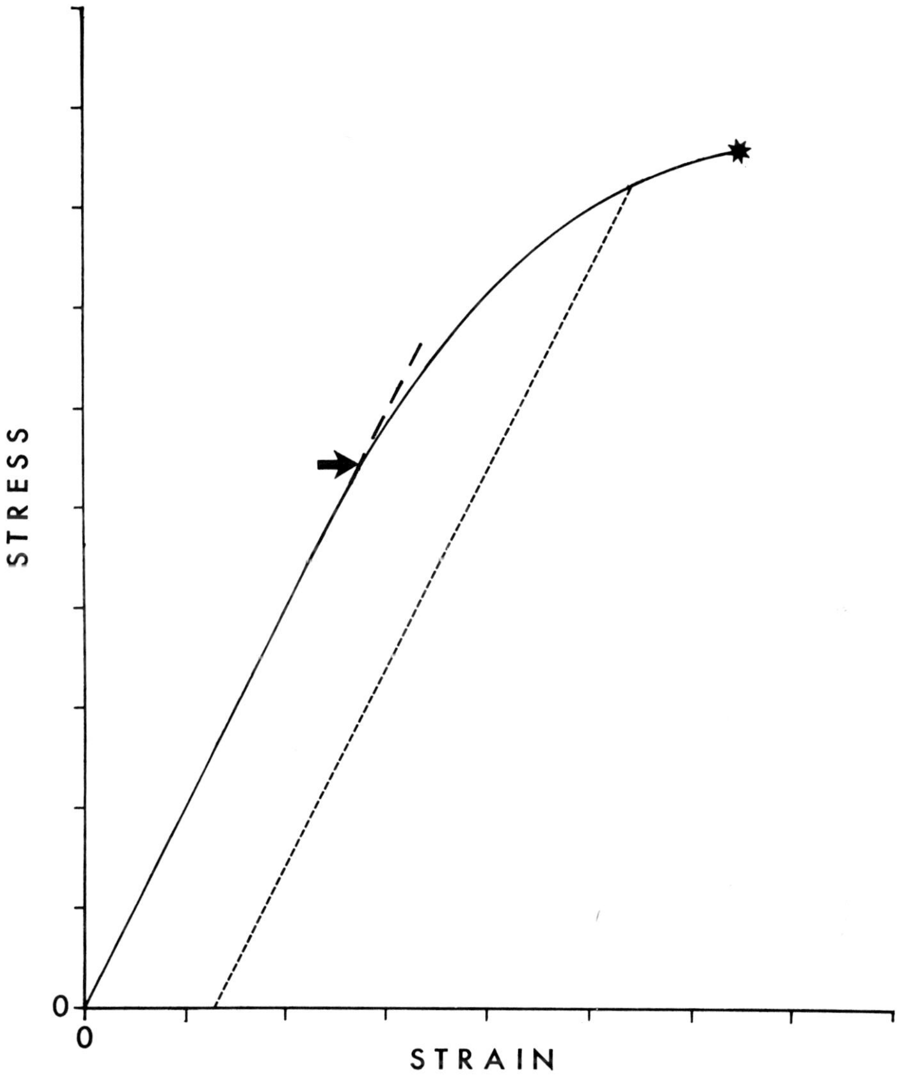

Fig. 8-2. The stress-strain diagram, showing the amount of deformation (strain) produced at each level of force (stress). The arrow indicates the elastic (proportional) limit, beyond which the material will be subjected to a permanent set. The star is the point at which the test piece fails (breaks).

and in certain engineering formulas. The large size of these values is due to the method used in their calculation; actual loads as high as the modulus expressed in pounds per square inch are never even approached in actual application.

The elastic modulus can be determined without even drawing an elastic curve; all that is needed are two pairs of figures from the tensile test—stress and actual length for two different stress levels below the proportional limit. This will indicate how far the test piece has been stretched by a specific force. To take a concrete example, an industrial test might be made on a steel bar with a cross-section of 1/2 square inch and a length of 2 inches between the points of measurement. If we know that a force of 7000 pounds has stretched this piece .001 inch, we have all the figures necessary to calculate the elastic modulus. Since the 7000 pounds was stretching a piece only 1/2 square inch in cross-section, it is multiplied by 2 to obtain the force that would be required to stretch a piece with a cross-section of 1 square inch. This would be a stress of 14,000 pounds.

The big increase in the size of the figure comes from determining how much force would be required to stretch the test piece to twice its length (for instance, to stretch the 2-inch piece to 4 inches). This is unrealistic as an ultimate objective because structural metal will break long before this point is reached, but the elastic modulus is merely a paper figure used for comparative purposes. In our example, if the 2-inch section stretched only .001 inch and stretching were continued proportionately according to Hooke's law, 2000 times as much force would be required to stretch the piece 2 inches. Therefore the 14,000 pounds must be multiplied by 2000, resulting in a value of 28,000,000 pounds per square inch. This is the modulus of elasticity for the test material.

Smaller test pieces can be used to determine the elastic modulus by merely multiplying the test values by appropriate factors to establish values per square inch of cross-section.

A surprising and very important characteristic of the modulus of elasticity is that it is usually one of the most invariable physical properties of any metal. Even heat treatments that soften or harden a metal have little effect on i[illegible] elastic modulus. These treatments make great differences in *how far* the metal [illegible] be deformed, but the force for a given deformation remains almost exactly the same.

The intermolecular and interatomic forces that hold the material together at stress values below those that cause slippage and permanent set are unchanged by the thermal and mechanical manipulations that influence such characteristics as hardness.

In orthodontics the modulus of elasticity is of practically no value as a criterion for selecting one material over another. It merely indicates ease of stretching, which is related to ease of bending. This is a measure of the stiffness of the material. If it were the only difference between two materials, one could completely compensate for it by an appropriate change in wire size. For example, the modulus of elasticity of gold wires is about one-half to two-thirds that of stainless steel, so a heavier gold wire of a size that provides sufficient increase in stiffness will be identical in stiffness to a steel wire. A gold wire .020 inch (.5mm) in diameter has about the same stiffness as a .018-inch (.45-mm) steel wire.

Proportional limit. The lower, straight-line portion of the curve represents a proportional relationship between stress and strain. The higher, curved portion shows strain increasing at a more rapid rate than stress, no longer a proportional response.

The point at which the straight line begins to curve is called the proportional limit (indicated by the arrow in Fig. 8-2).

This is an important point, because it marks the limit to which the material can be stressed without taking a permanent set and work hardening. Below this point the material is not permanently changed by applied stress; beyond this point it is subjected to irreversible changes.

In concept the proportional limit would seem to offer an ideal index for the practical comparison of materials, but in practice it is fraught with complications. The biggest stumbling block is its accurate determination. Carefully plotted stress-strain curves for stainless steel begin to curve so imperceptibly that no one point can be identified as *the* proportional limit. In fact, many such curves will show a small trace of curvature throughout, due largely to residual internal stresses.

This characteristic of the curves for stainless steel makes the proportional limit a more or less arbitrary value, based on an estimation or on some arbitrary standardized value for the amount of deflection.

Most gold alloys show a much more clear-cut break in the curve at the proportional limit.

Resiliency. As noted earlier, orthodontic appliances must make the most of the spring properties of the metal, and with stainless steel and chrome-cobalt this often means stressing up to or even beyond the proportional limit. Resiliency is the term used for total energy storage capacity, so a meaningful measure of this property depends on the level of loading (or overloading) that is considered to be acceptable.

Mechanical devices are usually rated for efficiency on the basis of the preservation of energy. If only part of the input is recovered, the loss represents a drop in efficiency, which is a disadvantage. In orthodontic appliances, energy for input is no problem—the hands of the orthodontist can provide it in abundance. The *recoverable* energy, regardless of input, is the important value in orthodontics, and judicious overstressing of our wires can significantly increase this value.

If a wire is stressed 50% beyond the proportional limit, perhaps 20% of the increase may not be recovered because of permanent set, but the 80% remainder will raise the overall total to 140% of that available at the proportional limit. Of course, consideration must be given to the resulting permanent set that will prevent the wire from reassuming its original form, but the loss of energy itself is of no consequence.

These considerations and the imprecision of the proportional limit suggest a need for a more meaningful point for the evaluation of resiliency for orthodontic applications. No such standards exist at this time, but two commonly used methods are available. One is the point of greatest curvature in the stress/strain curve, and the other is an arbitrary percentage of deflection beyond a straight-line response (5% or 10% are reasonable values for most materials).

In this connection it should be emphasized that any such value is *only* a measure of energy storage capacity (resiliency). Other qualities such as stiffness, formability, and lack of brittleness (durability) are also important, and these must often be compromised to achieve maximum energy capacity. Wires should always be selected for their *combined* properties, not just for one single characteristic.

THE SUPERFLEXIBLE WIRES

Superflexible alloys such as the Titanium alloys (including Nitinol) obey all of the same rules, but their numbers are so different that the various segments of the stress-strain curve take on different significance. The straight proportional part of the curve has a much lower slope, and it is so long that most applications do not reach the plastic deformation zone. All energy input over a broad range of deflection is stored elastically and is available for delivery, so these materials provide a high level of resilient storage capacity. The upper limit of energy storage is usually marked by deflection limits rather than by the proportional limit as is the case with steel and gold.

These properties are desirable in the working range, but there is a trade-off in more difficult adjustment and brittleness. A high proportional limit means that extreme deflections are required to achieve the plastic deformation that is required for clinical adjustment. A proportional limit that greatly exceeds clinical requirements offers no advantage to compensate for the difficulty or impossibility of forming the wire to best accomplish required movements. Careful evaluation of these properties in relation to individual patient needs should be routine when these materials are being considered.

Brittleness is typical of materials with extended elasticity. Ultimate strength is not extended in proportion to the extended elastic range; this range is extended largely at the expense of a reduction in the range of plastic deformation. This means that the margin of safety between the working range of adjustability and brittle failure is severely compromised by the abbreviation of the upper part of the curve. It also means that when these wires are subjected to work-hardening deflections, however slight, fatigue will progress rapidly through almost imperceptible plastic deformation to brittle failure.

RESPONSE OF ATOMIC STRUCTURE TO STRESS

Metals are crystals made up of atoms arranged in regular characteristic patterns. These regular patterns are interrupted by atoms of impurities and alloying metals

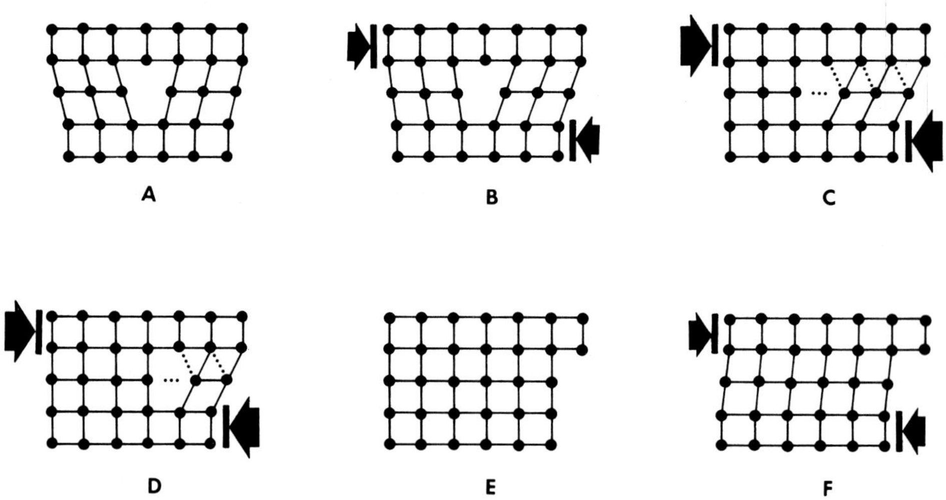

Fig. 8-3. Progressive crystalline lattice changes in elastic deformation (**A, B**), plastic deformation (**C, D**), and work hardening (**E, F**).

as well as by voids. Such irregularities are plentiful in all metals, and they account for several important physical characteristics.

Fig. 8-3 shows schematically how a void can contribute to workability. Fig. 8-3, *A*, shows a section of a crystal with a void in the center. In Fig. 8-3, *B*, this crystal is subjected to two forces that apply a shear stress. Comparable effects are produced under tension and compression, but a shear stress is shown here for simplicity of illustration. These forces stress the atomic bonds that are responsible for the elasticity of the crystal and so produce an elastic deformation.

If the force is removed, the crystal will return to its original form (Fig. 8-3, *A*). This same distortion could be applied repeatedly without causing any permanent change in the crystal. Forces at this level are within the straight-line elastic range of the metal.

Higher stresses: plastic deformation and work hardening

The important characteristic of most orthodontic wires is not how difficult they are to stretch or bend but *how far* they will stretch or bend. This requires examination of the upper reaches of the tensile curve.

In the straight-line portion of the curve the grains of the metal as well as the atoms within the grains shift only slightly; they do not move far enough to prevent the electromagnetic forces holding the atoms together from returning them to their original relationships when the force is released.

Further increases in force produce the situation represented in Fig. 8-3, *C*, in which some atoms reach a point where they can move to a new position as easily as they can return to their original position. At this point these bonds are no longer offering effective resistance to the force, and the material is more easily deformed. This point is where the elastic curve begins to deviate to the right. If the force is increased to move the atoms just past this midway point, they shift to new positions as shown in Fig. 8-3, *D* and *E*.

The metal has now undergone a permanent change at this spot; it will no longer return to its original form when the stress is released. This permanent change in shape is called *plastic deformation,* the process which produces a permanent set in a material. Fig. 8-3, *E*, shows the crystal after the remaining atoms have been moved by added stress and that stress has been removed. The crystal is again at rest, but in a new shape.

Plastic deformation of wire is not a cataclysmic change, like the breaking of glass; it is a gradual, piecemeal process in which little spots yield here and there as stress is increased. At first only the weakest areas are changed. Under increased stress, progressively stronger bonds yield and the elastic curve bends more and more to the right. This continues until the material finally fails, as shown by the star in Fig. 8-2. Some extremely plastic materials may deform until the line of the curve is horizontal, but structural metals will break before this point is reached.

Work hardening. Plastic deformation also brings about the work hardening mentioned in Chapters 6 and 7. As many of these voids and other irregularities yield under plastic deformation, they shift to new and stronger relationships that are less susceptible to further change.

The deformed crystal shown in Fig. 8-3, *E*, has been work hardened in this way. Elimination of the void and realignment of the atoms have stiffened its resistance to additional force. If the same forces are applied once more, as in Fig. 8-3, *F*, all of the intervening bonds will also offer resistance.

Elastic behavior after plastic deformation and work hardening. Plastic deformation and the resulting permanent set *do not* weaken a wire or reduce the amount of force that it can exert. Force storage continues to increase through this stage, though at a slower rate than in the straight-line region of the curve.

If force is released after plastic deformation, the material goes back *toward* its original form. It cannot return completely, because of individual crystals that have undergone changes like those shown in Fig. 8-3, *E*. Behavior in this situation is shown by the dotted line in Fig. 8-2. This line is parallel to the original straight portion of the curve, indicating that stress and strain maintain a straight proportional relationship through the entire range of decreasing force. In other words, force is released exactly the same as though no plastic deformation had occurred, but it begins at a higher level than could have been attained without the plastic deformation.

Individual bonds in the metal show one of two responses to stress. Either they behave elastically or they are broken. In elastic behavior they "give" in response to the stress, in the straight-line fashion of Hooke's law. If a bond is broken, there is a repositioning of the atom in the crystal lattice and a permanent change in the material.

When force is applied above the level of plastic deformation and permanent set, the straight-line stress-strain relationship will arc into a curve. When that force is released, there is no reversal of the permanent set, so there is no curve in the unloading line. The working bonds respond with a purely elastic behavior, so the curve descends down the dotted line parallel to the original elastic curve. Those bonds and atoms that have permanently changed their positions are responsible for the change in dimension of the material represented by the shift of the entire line to the right.

In reloading after these changes, *the curve will ascend the same dotted line until it reaches the original curve.* There will be no further plastic deformation at the force level where it first occurred, because all of the most susceptible areas have already been changed. In one very real sense the material has been strengthened by the plastic deformation and this increase in the proportional limit.

When force is increased further, beyond the original highest point, the curve continues along an extension of the original curve, just as it would have done without the interruption.

The effect just described takes place at any stage up to failure of the material. It is this effect that makes it possible for an orthodontist to make severe bends in a wire and still elicit useful elastic behavior.

Brittleness

As a material undergoes plastic deformation and work hardening, the proportional limit is increased but it also lies closer to the point of failure. The increased proportional limit brought about by work hardening makes the material more brittle.

Brittleness is the condition of a material that, while elastic, cannot undergo plastic deformation. Glass is an example; if it is bent, it will behave elastically but it will not take a permanent set. When the load reaches a certain level, a whole series of bonds gives way at once and the glass breaks.

Brittle materials can be extremely strong. Perfect crystals of a pure metal may be a thousand times as strong as ordinary commercial forms, but they behave in a brittle fashion. Used within their limits, these materials can be very useful, but the increased possibility of cataclysmic failure rules them out for many applications.

The elastic curve of a brittle material goes up the straight initial section, the same as the curve shown in Fig. 8-2, but it ends in failure without any curving of the line.

In work hardening the line shifts to the right, as shown by the dotted line in Fig. 8-2. With enough work hardening, this line will shift so far to the right that it also ascends directly to the point of failure without any intervening plastic deformation. This is what occurs with highly resilient stainless steel wires that can tolerate only limited adjustment without breakage.

Brittle fracture. Brittle fracture is characterized by a clean break, with no deformation of the material on either side of the break. The broken ends will fit back together, like broken pieces of glass or crockery. Plastic failure occurs when material is pulled apart by brute force, as in a tensile test. This type of failure is accompanied by distortion of the material at the point of failure because it pulls apart progressively.

Failures of orthodontic metals, like most metal failures, are brittle fractures. These are usually the result of fatigue, which is actually nothing more than excessive work hardening.

Fatigue of metals

Fatigue is the result of repeated stress at a level below that which would normally cause failure. These stresses, usually in the low plastic-deformation range, gradually bring about additional work hardening until the metal finally fails in a brittle fracture.

Below a certain stress level, a material can be subjected to repeated stresses almost indefinitely without failure. A good example is a watch spring, which is carefully designed to flex evenly throughout its length to maintain the lowest possible stress level on all parts. In this way no part of the spring is called upon to carry more than its share of the load. These springs are designed to operate only in the lowest end of the straight portion of the elastic curve, never even remotely approaching plastic deformation.

As bending reaches higher on the elastic curve and a material is bent repeatedly, a few failures may occur among a large number of samples. Increasing the force or increasing the number of bending cycles beyond this point causes additional failures until, at a high level, all samples of a particular type will fail.

This is an important aspect of fatigue failure; it may be predicted only approximately on a statistical basis. A certain proportion of samples can be expected to fail under any particular set of conditions, but failure cannot be predicted with accuracy for an individual piece. Too much depends on unknown details in the microstructure and minor undetectable flaws that can hasten failure.

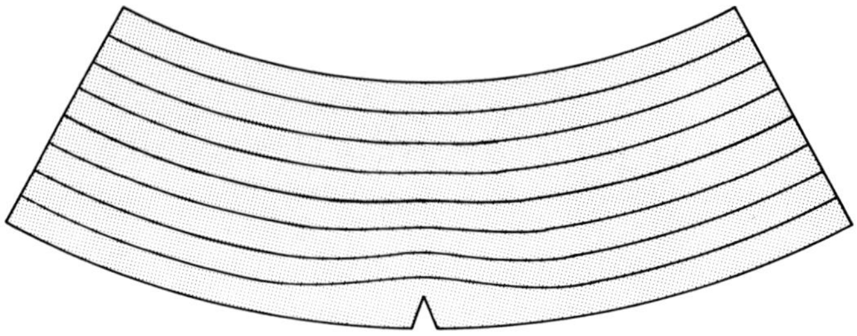

Fig. 8-4. A surface defect reduces the material available to carry the (bending) load, thus concentrating the stresses in the underlying material. This stress concentration accelerates work hardening and progressive failure in this overload region.

Fatigue failure of metal is hastened tremendously by flaws of any kind, even minute scratches. How the outer part of a bending wire is stretched and the inner part is compressed has already been shown in Fig. 4-1. If the material is perfectly uniform, these effects will also be uniform and all parts will carry an equal load.

If there is a defect in the material, such as a scratch or an internal flaw, the metal remaining around the defect will have to carry an added load. The result, as shown in Fig. 8-4, is that this part is stressed (and strained) more than the rest of the wire. The overstrained region will be higher on the elastic curve, so it will be work-hardened more than the rest of the wire. Each time it is bent again, the work hardening will increase further until finally the metal can no longer deform enough to adjust to the strain. This will occur first at the defect, enlarging it further and accelerating the process by further increasing the load on the remaining material, so eventually the crack will grow to the point where the wire breaks.

Stress raisers. Anything in the structure of a piece of metal that can cause such a local increase in stress is called a stress raiser. It may be a sharp notch, the scratch of a glass cutter, the thread of a screw, or a hatch on a ship. Brittle fracture can start at any such stress raiser. Even a slight surface roughness can be enough to initiate this type of failure; therefore critical parts in many manufactured products are carefully polished, shot-peened, or otherwise treated to produce a surface that is as free as possible from irregularities. Some common stress raisers in orthodontic wires are nicks from pliers, intergranular corrosion, soldered joints, and spots worn by occlusion. A worn spot is the least likely of all of these to initiate failure, at least in its early stages, because of the highly polished condensed surface produced by the wear. These and other stress raisers are shown in Fig. 8-5.

Wires can still fail because of fatigue in the absence of any initial stress raiser, but only after much greater stress or over longer periods of time. Such failure occurs as work hardening finally progresses to the point where fine cracks are formed on the surface. These then act as stress raisers, and the already work-hardened wire fails rapidly.

Prevention of fatigue failure. Broken wires can add much time to treatment, so it is important that all possible preventive measures be taken. Care should be taken in wire selection, even though really adequate information on fatigue resistance is not yet available. Most suppliers offer wire in which every effort has been made to

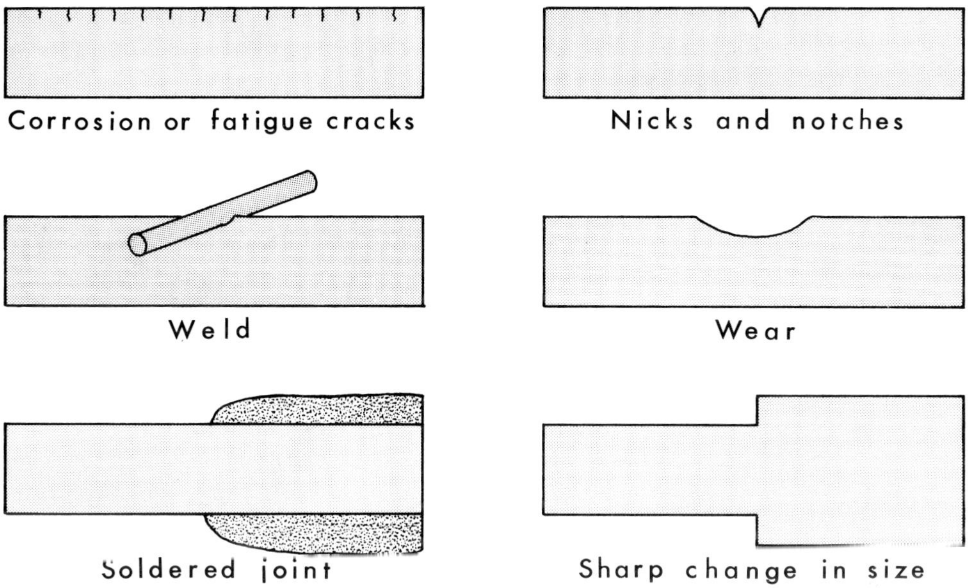

Fig. 8-5. Some common stress raisers in orthodontic wire.

keep breakage low, but this is difficult to control completely. Certain lots from any supplier may occasionally prove unusually resistant or susceptible to breakage.

Metals that work harden rapidly may fatigue more easily, but their higher resistance to deformation under stress helps to balance this disadvantage in some applications. Hard wires are more brittle than soft wires of the same material. Hardness level should be selected on the basis of individual demands—hard enough for needed resiliency but not so hard as to be excessively brittle. Experience with specific materials is often the only criterion in this regard.

Smaller diameter wires have a broader working range and so may not be so easily stressed to the proportional limit as a larger, stiffer, and seemingly stronger wire. For this reason a change to a smaller wire may be the answer in some cases of recurrent breakage.

Stress relieving can make the microstructure of steel more uniform and raise its resistance to deformation, both of which will be helpful in reducing breakage.

Good surface finish eliminates many of the small stress raisers that can initiate the process of failure.

The most important preventives lie in careful handling and in arch design. A wire should never be marked or notched with a file or other sharp instrument. Smooth-beaked pliers should be used to avoid unnecessary damage to the surface, and pliers should be selected and manipulated so as to avoid marking the wire with sharp edges of the beaks.

Sharp bends should be avoided wherever possible, especially if the bend will be subject to additional bending forces in the mouth. Sharp bends cause much more work hardening than large radius bends and bring the wire much closer to failure.

Rapid bending can also damage a wire. Wires should be bent at a steady rate, not in jerks, to give the small amount of additional time needed for the internal structure to adjust as the bend is being made.

Of course, repeated bending in the same spot will cause a tremendous increase in work hardening. If a bend must be reworked in a new arch, it is often better to begin with another piece of wire than to run the increased risk of later breakage. Ligature wires should be bent only once in tying; if it becomes necessary to readjust a ligature wire, it is best to begin again with a new wire rather than to untwist and retwist the same wire.

All adjustments should be made away from high-stress areas and previous bends. Bends at soldered joints should be avoided. This is not because the wire has been weakened by the heat but because the rigid solder causes the adjacent wire to bend more sharply. The situation is frequently the same as that shown in Fig. 4-1, in which the bending moment is highest at the junction of the wire with the more rigid soldered area. Sharp changes in cross section are notorious stress raisers that should be routinely avoided in all areas of stress. Full fluxing and careful soldering to produce a thin featheredge on soldered areas can also help to prevent this breakage.

Wire adjacent to soldered joints may be subject to intergranular corrosion initiated by the heat of soldering. This can be minimized by careful soldering, but additional protection will be provided by careful cleaning and electropolishing. This removes the outer surface of the metal that is most highly sensitized to corrosion. This same precaution should be taken after welding.

Another potential source of corrosion is contact with carbon steel. Stainless steel should not be polished with a wire-brush wheel or filed with a steel file without later electropolishing to remove the iron and carbon that are embedded in the surface.

9

Elastic action in bending and torsion

Elastic response of metal is the means by which tension, compression, and shear in the working wire are utilized to activate an orthodontic mechanism. An understanding of this elastic response provides an understanding of most of the subtle effects that can enhance or limit the effectiveness of an appliance in clinical application.

BENDING

The entire response to bending can be considered for this purpose as a response to equal tension and compression on opposite sides of the wire. Fig. 9-1 shows a bending wire loaded like that in Fig. 5-1. Shown with the wire is a diagram that looks something like an angular hourglass. This is a graph of the tensile and compressive forces induced by the bending inside a section of the wire. Compressive forces are greatest at the top. These taper off toward the middle (neutral axis), where there is no stress at all, and below this point the tensile stresses appear. The tension at the lower surface is equal to the compression along the top.

The shaded area in this diagram shows the total amount of stored elastic energy. Fig. 9-2 shows a series of bends in a wire, with tension-compression diagrams for each stage. In Fig. 9-2, *A*, a light force is applied to the wire, resulting in a picture similar to that shown in Fig. 9-1. The force is released in the wire shown in Fig. 9-2, *B*, and the wire returns to a straight form without any residual stress.

A heavier force is applied in Fig. 9-2, *C*, bending the wire enough to stress the upper and lower regions beyond their elastic limit. These areas deform plastically, and thus they are limited in their relative capacity to store energy. There is a curve in the graph in these areas as a result of the curved stress-strain relationship under the excessive forces. Stored forces no longer increase in proportion to the deflection, though they do continue to increase at a lower rate.

This force is *partially* released in Fig. 9-2, *D*. The extreme fibers have returned to an unstressed condition, but the intermediate fibers are still under tension and compression.

When all of the force is released from the wire (Fig. 9-2, *E*), these internal stressed regions still exert a straightening action. This puts the extreme fibers under reversed stresses as the internal fibers carry them past their new (bent) neutral

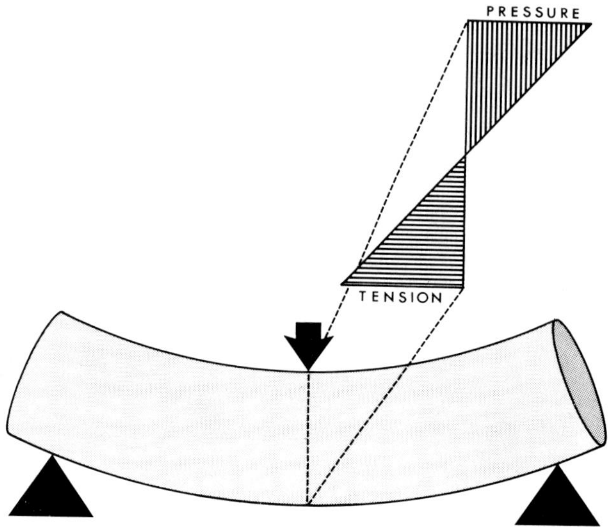

Fig. 9-1. Diagram showing levels of tension and compression across a section of bending wire. These stresses are greatest in the extreme fibers (top and bottom) and zero in the center.

state. At this point the wire is slightly bent as a result of the plastic deformation of the outer fibers. Because the outer fibers were plastically deformed and the central section was not, the final passive (unloaded) condition of the wire leaves these two regions opposing each other in a state of balanced internal stress.

Restressing the wire in the original direction brings a response very similar to the first one. The upper and lower sides do not help in resisting the new stress at the start, for they are moving toward a neutral condition and actually working in the same direction as the load. The central region is prestressed enough to offer increased resistance, which partially compensates for the ineffective extreme fibers. The reversed outer stresses are soon eliminated as the wire bends farther, and the wire will then continue to bend much as before. The only difference is that the elastic limit of the outer fibers has been increased by the previous plastic deformation, so that the wire will not take any additional permanent set until the earlier maximum load is exceeded.

Applying a reverse force to straighten the wire (Fig. 9-2, *F*) will unload the residual stresses in the center. The central section will still be unchanged from its original condition, but the plastically deformed outer regions will be under even greater reversed stress.

Bending the wire even farther in the reversed direction puts the entire wire under reversed stresses, but the outer fibers have such a head start on the inner fibers that they reach the plastic-deformation level in this opposite direction with much less bend in the wire than was required originally. In this reverse bend the original plastic deformation of the outer fibers has shifted more of the load to their area; the inner (undeformed) fibers behave exactly the same in either direction, but

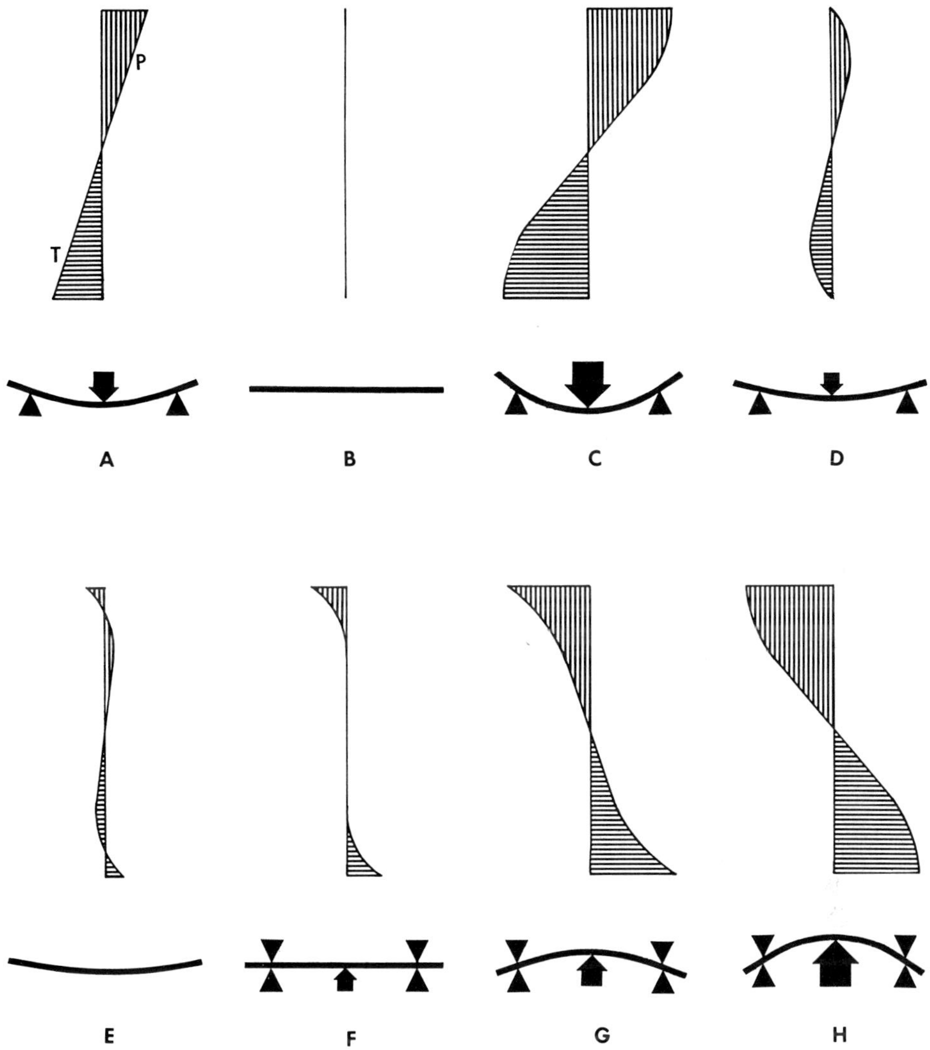

Fig. 9-2. Distribution of tension and compression stresses under different conditions of bending. Shaded areas show total stored energy, both elastically recoverable energy and unrecoverable internal stresses. **A,** Application of working load; maximum tension at lower surface and maximum pressure at upper surface, similar to Fig. 9-1. **B,** Load removed; no residual stresses. **C,** Overload; plastic deformation at upper and lower extremes reduces stored energy below that which would be available with a proportional response. **D,** Load partially removed; regions of maximum deformation returned to zero stress; interior regions still under stress. **E,** Unloaded; permanently bent, internal stresses balanced by reverse stresses in plastically deformed region before the wire can reach its original straight form. **F,** Reverse load is required to straighten wire, increasing reverse stress in plastically deformed regions as the interior stress returns to zero. **G,** Moderate reverse bend brings outside fibers to the proportional limit while interior fibers still carry a relatively small part of the load. **H,** Reverse overload results in mirror image of the stresses produced at **C.**

the outer (deformed) fibers are working from the new neutral point established by the original plastic deformation (Fig. 9-2, *G*). A greater part of the resistance is in the extreme fibers that rapidly approach plastic deformation; thus the wire is bent much more easily at this stage, and total stored force when outer fibers reach their proportional limit is less than that shown in Fig. 9-2, *C*.

Loading the wire with reverse stress equal to the original stress shown in Fig. 9-2, *C*, produces a situation that is an exact mirror image (Fig. 9-2, *H*).

The force required for the reverse bend from the bent wire shown in Fig. 9-2, *E*, past the straight condition to that shown in Fig. 9-2, *H*, is the same as that required to bend the original straight wire to the condition shown in Fig. 9-2, *C*. In each case the force, the final bend, and the permanent set are the same in spite of the fact that the reversed bend brought about a greater deflection by the amount of the original permanent set.

This whole effect means that for moderate loads a reversal of the force will carry the wire an additional distance equal to the original permanent set without any increase in force; the wire is less stiff in the reversing bend. For heavy loads the region of this effect is passed, and force requirements once more reach original levels as in Fig. 9-2, *H*.

All of these effects add up to the fact that a plastically deformed wire offers less elastic resistance and is less resistant to plastic deformation under a reversed stress than under a new stress in the original direction. This is one reason why springs are usually manufactured to carry their load in the same direction in which they were wound or formed.

Utilizing reverse bending actions

Orthodontics, it seems, must always be different. In spite of the fact that a wire may not perform at its very best under a reversed stress, it can still turn in a creditable performance. The differences are often small, and many orthodontic considerations can override this efficiency problem and still make a reversed-stress application the most desirable. This may sometimes be true in the use of arch loops.

Two very effective means are available for countering the reduced resistance to reverse bending. One is overbending when forming the wire to permit some adjustment in the reverse direction *before* activation. This can bring the wire to the condition shown in Fig. 9-2, *H*, in which its effectiveness is practically unimpaired. An increase in work hardening is the only important difference, and this is not serious for most wires.

The second means of increasing efficiency under reversed stress is stress-relieving heat treatment. This eliminates a great part of the internal stresses that are responsible for the problem.

Either or both of these measures will so reduce the detrimental effects of reverse bending that other advantages need not be sacrificed in an effort to avoid it. Where one has a choice, use a design that loads the wire in the direction of forming; where other requirements dictate reverse loading, design and compensate accordingly.

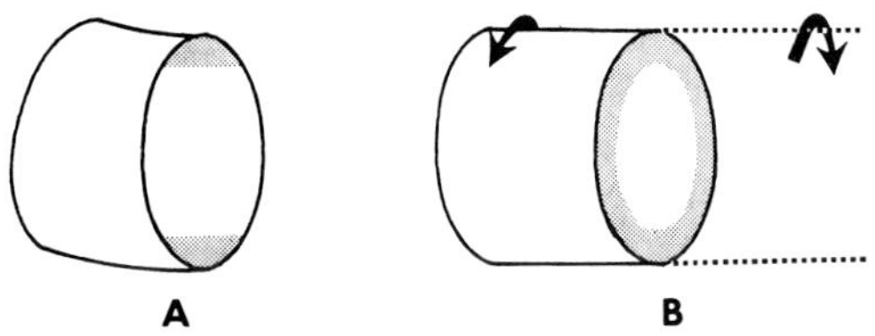

Fig. 9-3. Distribution of extreme fiber stresses in bending, **A,** and in torsion, **B.** When the outer 25% of the diameter is overstressed in bending, only 14% of the material is affected. A comparable overload in torsion will affect 44% of the material.

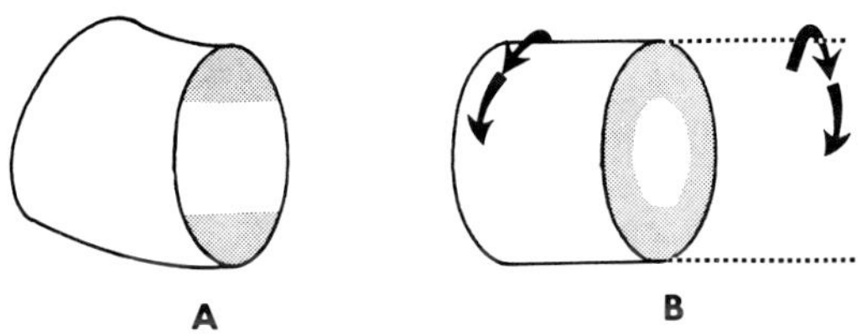

Fig. 9-4. Overstressing the outer 50% of a wire as in Fig. 9-3 will overstress 39% of the material in bending, **A,** and 75% in torsion, **B.**

TORSION

The response in torsion follows the same pattern as that in bending, but with some very important differences. The same effects shown in Fig. 9-2 apply, but the allowable working range in torsion is much shorter and more critical than in bending. The margin between working range and failure can be very narrow in some applications.

More of the material in a wire under torsion lies in the region of extreme stress, making failure a more precipitous event. Fig. 9-3 shows cross-sections of the same wire in bending and in torsion, with the outer 25% (shaded area) plastically deformed by a moderately heavy stress.

Bending a wire to plastically deform the outer 25% of its diameter will overstress only 14% of the wire. Stressing to include the next fourth of the diameter adds 25%, for a total of 39% of the wire overstressed when half of its diameter is overstressed in bending (Fig. 9-4).

The neutral axis of a round wire in bending is a flat section coinciding with its entire diameter, so most of a round wire lies in the area closest to the neutral axis in bending, where it is the last to be overstressed.

The neutral axis of a round wire in torsion is a line coinciding with the center axis, so the greatest area of the cross-section lies farthest away from the neutral axis, where it is the first to be affected. The outer fourth of the cross-section includes 44% of the entire wire. The next fourth includes another 31%, so that when half the diameter of a wire is overstressed in torsion, it will affect 75% of the material compared to 39% in bending.

The final reserve strength in torsion is virtually nil, since the neutral axis is merely a line, with very little surrounding material available to resist any ultimate stress. This rapid depletion of reserve strength in torsion as compared to bending is what accounts for the rapidity of failure once it begins. Each successive increment of overload affects a smaller volume of material as it approaches the center, so it has a progressively larger effect.

An added problem in torsion is the ease of overloading. It is impossible to bend a wire more than 180 degrees (doubling it on itself), but a twist can be applied through many revolutions.

STIFFNESS IN BENDING AND TORSION

The abruptness of failure in torsion is another example of an advantage in one area proving to be a disadvantage in another. The large proportion of material that lies in the area of extreme stress also provides greater stiffness in torsion. As will be seen in Appendix A, moments of inertia in torsion are twice those for the same wires in bending. This is because more of the wire is working at its maximum in resisting even low-level stress. But as the range of plastic deformation is entered, this same material is already working at capacity; there is more available initially but less in reserve.

Coil springs are an excellent example of designing for optimum utilization of physical properties. They function through a torsion stress in the wire, which will deliver orthodontically useful forces with wire sizes much smaller than those used for archwires. Their configuration limits the range of deflections to the lower part of the elastic range for most applications, and this combines with relatively long wire length to protect them from overstress while still providing ample working ranges.

PART II

Teeth in motion and moving teeth

■ To the casual observer the teeth merely sit motionless in the mouth, moving only as the jaws move to carry out their active functions. Dentists are well aware that teeth also move within the jaws, but little attention has been paid to the phenomena surrounding these essential small movements and their importance to both orthodontic and restorative dentistry.

The periodontal membranc that occupies the space between tooth root and supporting bone has numerous vital functions, both mechanical and physiological. Of special interest here are the mechanical ligamentous functions related to response to outside forces. These responses are the basis for all orthodontic and functional effects. Orthodontic movement is a secondary effect of the small intra-alveolar movements that transmit appliance and other forces to the tissues.

The dental mechanism provides the most direct application of outside forces to bone that can be found anywhere in the body, and the periodontal membrane provides the critical link.

Just as a wire responds to external forces by distortion and resultant internal stresses, so the supporting tissues respond to forces on the teeth. Stresses and strains within the supporting structures are natural phenomena that transfer outside loads to deeper structures and at the same time stimulate physiologic responses that can ultimately result in tooth movement.

The general characteristics of these tissues have been known for years, usually studied and presented in a context far removed from orthodontics. The supporting tissues will be examined here in relation to their major function of support and the vital role that they play in establishing, maintaining, and altering tooth position.

10

Dental support under mechanical stress

The periodontal membrane is a dual mechanical system whose description often ends with the fibrous component. This preoccupation is so strong that this tissue is often called a ligament, while its other vital components and functions are completely ignored. The ligamentous component is actually many small individual ligaments that make up one part of the dual system that can be crudely compared to the combination of springs and hydraulic shock absorbers used in most automobiles.[9,10] The fibrous system provides primary attachment comparable to the springs, while the hydraulic system furnishes protection from high instantaneous or brief loads. Neither of these components can function effectively by itself; they form a coordinated system in which each responds in its own way to every outside stress.

THE FIBROUS DENTAL ATTACHMENT MECHANISM

The tooth is retained and supported in the alveolus by a fibrous suspension system in which the bone plays a secondary part. The collagenous fiber bundles embedded in the cementum of the root pass through the periodontal membrane (as periodontal fibers) and then into the bone (Sharpey's fibers) in an uninterrupted pattern, forming the basic structural matrix for both periodontal ligament and bone. The flexibility and tensile strength of these collagenous fibers provide a secure yet flexible attachment that serves as the primary support and adjustment mechanism of the tooth, adapting on demand to the varying stresses to which it may be subjected.

At some distance away from the root this fibrous structure is stiffened and reinforced by calcification to form alveolar bone. The basic fibrous structure remains, but some of the space between the fibers is infiltrated with mineral that provides rigidity and a means of attachment to the underlying skeletal structures (Fig. 10-1).

This unique continuity of support from tooth to bone is what gives the alveolar complex the adaptability with which it meets the many varied functional demands of the environment, providing resistance to forces from all directions while at the same time providing shock absorbing and fine adjustment capability.

The key to this design is the primary structural component in the alveolus, the collagenous network that provides direct attachment to the tooth and structural

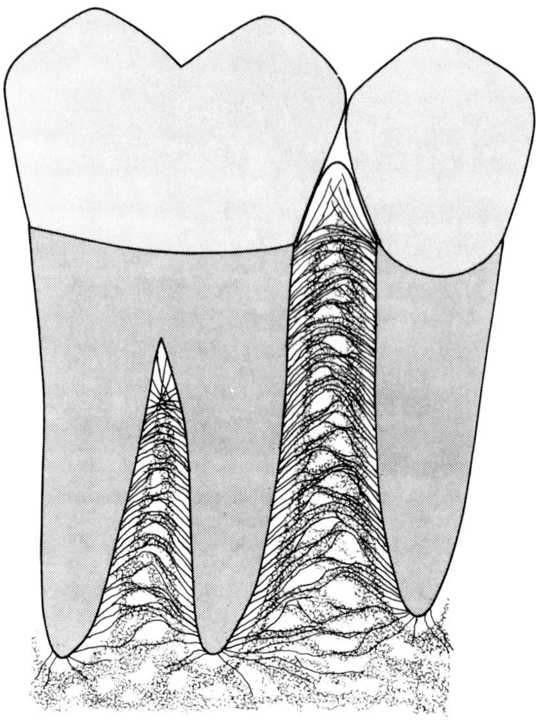

Fig. 10-1. The pattern of the fibrous matrix is continuous from tooth into bone, oriented to the prevailing stresses. Calcification is a secondary phenomenon adapted to the demands of support and mobility.

integrity to the bone. Calcification is a secondary phenomenon, which occurs only some distance from the teeth, where the need is for rigidity rather than flexibility. Function will always prevail, with calcified bone advancing and retreating in response to its stimulation. That response is the basis for orthodontic tooth movement as well as many other periodontal phenomena.

Orientation of periodontal fibers

The periodontal attachment fibers tend to assume an orientation that provides maximum resistance to stress. The collagenous fibers align along the direction of stress so that individual fibers are subjected to minimum loading under the stress of function.

Two conflicting factors must be reconciled in establishing the most efficient angulation at the root surface.[11] One is the orientation of the fibers to the force and the other is the number of fibers that can be attached to the root (Fig. 10-2). The fiber orientation that most efficiently balances these two factors is the bisector of the angle between the periodontal walls and a line perpendicular to the force, as shown in Fig. 10-3. Microscopic sections such as that shown in Fig. 10-4 demonstrate the tendency of the fibers to assume this optimum orientation.

It is important to note that while the bisector is the most efficient angle attain-

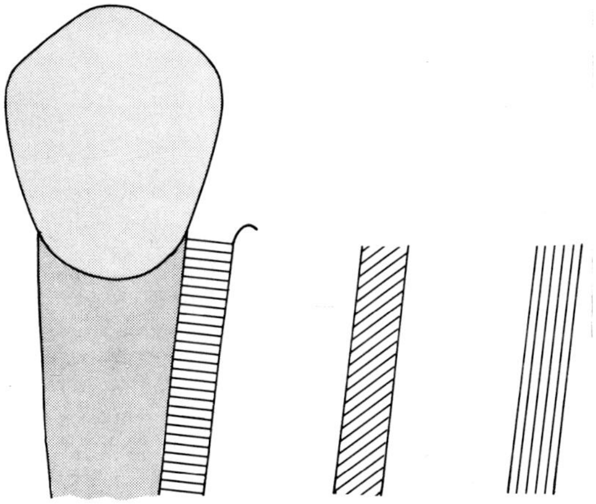

Fig. 10-2. Orientation of periodontal fibers affects the number that can be attached to any given area. **A,** Orientation perpendicular to periodontal walls provides attachment for maximum number of fibers. **B,** Angular orientation reduces this number. **C,** Parallel orientation makes attachment from tooth to bone impossible.

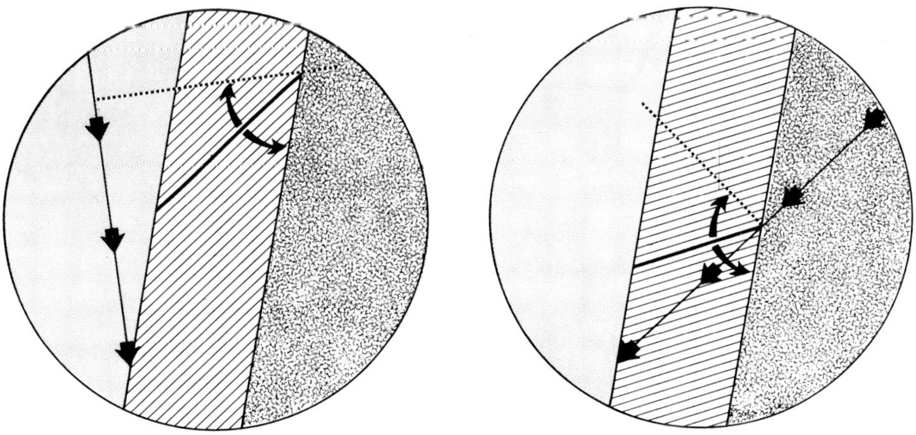

Fig. 10-3. Optimum fiber orientation is the bisector of the angle formed by the periodontal walls with a line perpendicular to the direction of the applied force. **A,** A force directed from tooth toward bone requires a small fiber angle. **B,** A force moving tooth away from bone requires a larger fiber angle that permits attachment of more fibers.

able for any given angulation of applied force, the maximum potential strength will vary with the angle of the force. Fig. 10-5 shows the relative attainable strength (efficiency) for all angles of force. Maximum strength (100%) is attainable only when the force is moving the tooth directly away from the bone, enabling a maximum number of fibers to work at the most efficient angle. Occlusal forces are usually about parallel to the alveolar walls, with a periodontal efficiency in the 50% range.

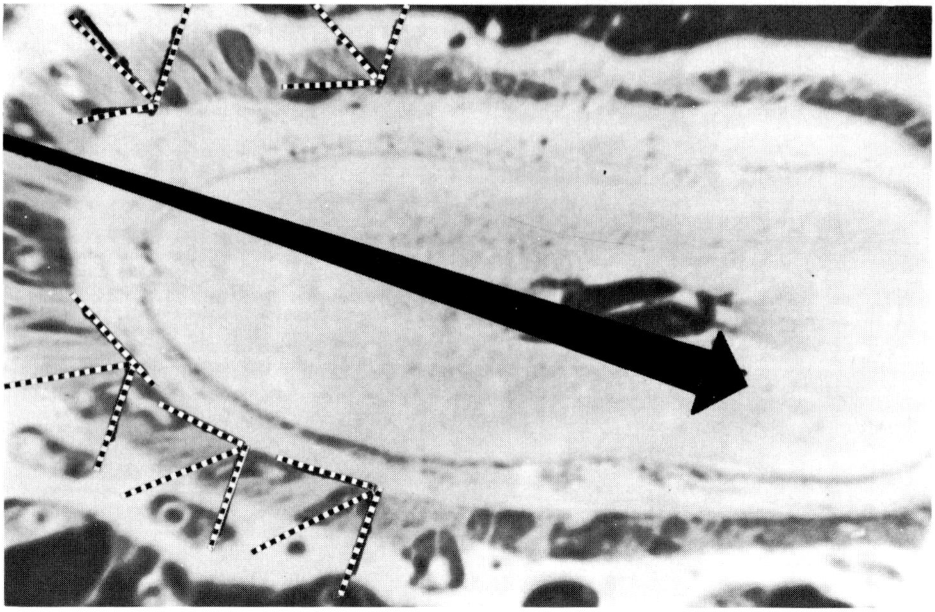

Fig. 10-4. Photomicrograph of root cross-section with optimum fiber angulation constructions superimposed.

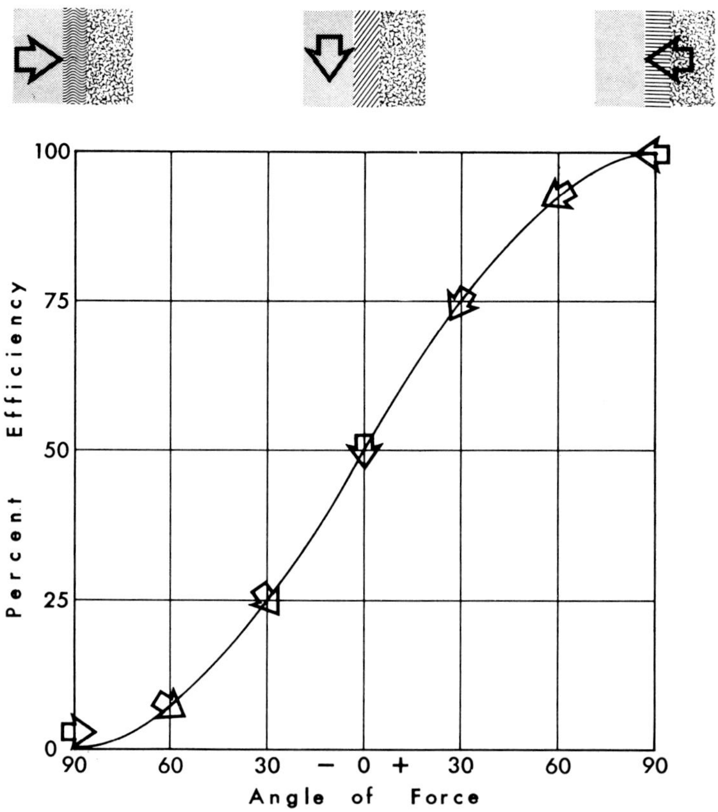

Fig. 10-5. Variation in maximum possible periodontal fiber resistance with the direction of applied force load. This resistance varies from zero with the force moving the tooth directly toward the bone, to 100% when the tooth is being moved directly away from the bone. Arrows indicate the direction of the force applied to the tooth, as in the three sections shown at the top.

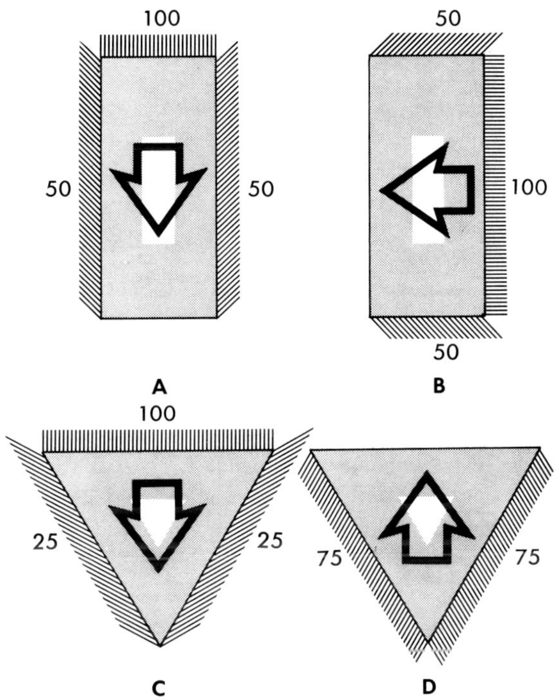

Fig. 10-6. Schematic root cross-sections, showing how the perimeter is the only factor affecting potential total resistance of the supporting ligament to applied forces. In each case the total overall resistance is exactly 50% of that attainable if the entire perimeter could function at 100% efficiency. Maximum available efficiency for each side of the root is based on Fig. 10-5, shown as a percentage. In **A** and **B,** opposite sides (top and bottom or right and left) always average 50%. In **C** and **D,** the average for all three sides is always 50%. Intermediate angles will also produce a 50% average efficiency for the entire perimeter.

Forces moving a tooth directly toward the bone (compression of the periodontal membrane) are met with zero resistance from the fibrous attachment on that side.

Effect of root size and shape on strength of periodontal attachment

The variation in attainable strength of the periodontal membrane with the orientation of the force provides an answer to the effects of root form. Is a flat-rooted tooth such as a bicuspid better able to withstand mesiodistal or buccolingual forces? Does the roughly triangular cross-section of upper incisor roots provide more resistance to labial than to lingual forces?

The shape of the cross-section of a root actually has *no effect* on the capacity of the periodontal ligament to resist lateral forces. This strength is *directly proportional to the perimeter of the section,* regardless of shape (Fig. 10-6). Root form is significant in the way that it affects both the perimeter available for support and the structural strength of the alveolar bone that lies between and around the roots.

The alveolar bone can often be more critical than the periodontal ligament in this structural complex. Labial and lingual bone is inadequate to carry the compressive loads imposed by the periodontal ligament, making the interproximal bone an essential contributor to dental support. Root form is directly responsible for the size and configuration of the space that can be occupied by this interdental truss-work.

Perimeter is equally important in the case of vertical loads such as occlusion, but here the taper of the root becomes an even more important factor. When the tooth is functioning under occlusal forces, all of the periodontal ligament is working at 50% efficiency or less—50% if the force is parallel to the periodontal space and less if root taper reduces that angle. The only exception is the upper anterior teeth, where occlusal forces deviate markedly from the long axis of the root; this loads the lingual gingival fibers in such a way that they can function well above the 50% efficiency level. There are no areas of the ligament working at 100% efficiency in occlusal function, as is often the case with lateral forces.

Greatest periodontal strength in axial (vertical) occlusion would be provided by a root with vertical sides and a flat (nonfunctional) tip. The sides of such a root would have equal resistance to both horizontal and vertical forces, each 50% of the maximum capacity of the total surface area (Fig. 10-7).

At the other extreme one of the most poorly supported root forms is a cone (Fig. 10-7). For a root with a working length twice its diameter, the alveolar walls will lie at a 15-degree angle to the force, and efficiency of the periodontal fibers will drop to 37% from the 50% available with parallel walls—a 25% drop in effi-

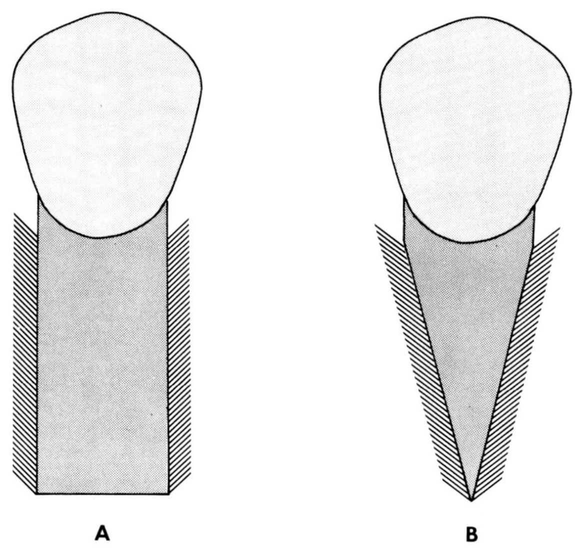

Fig. 10-7. Conical root form, **B,** compared to a cylinder, **A,** under vertical stress. Fibers on the cone with sides inclined at 15 degrees have a potential for 37% efficiency, compared to 50% for the parallel sides. Added to this effect is the fact that the cone provides only half the attachment area available on the sides of the cylinder, so the maximum strength of the supporting ligament for such a conical-shaped root cannot be more than three-eighths that of the cylindrical root.

ciency! In addition, the total area of such a root is only half that of a cylinder of equal overall dimensions. The combined effect of half the area working at three-fourths efficiency is a periodontal support for the pointed root only *three-eighths* as strong as the comparable cylindrical or parallel-sided root. This difference will be somewhat less for roots of longer (more slender) proportions.

The importance of cementum apposition in the periapical area becomes clear when these two root forms are compared. Such apposition alters the form toward a cylinder, simultaneously increasing the attachment area *and* the effectiveness of that attachment, for a twofold advantage.

A gentle root taper results in a tapered form in the surrounding bony framework, providing good support for the adjacent roots. Parallel root surfaces leave inadequate space for supporting bone, while a conical root leaves unnecessarily large space available for bone in the apical region. Normal root form produces a design that optimizes crown support, periodontal fiber support, and alveolar bone support in an integrated structural complex.

Note that the discussion thus far has been based on functional forces applied to a stable tooth in which the tissues have had time to adjust to the direction of forces. Orthodontic forces are usually applied from new directions, loading the fibers under less than optimum conditions that stimulate change as the force is continued over a period of time.

THE PERIODONTAL HYDRAULIC MECHANISM

Attention is usually focused on the ligamentous support system, probably because its function is so obviously clear in microscopic sections. Most slides show the hydraulic component of the supporting mechanism only as a collection of voids and isolated segments of blood vessels, difficult to recognize as an important mechanical component.

Virtually all of the periodontal space not occupied by attaching fibers is a part of the hydraulic system, and under extreme stress even the fibers may make a hydraulic contribution. Blood vessels are filled with blood, and the remaining space between the ligaments in the periodontal membrane contains various cells and fluid ground substance.

In the resting state the highest pressure in this region is the blood pressure, with the tissue fluid at a much lower pressure. The low ambient fluid pressure in the periodontium is the base level on which functional forces and pressures are superimposed. In function all of these normally low hydraulic pressures undergo rapid and extreme changes.

As a hydraulic mechanism the entire contents of the periodontal space can be viewed as a heterogeneous fluid of mixed viscosities. In this light we can temporarily ignore the mechanical attachments of the fibers and think only in terms of the fluid pressures that result from dental forces. These fluid pressures are the first response to outside force, increasing markedly before the tooth moves far enough to tense the fibers.

The basic hydraulic law that applies in this situation states that a fluid under pressure (positive or negative) will exert the same pressure per unit area *in all directions* (Fig. 10-8). Equilibrium of forces is just as basic in hydraulics as in me-

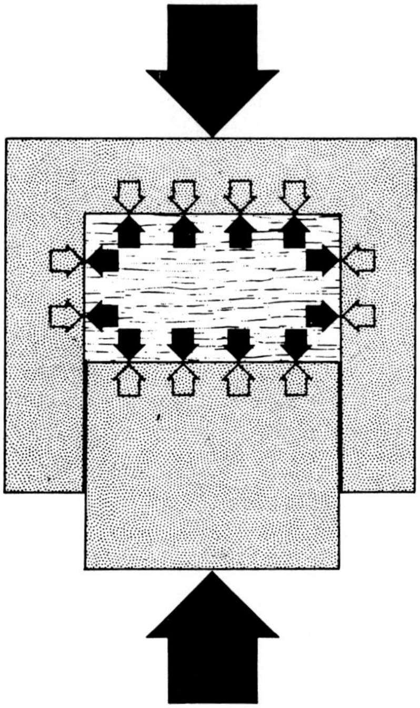

Fig. 10-8. Compressed fluid exerts equal pressure in all directions. Large vertical arrows show external forces on piston and cylinder. Small solid arrows show fluid pressure on containing walls. Open arrows show balancing forces of container on fluid. Horizontal forces are completely balanced within the cylinder walls; they have no external effects.

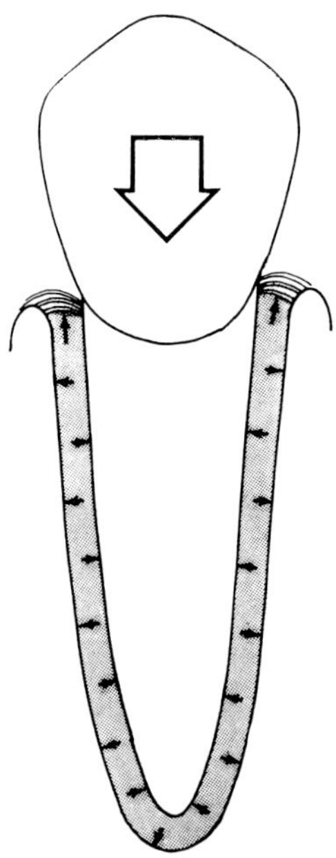

Fig. 10-9. Vertical force on a tooth places the fluid periodontal structures under hydraulic pressure. At the alveolar crest the transverse fibers serve as the "seal" to contain this pressure and prevent extrusion of the contents of the periodontal space.

chanics, so these evaluations follow a pattern very similar to the previous mechanical analyses *except* that time becomes an important consideration. Much of the fluid pressure in the periodontium is rapidly dissipated as the pressurized fluid is forced out.

The rapid dissipation of hydraulic pressure serves a shock-absorbing function. Hydraulic forces should be considered both on an instantaneous basis and with an evaluation of the relatively rapid changes that will be brought about by that instantaneous force picture.

A tooth functions as a loosefitting piston in which the gingival fibers of the periodontal ligament perform a sealing function comparable to that of piston rings. The dense collar of gingival fibers is essential for prevention of excessive fluid loss in function *and* for protection of the entire periodontal ligament from excessive trauma. By blocking the "easy" gingival escape route these fibers bring about a diffuse escape of fluid through the entire alveolar wall. Loss of this gingival seal makes the long vertical escape route the path of least resistance, resulting in a heavy flow in this direction instead of outward into the bone. Such a flow reduces the shock-absorbing capability of the hydraulic mechanism, and the increased vertical "pumping" tends to traumatize the contents of the periodontal space and extrude them out of the gingival crevice as the tooth moves down with function (Fig. 10-9).

A vertical load on a tooth that forces it into the socket places the entire contents of the periodontal space under uniform fluid pressure. A sudden biting load of 1000 gm on a tooth with a cross-sectional area at the cervix of 30 mm^2 will produce a pressure of $\frac{1000}{30}$ or 33 gm/sq mm^2. If the periodontal ligament is .25 mm thick, the free area around the 20-mm periphery of the tooth will be 5 mm^2; so the gingival fibers will be restraining a hydraulic load of 166 grams. If the thickness of the ligament is doubled to .5 mm, the free area and the total hydraulic load on the same fibers will also be doubled. It should be noted that this is an *upward* load, essentially perpendicular to the fibers, so actual tensile load on the fibers will be much greater. The deleterious effects are increased even further by the increased mobility with the thicker ligament and by the increased volume of movable fluid in the periodontal space.

The above forces are the instantaneous hydraulic load at the moment of contact. At this time the entire biting load is carried by the hydraulic system because the tooth has not yet moved. The function of the hydraulic system as a shock absorber is to absorb these high instantaneous loads and smoothly transfer them to the fibrous suspension system as the periodontal fluid escapes. *The fibers cannot carry any load until after the tooth has moved.*

The transfer of forces from the hydraulic to the mechanical is accomplished by the controlled escape of fluid from the periodontal space, permitting the tooth to move and therefore tense the periodontal fibers. This graduated transfer of the load applies to all fibers, even the gingival fibers. The original load cannot tense the fibers until the tooth moves and some fluid flow takes place, so under normal circumstances the load is diminished by redistribution before these fibers are fully tensed. For purposes of this discussion we can divide the periodontal fluids into

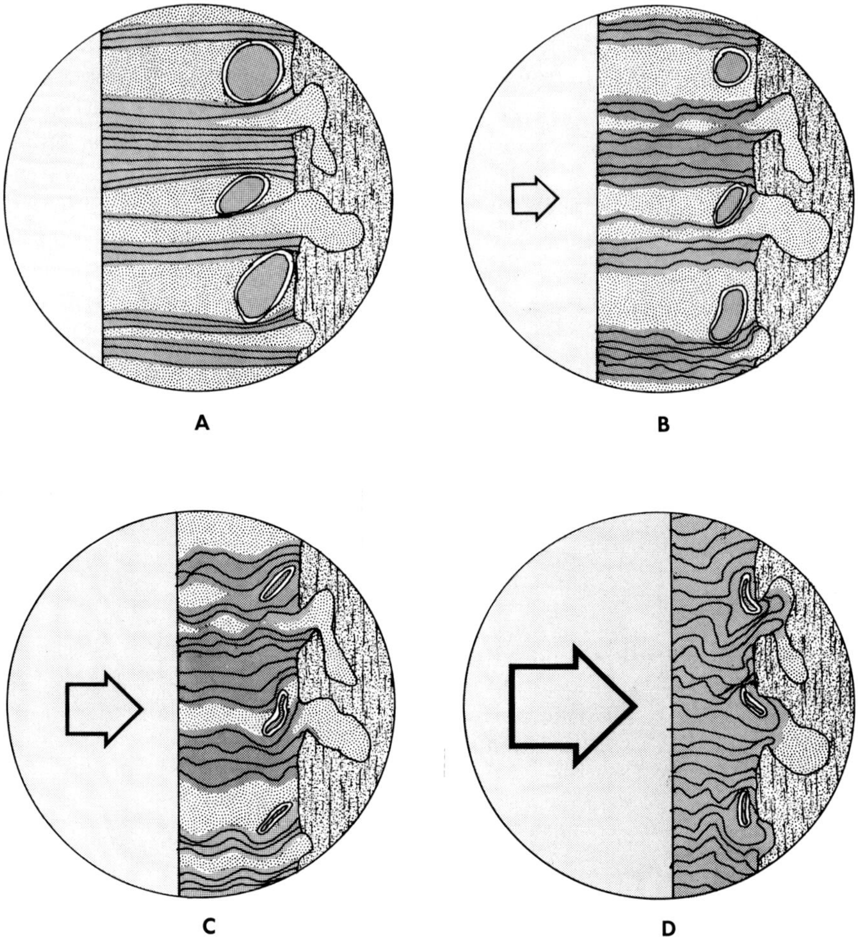

Fig. 10-10. Stages of hydraulic pressure effects on the periodontal structures. **A,** Passive. **B,** Light force, partially collapsing blood vessels. **C,** Heavier force, extruding intercellular fluids. **D,** Extreme force, extruding cellular and fibrous structures.

three groups on the basis of ease of escape: blood, interstitial (tissue) fluid, and cells (Fig. 10-10).

First stage: blood movement

Blood is the most mobile of the periodontal fluids because it is already contained in a system of tubes that provide a direct route for escape. Blood pressure is normally the highest of the fluid pressures within the periodontal space, but this does not mean that it is the last to be forced out. In the normal equilibrium state, the blood pressure is balanced by the combination of tissue fluid pressure and restraining elasticity of the blood vessel walls, so it is in pressure equilibrium with the local environment even in the unloaded state.

Any increase in tissue fluid pressure such as that produced by a load on a tooth

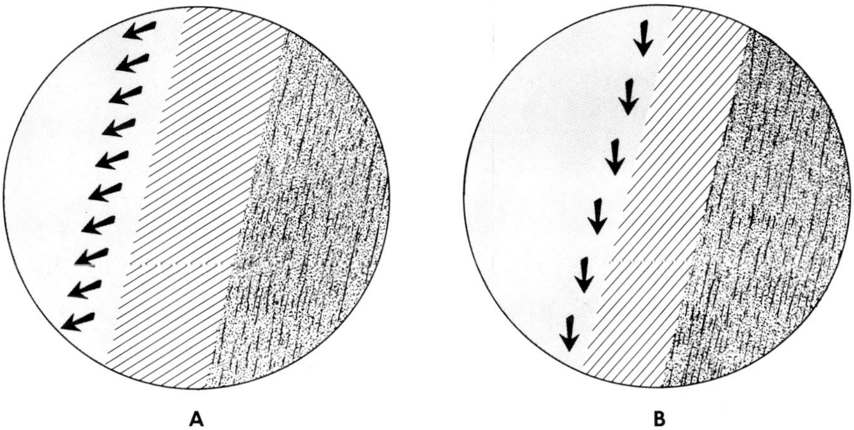

Fig. 10-11. A, Nonaxial forces tense fibers (positive tension) at the same time the tooth is moved away from the bone (negative pressure). Reversal of the force will reverse these effects. **B,** Axial force on the tooth places fibers under tension (positive tension) at the same time that the intruding tooth narrows the periodontal space (positive pressure).

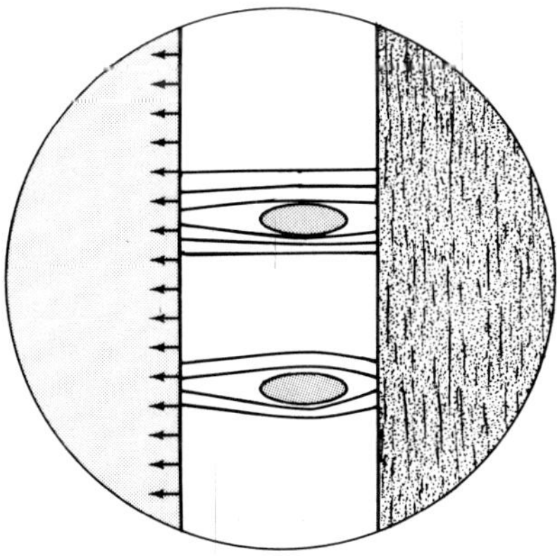

Fig. 10-12. Tensed fibers can compress blood vessels and so produce a localized pressure increase.

will cause an immediate blood vessel collapse with expression of blood out of the periodontal vessels and into the connecting vessels in adjacent structures. This *does not* require a force in excess of the blood pressure, as has often been suggested, because the blood pressure is already balanced under normal unloaded equilibrium conditions; any increase in the pressure around the blood vessels will cause some degree of collapse with expression of blood.

Nonaxial (tipping or horizontal) forces produce essentially the same effects on the blood supply in areas where the periodontal ligament is narrowed (pressure areas). Widened (tension) areas of the ligament are under reduced pressure, with a resulting influx of fluids.

For nonaxial forces the sense of the load on the fibers is the same as that of the fluid pressure on the attaching tooth and bone—either negative (tension) or positive (compression). On the other hand, a direct axial load (intrusion) places the fibers and their attachments under tension at the same time that the fluids are under positive pressure (Fig. 10-11).

The relationships between the nature of the force on the supporting fibers and positive or negative hydraulic pressure *are exactly opposite* for axial and nonaxial forces.

Another anomalous situation occurs in areas under tension from nonaxial forces. Here the fibers are tensed and the overall hydraulic pressure is reduced, yet many blood vessels are compressed by the tensed fibers that surround them. This effect can be balanced only by an increased tissue fluid flow into the area (Fig. 10-12).

It has been suggested[12] that the ease of blood flow makes it unimportant as a hydraulic cushion, but this does not consider the time factor. It is true that this free flow prevents the actual buildup or retention of high hydraulic pressures, but it buys essential time for the fibers. Even a fraction of a second can make a significant difference in traumatic effect on the fibers and on the cellular contents of the periodontal space.

As the tooth moves, the periodontal membrane is compressed and blood is forced out. This progressively transfers the load to the supporting fibers with a proportionate reduction in residual force available to maintain fluid pressure within the periodontal ligament. With normal functional forces this transfer may approach completion, but loads are usually so brief that the entire system rapidly returns to its original resting state.

Second stage: tissue fluid movement

Interstitial fluids become an active part of the hydraulic mechanism when the time or magnitude of force application overloads the blood supply and fibrous support system. This is often the case with orthodontic forces or other prolonged imbalances.

In these circumstances fluid pressures will still be elevated after the blood has been expressed from the periodontal vessels, so interstitial fluids will also be forced out. This is a somewhat slower (but still rapid) process, because these fluids do not lie in a system of freely communicating ducts, as the blood does. Tissue fluid must pass through circuitous routes by a combination of direct flow and diffusion, moving through either interstitial spaces or blood vessel walls.

Loss of tissue fluid in this manner *cannot* fully restore the normal pressure equilibrium because *these fluids themselves are a part of that equilibrium.* The net effect of this fluid loss is a literal dehydration or hyalinization of the tissues, plus a continuing elevation of pressure. The elevation of pressure must continue as long as the fluid imbalance persists, because of altered osmotic and chemical equilibriums.

Third stage: cellular movement

Cellular structures may also be squeezed out of the periodontal space if forces are sufficiently heavy and protracted. These structures are much more viscous than blood and tissue fluid, and their movement is restricted by fibrous elements as well as by the small size of openings in the alveolar bone. Forces at this level are well above optimum orthodontic forces, seriously impeding circulation and osteoclastic activity in the immediate area.

ORTHODONTIC EFFECTS

Orthodontic forces, with their wide variations in force levels and directions, can produce any conceivable combination of the stages just described.

These small movements of the tooth in the alveolus, with their resulting tissue strains, provide the stimulus for the histologic changes that follow and ultimately result in orthodontic tooth movement.

Natural functional forces are equally capable of stimulating orthodontic tooth movement whenever they cause a change in the status quo of tooth position and tissue strain.

11

Tissue adaptation to functional and orthodontic stresses

The most distinctive feature of orthodontic tooth movement is the mechanical appliance. As the intraoral force storage and distribution mechanism for orthodontic movement, the importance of the orthodontic appliance is obvious, but it is still only a means to an end—the stimulus for the ultimate objectives of orthodontics. Orthodontic tooth movement actually occurs out of sight, deep in the supporting tissues as they respond to the external stimuli, and effective application of these stimuli requires an understanding of such responses.

External forces reach a tooth only through the crown, and they are transferred from tooth to supporting tissues only through the root. When the crown of a tooth is subjected to any kind of force, the resiliency of the periodontal ligament permits the minute root movements described in Chapter 10. These immediate movements are not orthodontic movements in any sense, but they *are* the essential stimulus to orthodontic movement.

The mechanical support of the teeth outlined in Chapter 10 underlies many areas of dentistry in addition to orthodontics. Operative dentistry, periodontics, and prosthodontics are all deeply concerned with problems related to the function of this mechanism.

As will be shown later, even though orthodontic forces may differ in some ways from other dental forces, they are far from unique in their capacity to induce movement.

THE PERIODONTAL SPACE AND TOOTH MOBILITY

Normally the calcification of the periodontal tissues approaches the tooth but never reaches it, maintaining the uniform layer of intervening soft tissue called the periodontal membrane.

Direct contact and union between calcified bone and tooth, even over a small area, is the pathologic condition of ankylosis.

The width of the uncalcified region (periodontal membrane) varies widely in response to function, with the calcification advancing and receding in response to the functional demands for mobility. The membrane is thinnest in embedded teeth, thickening progressively with eruption, increasing function, and traumatic overloading.

Need for mobility

Tooth mobility is a normal physiologic response to stress. Even in extreme cases with pathologic bone loss, the mobility is only a symptom of the pathologic stress condition. *The periodontal loss in such cases is not a result of the mobility but rather of the undue stress exceeding the adaptive capacity of mobility.*

Mobility literally softens the blow of dental forces, slowing and smoothing the transfer of force to the fibers. If occlusal forces are light or nonexistent (as in an open bite), there is no need for such a cushion. The periodontal space under these conditions can be extremely thin, the attachment rigid, and mobility difficult to detect.

Normal occlusal stresses on such a tooth over a period of time will cause a retreat of the bone and more mobility. This mobility extends the range of movement available in the first and second stages of hydraulic adjustment and so provides a gentler transfer of forces to the fibers without the traumatic effects of third-stage responses. When mobility reaches a level where the protection of this thickening is sufficient to prevent damage to the supporting tissues, a physiologic equilibrium should be maintained at that level of mobility.

Excessive stress beyond the adaptive capacity of the periodontium will result in periodontal loss. The tooth in this condition will be highly mobile with the adaptive thickening of the periodontal ligament at its maximum. This coincidence of greatest mobility with periodontal loss may give the impression that the mobility has caused the loss, when in fact both have occurred concurrently as separate responses to the excessive stress.

Traumatic occlusion is a special case of this type, in which a tooth is subjected to *two or more different forces* that prevent an orthodontic response that would provide a retreat from the increased stress. Excessive force from one direction alone will cause a tooth to move away from that force—the typical orthodontic response. A concurrent force from another direction can prevent that retreat, trapping the tooth in an overloaded state of dynamic equilibrium, much like the "bird" in a badminton game. The result of this situation is a marked increase in mobility, and if this does not provide adequate relief for the periodontium, the next response will be some degree of periodontal destruction.

Contact tightness

In the normal dentition there is *no space* between the crowns of adjoining teeth; they lie in intimate contact, but with *no pressure* between teeth at rest. In this resting state with teeth in contact, the term *contact tightness* has no meaning. Contact tightness, as it is determined and used clinically, is an index of the combined effects of the thickness and strength of the periodontal membranes and the integrity of the arch. This is usually evaluated on the basis of the ease of separation of the teeth (Fig. 11-1, *A*), which is actually an indicator of mobility.

If two teeth in contact are ankylosed, they cannot be separated at all; their

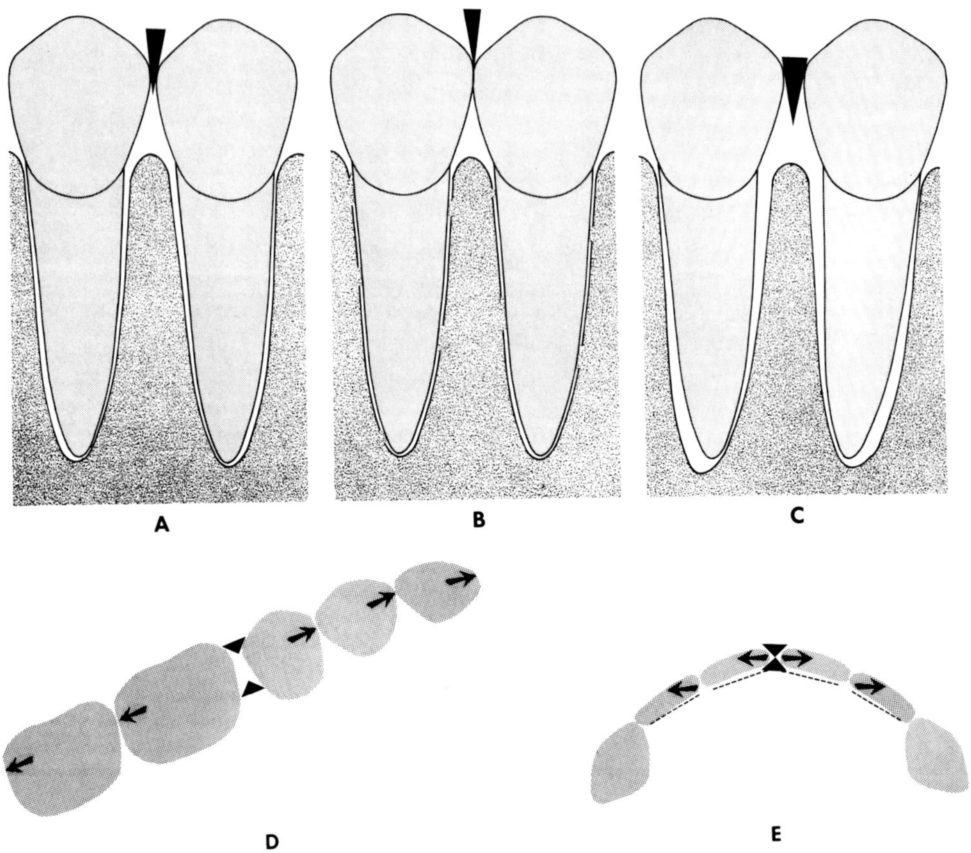

Fig. 11-1. *Contact tightness* is a function of periodontal thickness (mobility) and tooth alignment. **A,** Thin periodontal membrane permits slight tooth movement and a clinically tight contact. **B,** Ankylosis will prevent *any* separation of teeth in contact. **C,** Thick periodontal membrane permits great mobility and a clinically loose contact. **D,** Separation of buccal teeth in good alignment meets with resistance from the periodontal support of all the teeth on that side of the arch. **E,** Labial movement of anterior teeth permits separation with much less movement of nearby teeth.

contact will be so firm (Fig. 11-1, *B*) that nothing can be inserted between them with any reasonable force.

If the two teeth in contact have unusually thick periodontal membranes, they can be separated easily and the contact will be "loose" (Fig. 11-1, *C*).

The same two teeth standing by themselves can be more easily separated than if they are part of a continuous arch. Separation of two buccal teeth in a continuous arch requires equal movement of *all* teeth on either side of the contact, up to the point where the arch curves at the cuspids; the periodontal support of all the buccal teeth on that side is active in resisting the separation (Fig. 11-1, *D*). In the curved anterior segments of the arch the teeth can move labially to provide added space with less effect on adjacent teeth, which is one reason why separation is more easily accomplished in the incisor segments (Fig. 11-1, *E*).

Each interdental contact has its own normal degree of mobility (tightness) for the existing functional conditions, and it is important that this not be violated in restorative procedures. Overzealous extension of dental restorations to "tighten contacts" merely separates the teeth by stressing the periodontal fibers, and then locks them into the new relationship shown in Fig. 11-1, *C*. The net result of such a procedure is an orthodontic movement of the teeth, with the periodontal ligaments soon reestablishing their original thickness and mobility in the new positions. Such unwarranted tooth movement may easily precipitate new problems stemming from the unnecessary disturbance of occlusal relationships. Dental restorations should restore contact tightness only to its original level, just as original tooth contours are restored, unless functional changes related to tooth mobility are also a part of the treatment.

EFFECTS OF FORCE ORIENTATION

Most of the discussion thus far has revolved around normal more or less axial functional occlusal loading, but this is only one of many possible force situations. The most common heavy nonaxial forces are those of traumatic occlusion and orthodontics. These two present many similar instantaneous force pictures, but there are many very important differences.

Under an outside force, whether it is orthodontic or functional, a tooth will transfer predictable forces on the periodontal structures. The various orientations of these forces are most easily classified according to their effects on the periodontium as expressed by the strains and movements that they induce.

Tension and pressure

Periodontal forces have been traditionally classified as either tension or pressure, based on effects on the alveolar bone. This oversimplification ignores the different combinations of effects that may be produced on fibers and in the hydraulic mechanism. As discussed previously, some forces can even produce the anomalous situation of bone subjected to tension from the periodontal fibers at the same time that it is subjected to hydraulic pressure from the fluid system.

For this reason, an adequate description requires that the effects of both the fibers and the hydraulic system be considered.

Effects on fibers can best be described in terms of tension, which may be positive (stretching), zero (passive), or negative (shortening). Hydraulic effects can be described in terms of pressure, which may also be positive (compression), zero (passive), or negative (less than passive pressure). These different loading conditions are shown in Fig. 11-2.

Individual tooth movements

Individual tooth movements fall into several broad types, each with its own unique effects on the different parts of the periodontium.

Apical movement. Apical movement is intrusive into the alveolus in the same direction that forces are imposed by occlusion.

The periodontal loading under orthodontic forces is essentially the same as in function. Positive tension is applied to the fibers and positive pressure to the contents of the periodontal space and bone (Fig. 11-3, *A*). This is the situation that is

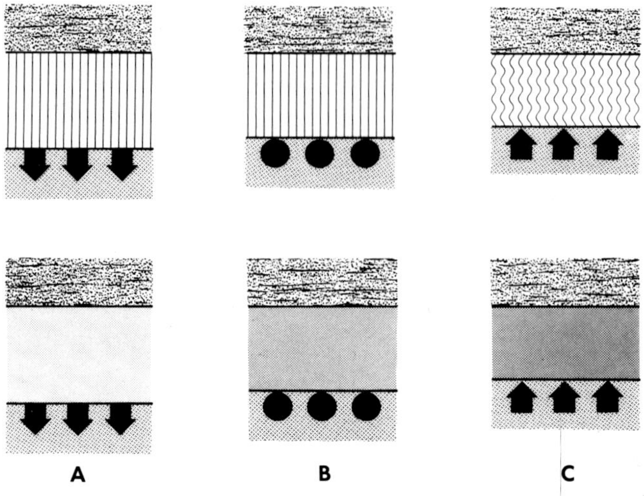

Fig. 11-2. Response of fibers (top) and fluid (bottom) under different loading conditions. **A,** Tooth moved away from the bone, producing positive tension on fibers and negative fluid pressure. **B,** Static condition. **C,** Tooth moved toward bone, producing negative tension and positive pressure. Angular movements may produce positive tension in combination with any fluid pressure condition.

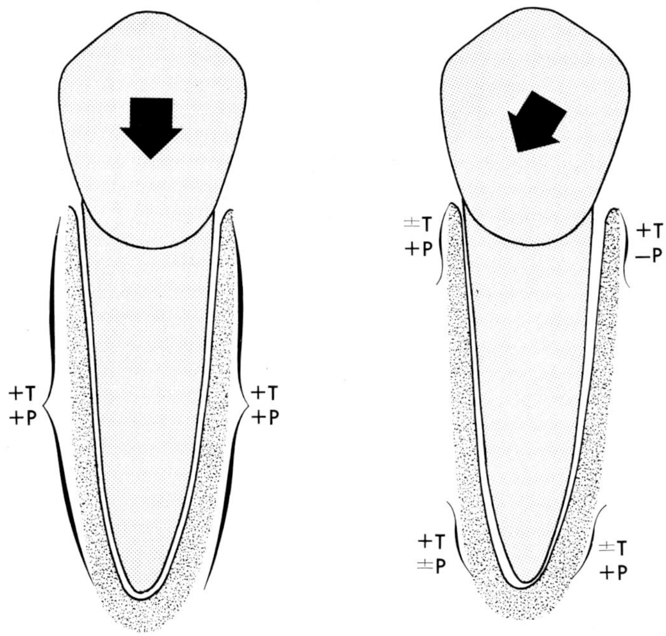

Fig. 11-3. A, *Direct apical movement* places the entire periodontal ligament under a unique combination of positive tension *and* positive pressure. **B,** Combining tipping with apical movement introduces negative tension or negative pressure into some areas, depending on the exact direction and the magnitude of force.

generally most resistant to orthodontic forces, and the explanation may lie in this unique combination of simultaneous hydraulic pressure and fibrous tension that is applied to the bone.

Very light forces applied continuously are most effective in the clinical accomplishment of apical orthodontic movement. This provides a stimulus for change through small increases in fiber tension without elevating hydraulic pressures beyond the first level, where cellular elements are not traumatized.

It should be noted that this unique pressure/tension combination exists *only* for pure intrusion. The introduction of a lateral force will significantly alter the picture in some areas (Fig. 11-3, *B*). This correlates well with the clinical observation that apical orthodontic movements are most readily accomplished when carried out in combination with other movements.

Occlusal movement. Occlusal movement operates in the same direction as eruption. Force on the periodontium is positive tension and negative pressure (Fig. 11-4). Orthodontic movement in this direction is one of the most easily accomplished, provided that it is not inhibited by opposing functional forces. It should be noted that in cases of open bite the opposing functional forces applied by soft tissues may prove very unyielding.

Horizontal tipping (rotation around a horizontal axis). Tipping and other horizontal movements that follow present a more complex force picture than apical or

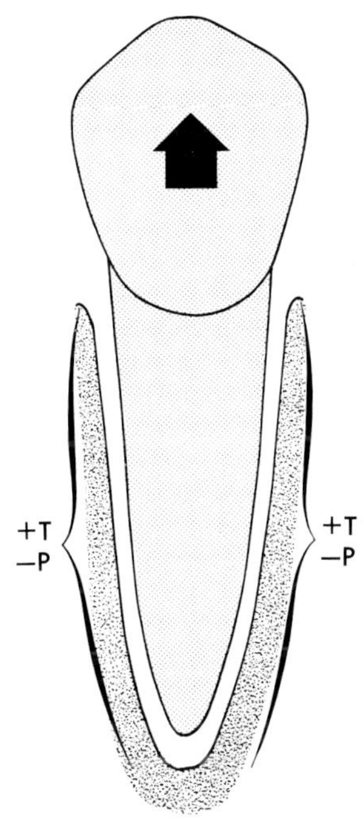

Fig. 11-4. *Occlusal movement* places the entire periodontal ligament under positive tension and negative pressure.

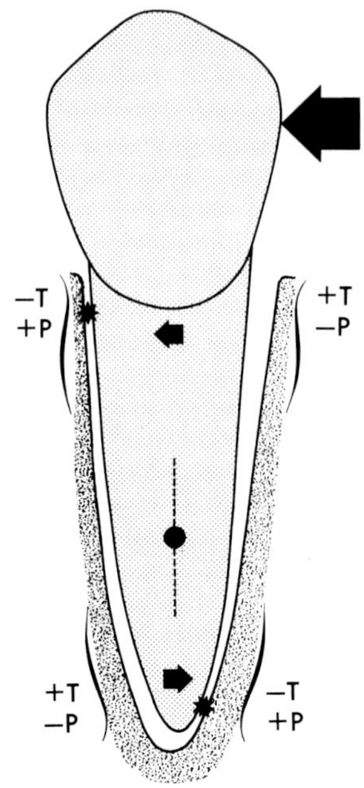

Fig. 11-5. *Simple tipping.* The root pivots on resisting fulcrums in the gingival and apical areas, rotating about an axis somewhere between. Pressure and tension effects are greatest in the fulcrum areas, diminishing to zero opposite the axis of rotation.

occlusal movements. Simple tipping is the elemental tooth movement that takes place when force is applied to the crown so that a tooth is free to tip around a horizontal axis. This kind of tipping can be in either mesiodistal or buccolingual directions. (Fig. 11-5). A rigid orthodontic attachment to the tooth is not required to accomplish this effect.

When a simple horizontal force is applied, the resistance of the gingival crest area causes the tooth to pivot there. The pivoting around the gingival region causes the apex to move in a direction opposite that of the crown. Both apical and gingival ends of the root encounter similar resistance and stimulate similar responses, but in opposite directions.

Positive tension and negative pressure occur together on opposite sides of the gingival and apical ends of the root. Negative tension and positive pressure occur together in the alternate areas, as shown in Fig. 11-5. As a result the final movement of the tooth is a tipping rotation around an axis somewhere in the middle or apical third of the root.

This axis around which the tooth rotates is correctly called the *axis of rotation* rather than the fulcrum. A fulcrum is a point of support or resistance, and in this case there is no support or resistance at the axis; in fact, the axis lies in the neutral transition area where net force is zero.

In such a tipping tooth there are actually two true fulcrums, located at the gingival and apical ends of the root. If the resistance at either of these ends were removed, the tooth would pivot around the other end. As long as both ends of the

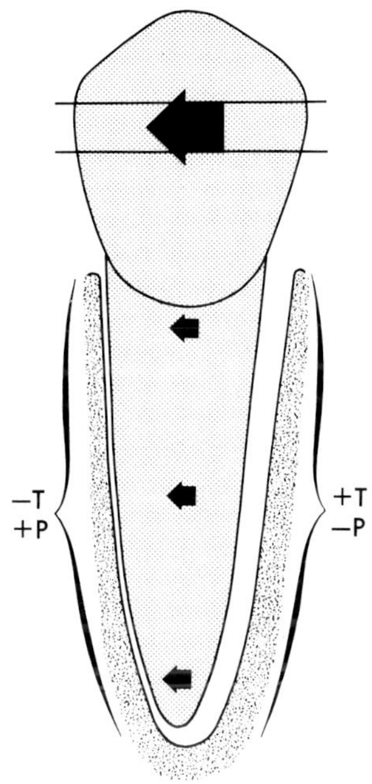

Fig. 11-6. *Translatory movement.* Crown and root are moved in the same direction. One entire side of the root is under positive tension and negative pressure, with the opposite effects on the other side.

root resist the force, the tooth will rotate around the neutral axis somewhere between them.

The actual location of the axis depends on the dimensions of the root, the condition of the supporting tissues, and the exact strength and point of application of the force.

Such tipping is the instantaneous effect of force application. Orthodontic tipping occurs initially around approximately the same axis in response to the resulting tissue forces, but this axis may shift as movement progresses and force patterns and responses change.

Horizontal translation. Pure horizontal translation (bodily movement) is accomplished with a nonpivoting orthodontic attachment to the tooth that prevents tipping by the application of a countertipping moment in combination with the horizontal vector. The tooth is moved horizontally in such a way that the crown and the root move the same distance without change in axial inclination (Fig. 11-6). Positive tension and negative pressure occur along one entire side of the root while negative tension and positive pressure occur along the other side.

Elimination of the inactive neutral area near the center of the root *doubles the active resistance* of the periodontal ligament to such a force when compared with tipping, one of several considerations that should not be overlooked in this type of movement. Also important is the change in blood supply, as extensive areas are subjected to simultaneous stress.

Root movement. Of course the root moves in all orthodontic movements, but

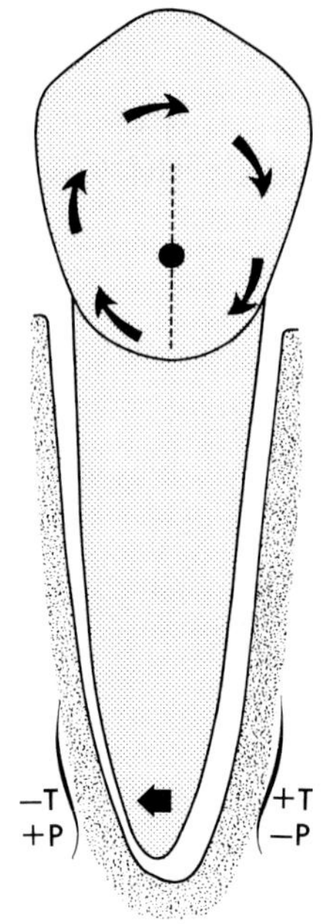

Fig. 11-7. *Root movement* (usually uprighting) concentrates forces near the apex while the crown is held relatively motionless. Periodontal stresses diminish to zero at the alveolar crest.

the term *root movement* is used in orthodontics to describe a situation in which the primary objective is to move the apical end of the root, with no appreciable crown movement (Fig. 11-7).

Mechanical requirements for root movement are similar to those for translatory movement, but with a change in the relative values of tipping rotation and horizontal vector. Forces on the periodontium are similar except that they diminish toward zero at the alveolar crest for root movement. Most orthodontic movements are actually a combination of these two, rather than pure translatory movement or pure root movement.

Other terms used to describe specific cases of root movement are *uprighting*, in which a tipped tooth is restored to normal inclination without moving the crown, and *torquing action*, in which a root is tipped in a labiolingual direction.

Describing tipping movements

The varied terminology used to describe tipping movements leads to many ambiguous situations when attempts are made to describe specific clinical procedures. In an effort to reduce this problem these movements will be described in this book by identifying both the tipping and translatory components of the movement.

Tipping action. Tipping action can be described purely on the basis of the change in crown position in relation to the root. For example, a distal tipping action on a molar is one where the crown is positioned more distally in relation to the

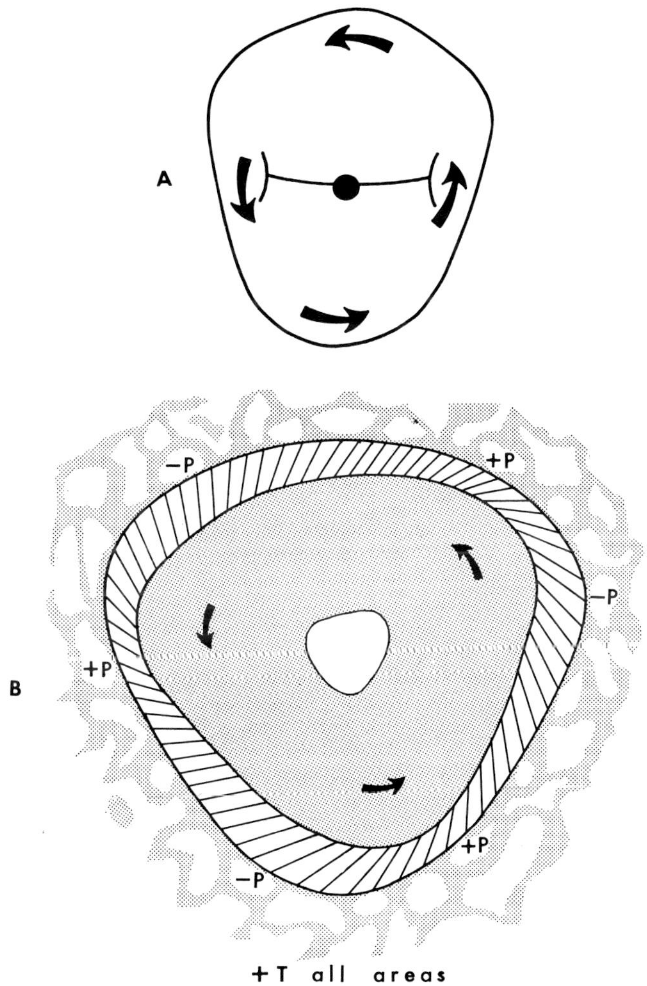

Fig. 11-8. A, *Rotation.* Tooth is rotated on the long axis of the root. **B,** *Rotation* in schematic cross-section. All fibers are under tension, with pressure effects dependent on the shape of the root.

root. If the crown is held immobile as this takes place, the root will move mesially. If the root tip does not move, the crown will move distally. Or a strong mesial vector applied from an outside source such as intermaxillary traction may move the entire tooth mesially as it is being tipped distally. In all of these situations the tipping mechanism is the same, and the final position of the crown will be more distal in relation to the root, so it may be described as distal tipping.

The same principle applies to mesial or distal, buccal or lingual tipping.

Concurrent translatory effects that combine with the simple tipping movement to accomplish uprighting, root movement, etc. are introduced by applying a horizontal vector to augment or resist the crown movement of the tipping action. These are described simply as mesial, distal, buccal, or lingual vectors.

Axial rotation. Axial rotation is the pivoting of a tooth around the long axis of the root without any translatory effect (Fig. 11-8). We often tend to think of rotation as involving only a pure sliding action between root and alveolus, but this would be true only if the root were perfectly round.

All periodontal fibers are under tension in rotation, but the bone may be under either positive or negative pressure in different regions, depending on the shape of the root. Some areas of the alveolar bone may be subjected to tension from the fibers at the same time that they are subjected to hydraulic pressure from tissue compression, as in apical movements, but the pressure areas are more limited in rotation.

Rotations must progress a considerable distance to produce significant changes in the ligament. The fibers of the rotated tooth will be oriented as shown in Fig. 11-8, *B*, ready to return it toward its original position. For this reason, teeth should be slightly overrotated and rotations should be carried out as early in treatment as possible. With early correction the remaining treatment time becomes a part of the retention period for the rotations.

Rotations can be described in a manner similar to that used for tipping. The movement of the buccal (or labial) crown surface in relation to the axis of the tooth is used to identify the movement. A distal rotation of the upper right central incisor would indicate that its labial surface moved distally in relation to the axis of the tooth. This would be counterclockwise as viewed from the occlusal, with the distal corner moving more lingually and the mesial corner more labially.

Concurrent translatory movements of a tooth may cause some surfaces to move more than others in relation to the dental arch, but the primary consideration in rotation is how the change relates to the tooth itself. This single-term phraseology avoids the ambiguities of clock references or compound terms that have contradictory meanings in different areas of the mouth.

Orthodontic tissue response

The general pattern of orthodontic response to forces is well known, consisting essentially of resorption in advance of the moving tooth and osteogenesis in its wake. That sounds simple, but many of the controlling factors are difficult to identify and correlate in specific situations. In all situations the response at the site of action, where root and periodontium interact, is dependent only on the local force picture where the tissues are healthy. Conditions in other areas of the dentition are irrelevant except as they interact with the appliance to contribute to this local force picture.

Positive tension on fibers. Periodontal fibers are not strictly elastic; they are woven together in a syncytium that makes the entire unit elastic in much the same way that the twisting of inelastic fibers in a rope allows it to stretch. As these weaving, twisting fibers are pulled they tend to straighten, allowing the entire ligament to stretch just as though the fibers themselves were elastic. This response to force gives very little stimulus for tissue changes without considerable protracted stretching.

Continued tension will stretch the fibers in a semielastic manner that requires relatively small forces to maintain the extension. These fibers have great strength in resisting short-lived forces, but will fatigue and extend under continuous loading. Increasing the thickness of the periodontal space by loading in this way can be expected to result in calcification advancing toward the tooth, with a tendency to restore the original space thickness. This is the usual response in horizontal orthodontic movement.

The effect of fiber tension on the alveolar bone is clearly shown in microscopic sections demonstrating osteoblastic activity and calcification. This is a surface activity, tending to follow the periodontal fibers, which in turn tend to align with the lines of stress.

This orientation of the fibro-osseous structure with the prevailing stresses presents an optimum structural design for withstanding these stresses.

The uncalcified fibers within the periodontal ligaments also respond to increased stress, but here the problems of direct observation have limited current knowledge. It is certain that the attachment is always maintained, and it is equally certain that the fibers elongate in some fashion; the question is "how"?

The picture of an intermediate plexus with fibers woven together, disconnecting and reconnecting as movement progresses, is probably an oversimplification. Histologic work tracing individual fibers from tooth to bone[13] casts more doubt on this view, but the nature of the collagen fiber itself should not be overlooked.

"Interstitial fluid" is actually a suspension of giant molecules, a macromolecular gel of mucopolysaccharides. There is a tendency even at the molecular level for these long molecules to align with the stresses in the gel. The details of fibrogenesis and the nature of the necessary stimuli are still incomplete, but there is little question that fibers form through a consolidation and interweaving of these molecules, with lateral chemical bonds adding to the strength of the ultimate structure. The entire fiber is nothing more than an accumulation or consolidation of this woven pattern repeated at molecular, fibrillar, and fiber levels.[14]

The molecular bonds that are the fundamental source of strength can be formed (fibrogenesis) or broken (fibrolysis) under many circumstances, and the action is not necessarily the same or simultaneous for all molecules in one area. It is not at all difficult to visualize fiber extension as a purely molecular effect in which the most heavily stressed bonds "slip" and reattach in new extended positions, in a manner not unlike that which occurs in plastic deformation and work hardening of metals.

In places where fibers are under tension but the root does not move away from the bone, these fiber alterations are the only orthodontic changes that can take place; calcification will not advance along an extended fiber if its alveolar end is not far enough away from the tooth.

Negative tension on fibers. On the "pressure side" of a moving tooth, the periodontal fibers obviously must shorten or otherwise adjust in order to maintain a normal attachment. Continued tooth movement in one direction without active fibrolysis would result in a massive accumulation of fibers piling up on the advancing side. At the same time, new fibers with a shorter length must form to maintain the attachment. Such changes must take place at the molecular level through ongoing simultaneous fibrolysis and fibrogenesis.

It is clear that these fibrous changes do not occur readily without positive and consistent mechanical stimulation. The stresses introduced into the alveolar space

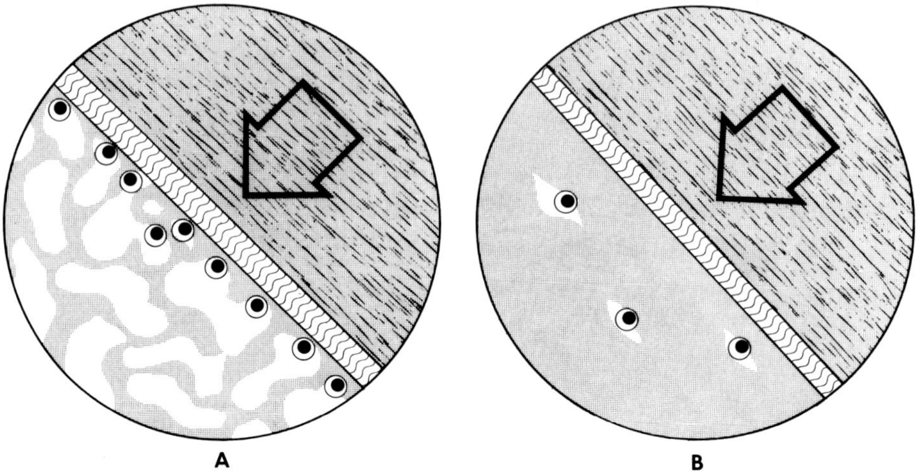

Fig. 11-9. A, Cancellous bone has many places in which resorption may take place when the bone is subjected to pressure from a tooth moving under orthodontic force. **B,** Dense cortical bone has few places in which resorption may take place when the bone is subjected to pressure from a tooth being moved by an orthodontic force.

are adequate to stimulate these adjustments, but a similar response is not found in the fibers of the gingival tissues.

Gingival tissues show a long-term propensity to return to their original form, as evidenced by persistent posttreatment relapse tendencies. The relatively longer length of the gingival fibers and the lack of hard, confining walls greatly reduces the strains that may be induced by outside stresses.

Positive pressure on bone. Bone response under pressure is generally resorption, although calcification (though not necessarily osteogenesis) has been demonstrated at some points of pressure application.[15] The nature of the resorption pattern and its rate depend on the force and on the bone itself. Even the lightest orthodontic force will grossly curtail or completely cut off the blood supply to tissues squeezed between root and bone. Removal of the alveolar bone by osteoclasis requires a flanking attack from areas that still have an adequate blood supply and a sheltered spot in which the osteoclasts may work. Such a situation in cancellous bone is shown schematically in Fig. 11-9, *A*. Here the bone is removed rapidly, and the tooth is soon free to move in response to the force of the appliance.

Fig. 11-9, *B*, shows the comparable situation in dense cortical bone. Here there are very few areas in which osteoclasis may begin, and removal of the bone will be a long, slow process. The dense bone around the lower molars causes these teeth to be especially resistant to orthodontic change in some patients.

Even in this dense bone pressures should be kept low. What is needed here, along with everything else, is patience. Great areas must be removed, almost as one giant spicule, and this takes *time*. Impatiently escalating force levels can slow progress even further.

After the bone nearest the tooth has been removed, the tooth will move into

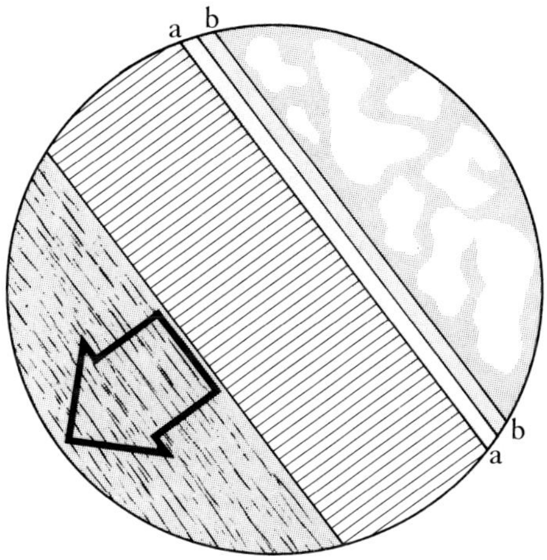

Fig. 11-10. On the tension side of a moving root, a layer of osteoid is laid down on the surface of the alveolus, *a*. This is slowly transformed into mature bone, *b*.

the space and the whole cycle is repeated. As movement progresses, the ligaments on the tension side take up part of the orthodontic force, reducing the pressure on the pressure side. In cancellous bone, pressure will tend to localize at the highest remaining spicules of bone, leaving resorption in other areas free to progress unimpeded. These factors combine to accelerate the resorption of bone and the movement of the tooth.

Tension and negative pressure on bone. Widening of the periodontal membrane by an outside force places the fibers under tension and applies negative pressure to both soft tissue and bone. This is the typical "tension side" situation under which new bone is laid down on the inner surface of the alveolus, tending to narrow the periodontal membrane toward its original width.

This apposition of bone takes place in stages. First a connective tissue matrix (osteoid) is formed, and this gradually ossifies into mature bone (Fig. 11-10). Under continuous tooth movement, the inner surface of the alveolus on the tension side is always lined with osteoid, whereas the deeper layers show progressive ossification.

Response to tension takes time, for the first application of force does not stretch the periodontal fibers enough to stimulate much bone apposition. The bone on the pressure side stops the movement too soon. Resorption must begin on the pressure side first to allow enough additional tooth movement to stretch the fibers on the tension side further. The typical thickening of the periodontal membrane with increased mobility of the tooth under orthodontic stimulation is partly the result of this lag in response to tension.

Once a tooth begins to move after the initial resorption on the pressure side of the root, the fibers on the tension side will carry a greater proportion of the orthodontic force. This helps to relieve the pressure side, which carried most of the load at first. This shifting of the load results in more even distribution of force, with greater comfort for the patient and steadier tissue response. This is especially true if the initial adjustment was gentle enough and if the appliance is designed, fitted, and activated to follow through for some distance without further adjustment.

Angle[16] stressed the importance of light continuous application of force many years ago, but at that time such force application could be attained only with frequent, extremely delicate adjustments. Light steel archwires, force-reducing loops, and elastic modules make this type of force application much more simple and effective today.

Reversal of direction. A serious clinical problem connected with the tension response arises when the direction of tooth movement is reversed, suddenly subjecting an area previously under tension to pressure. Moving the root in this new direction requires resorption in an area of the alveolus that has recently become lined with osteoid in response to the previous tension.

Resorption of bone and movement of a tooth are impossible in such an area until there has been time for the completion of the transformation of the osteoid to mature, resorbable bone. This means a delay in the progress of treatment that can vary from serious to devastating in its effect.

A typical situation in which this condition can arise is the case in which a tooth, such as a cuspid, is moved by tipping and then uprighted. If the initial tipping is

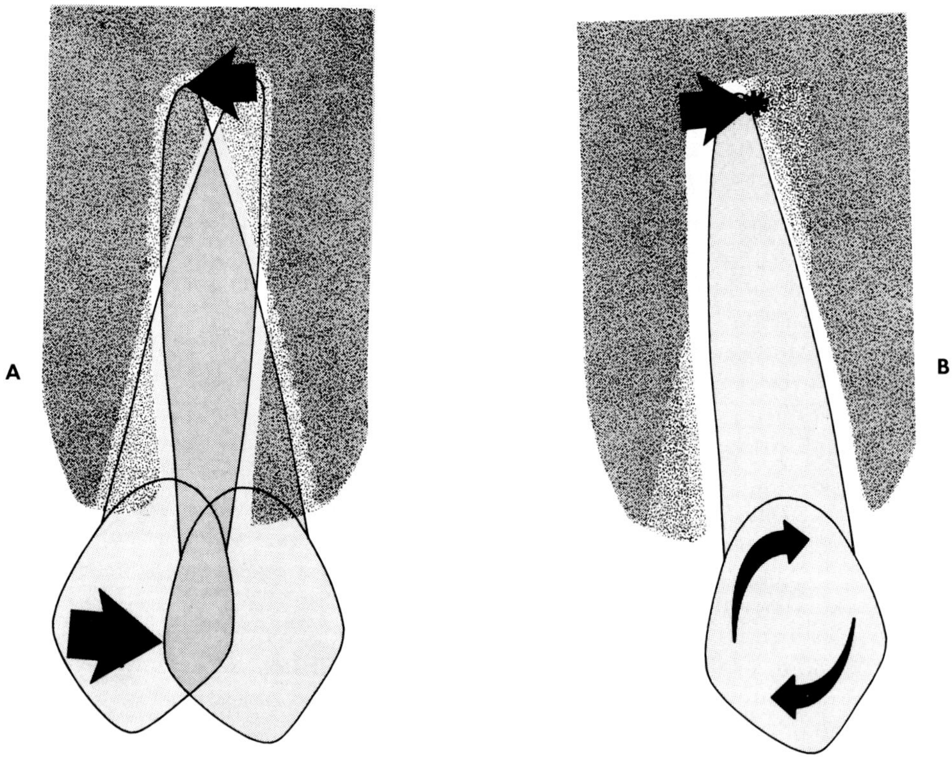

Fig. 11-11. In simple tipping, osteoid will be formed on opposite sides of the root at gingival and apical levels, **A.** This may retard any attempt at immediate uprighting, **B.**

uncontrolled (without any uprighting moment), the apex can be expected to shift in a direction opposite that of the crown (Fig. 11-11, *A*). This results in the formation of osteoid on the distal side of the apex. When an uprighting moment is applied to this tooth at a later adjustment (Fig. 11-11, *B*), the objective is to return the apex back in the direction of the new osteoid. This region is not resorbable until after the osteoid has matured, so the forces directed at moving the root tip distally will be dissipated in mesial movement of the crown or of the resistance units (anchor teeth). This can be avoided by controlling the initial tipping or by a delay in the uprighting action in cases in which this condition may have developed.

Short-term studies by Reitan[17] indicate that delay from this cause may be only a matter of days, but even this can stop virtually all progress if a patient does not follow instructions in the wearing of elastic traction or similar removable sources of force. If elastic traction is removed for a period of time, either willfully or forgetfully, the elasticity of the appliance and the supporting tissues can be sufficient to reverse the direction of tooth movement and initiate osteoid formation on what should be the advancing sides of the roots. Later, when traction is resumed, the layer of osteoid will retard the movement of teeth into these areas. Regular repetition of such episodes can add to treatment time far beyond the actual time that the necessary traction is not applied, so it is easy to see how continued spasmodic efforts can cause an almost endless delay in progress and threaten the ultimate success of treatment.

No effort should be spared to impress patients with the important fact that days of negligence can mean extra weeks and months of treatment. Every orthodontist is familiar with the situation in which a slowly responding correction suddenly progresses miraculously as the patient finally sees the light and begins to follow instructions faithfully.

Sliding (positive tension, zero pressure). In sliding movements the root moves more or less parallel to the adjacent bone surface (Fig. 11-12). This condition exists

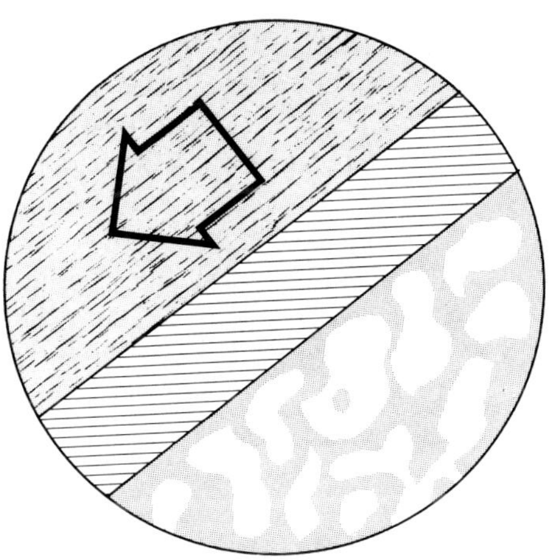

Fig. 11-12. When a root surface is moved parallel to the adjacent supporting bone in a sliding action, there is no occasion for bone change, either apposition or resorption, in spite of the fact that the periodontal fibers may be under extreme tension.

to some degree in all movements, but is most prominent in axial rotation and apical movements.

Bone changes can contribute little to such movements where there is no change in periodontal width. This minimal bone response, together with the need for considerable change in the fibers, combines to make these some of the most difficult movements to attain and to retain.

Gingival tissues

Gingival tissues usually exert only mild resistance to orthodontic movements, but they loom large in the relapse problem.

The gingivae are heavily laced with connective tissue fibers, and many of these are directly attached to the teeth. When a tooth is moved, these tissues are distorted and behave almost like rubber in their tendency to return to their original contours and positions.

In addition to their stretching action, the gingivae can create an additional problem through sheer bulk. The frenum between the central incisors is a familiar example, but the tissue in any space, including extraction spaces, presents a similar problem. A fully healed extraction site will contain two complete interproximal papillae plus the new gingivae covering the alveolar ridge. When this space is closed, all of that tissue is compressed to the dimensions of one interproximal papilla and must then adjust accordingly. This adjustment cannot begin until after the teeth have been moved, so it is often a part of posttreatment adjustment.

These characteristics of the gingivae call for countermeasures similar to those required for rotation. Early correction of the relationships subject to these gingival relapse forces, together with overcorrection to stretch fibers past the desired positions, will do much to ensure later stability. Spaces should be closed and rotations and overlapping teeth corrected in the first few months of treatment whenever possible. In extreme cases surgical measures may be beneficial.

Gingival inflammation. During orthodontic therapy the gingivae sometimes show an inflammatory reaction. This is often due to inadequate oral hygiene combined with the irritation of band or adhesive margins, and the condition will normally improve rapidly after the appliances are removed. Gingivae compressed in the course of tooth movement may also react with an inflammatory or proliferative response.

Although most gingival changes during treatment are transitory, it is still important to minimize them as much as possible. Any gingival conditions that exist before treatment will usually be aggravated by the additional insults of appliances and more difficult hygiene. If these conditions are brought under control before treatment is begun, it should be a rare case indeed in which interruption of treatment is required to relieve a gingival problem.

Pain

Pain is often a consideration in orthodontic treatment, but with careful attention it can usually be limited to an occasional minor annoyance.

The source of most pain sensations in orthodontic treatment is the periodontal membrane. Increasing force or trauma or increasing the area of the membrane subject to those forces can cause or increase pain.

A simple tipping action subjects relatively small areas to pressure and tension, and pressure anesthesia tends to reduce the pain response in the areas under greatest pressure.

Rotation represents the other extreme. It involves the entire membrane surrounding the root. There are few parts of the membrane in which pressure anesthesia can reduce the pain response. Circulation is not appreciably reduced; in fact, a membrane under a heavy rotational force may actually be in a state of circulatory congestion that can further increase the patient's discomfort. Many rotation mechanisms work over a long period of time, keeping the ligaments under constant tension.

Gentle continuous forces offer the most effective control of pain in rotations, as in most other movements. Carefully applied, these forces will not prove unduly uncomfortable for the great majority of patients, and the correction will proceed with gratifying speed.

FORCES

The repeated references that have been made to orthodontic forces call for some discussion of just what forces should be used.

The important variables in orthodontic force are direction, intensity, and application cycle. The importance of direction is obvious, since it determines the direction in which the tooth is to be moved. The remaining two variables can make all the difference between uncertain and optimum responses to treatment.

Intensity

Little is known about the minimum force requirement for tooth movement, except that it is very, very low—probably only a few grams. Certainly, a pressure of 1 ounce (28 gm) is more than adequate to move most teeth. The lower limit of clinically effective orthodontic force probably depends more on the counterforces acting on the tooth than on the responsiveness of the tissues themselves.

Teeth under orthodontic therapy are simultaneously subjected to the forces of occlusion, to those of tongue and lips, and sometimes to other forces from intraoral or extraoral habits. These forces vary greatly, and for any individual tooth the orthodontic force must be considered together with these other forces to determine the net force acting to move the tooth. Forces acting in opposite directions will tend to cancel each other, and failure to recognize balancing environmental forces can easily result in a stalemate. The supporting tissues will not react selectively to an orthodontic force merely because it has been applied with conscious intent to bring about tooth movement.

In general most individual teeth will respond favorably to an orthodontic force in the 25- to 100-gm (1-ounce to 4-ounce) range. The lower end of this range is adequate and preferable for the smaller teeth. Cuspids and molars require more force because of the larger area of periodontal attachment. On the other hand, a continuous intermaxillary force in the range of 100 gm (2 ounces each side) can move all of the teeth in an arch.

Force distribution within the periodontal membrane cannot be overlooked in considering force levels. It is the force at the cellular level that is responsible for the tissue changes of tooth movement, and this depends not only on the area of the root of the tooth but also on the way in which the loads are distributed over that root. Translatory movement requires considerably more than twice as much applied force to produce the same force in the large resisting areas of the supporting tissues as is required by the more localized distribution in tipping. Figs. 11-5 and 11-6 show the distributions of force in these two situations, with only the gingival and apical fibers approaching a full load in tipping while all of the fibers on one side of the tooth share the load in translatory movement.

The use of gentle forces was stressed over and over again by Angle, but the design of the edgewise appliance is such that it is capable of applying extremely high forces.

The introduction of stainless steel has increased the level of force potential so that great care is required to keep force levels in an optimum range. Direct substitution of steel for gold can double and even quadruple force levels, but designs based on the properties of steel in everyday use today can effectively apply forces well below those that were possible in Angle's time. The difference lies in the skill of the clinician, not in the materials.

Light forces have become so popular that the term *light* is applied indiscriminately to forces varying from a few grams to several pounds. In this book the term *light* will be reserved for forces below 100 gm. The light force concept is a valuable one, but its effective use requires a thorough understanding of the mechanics of the appliance and the supporting tissues.

Light forces can move teeth rapidly over great distances, and a single adjustment can have a significant effect on teeth far removed from the area of adjustment. Careful control is of paramount importance when operating an appliance with such great capacity for energy storage and delivery.

Force application cycles (rhythms)

Much more has been written and said about the level of orthodontic force and its effect on tooth movement than about the equally important time factor. Vague references to continuous and intermittent forces have given lip service to the concept, but this division hardly scratches the surface.

In the strictest sense, *all* orthodontic forces are intermittent; they have a beginning and they have an end. Differences lie in the form and the number of cycles of application—the rhythms of force application.

The variables of the individual cycle that contribute to these rhythms are (1) period of force application ("on" period), (2) level of force during "on" period, and (3) period of rest ("off" period).

It would be a rare situation that was fully corrected in a single cycle—a one-adjustment treatment. Most of our work involves multiple cycles, with all conceivable variations in the three parameters.

The force rhythms for a single day with each of the major classes of appliances are shown and described in Figs. 11-13, 11-15, 11-16, and 11-19. Forces shown in these illustrations are arbitrary selections presented only to suggest relative force values, but the principles are equally applicable throughout the range of orthodontic forces.

The important differences here lie in the relationships between force levels and

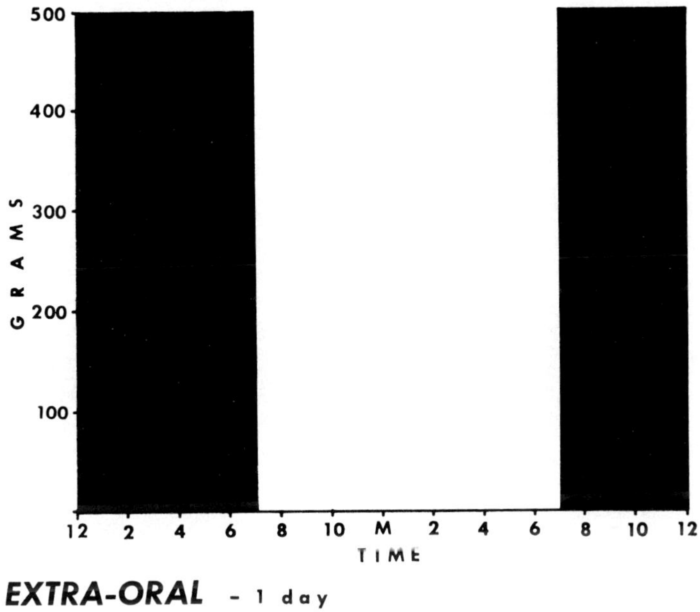

Fig. 11-13. Typical daily force application cycle for an extraoral appliance. Force is applied continuously at the preset level while the appliance is worn, with intervening periods free of force when it is removed.

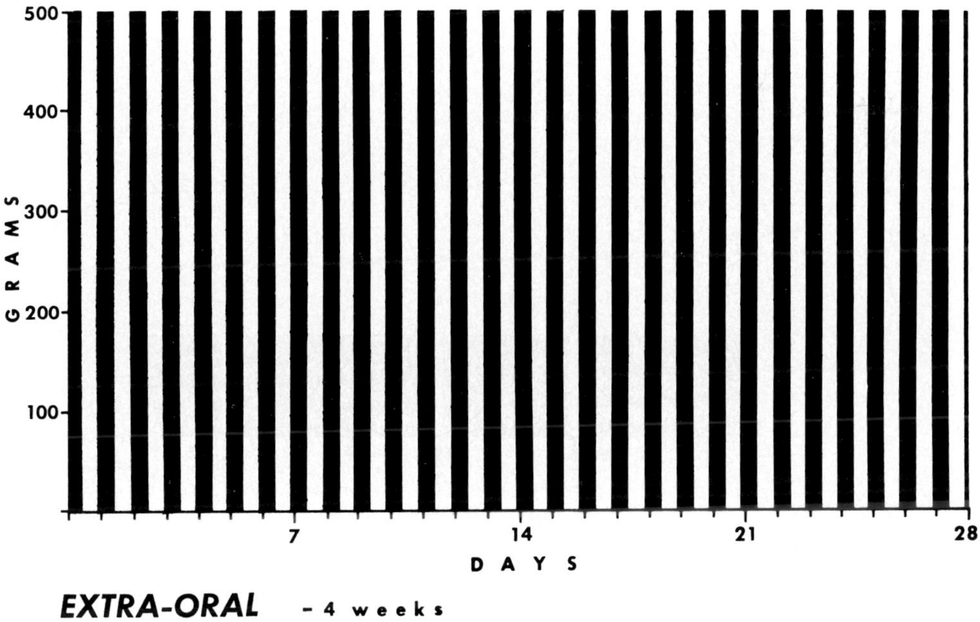

Fig. 11-14. Four weeks of extraoral traction such as shown in Fig. 11-13.

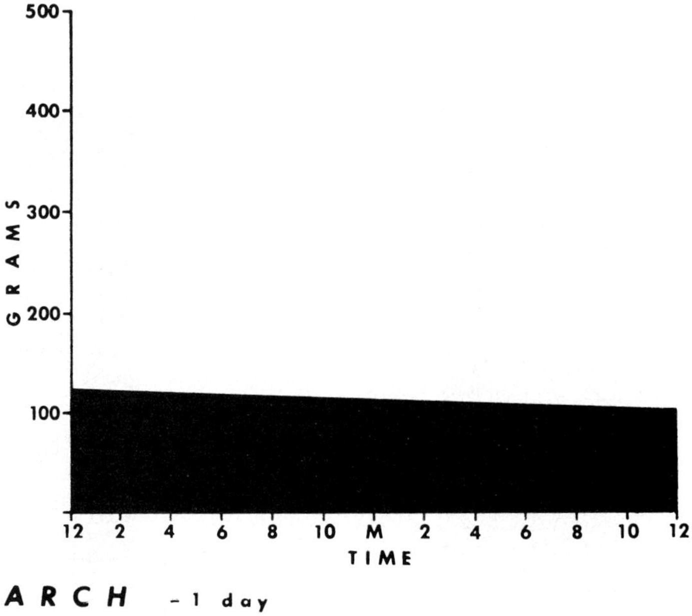

Fig. 11-15. Daily force cycle for an archwire. Force is continuous, with a slow reduction (exaggerated for purposes of illustration) as the tooth moves and the arch returns toward a passive state. Actual force levels may vary widely from those shown.

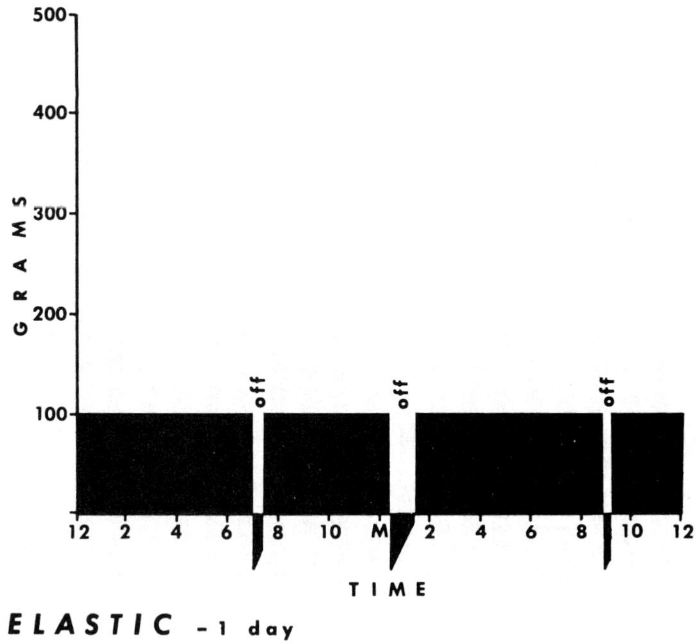

Fig. 11-16. Typical daily force cycles for rubber elastic traction. Removing elastics for meals, toothbrushing, etc. can subject some teeth to a force reversal from the elastic deformation of the archwire.

"on" and "off" periods. The "on" period provides the necessary stimulus to movement. The "off" period provides time for what can be either rest, recovery, or relapse.

In a diurnal cycle with relatively strong forces such as those applied by an extraoral appliance, the "off" time can best be regarded as a rest period. Removal of the force permits restoration of circulation in the stressed tissues, providing the nutrition necessary for the changes incident to tooth movement. The activating force is sufficiently strong for its effects to carry through this period so that the interruptions are actually an essential part of the treatment cycle. Continuous force application requires a reduction in force level for these desired tissue responses to take place.

Interruptions in lighter forces that themselves do not seriously impede circulation merely interrupt the necessary stimuli without any compensatory benefits. These interruptions can retard tooth movement out of all proportion to their duration because the tissues rapidly resume a stable state from which the stimulus must start anew on the next application.

This effect may be compounded in practice by the fact that appliances are usu-

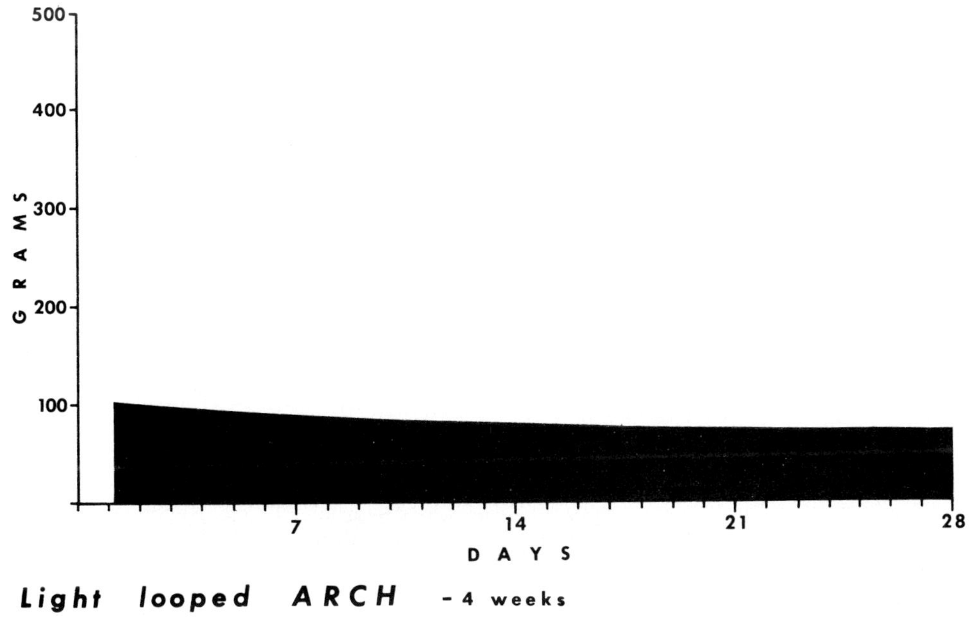

Fig. 11-17. Schematic representation of force application with a light archwire. Force values shown are arbitrary and far below those often described as "light forces." The high resiliency and added loops in these arches provide an extended range of activation with relatively small reductions in force as the tooth moves. This subjects the tissues to long periods of force without relief. Actual "gram-days" of force application, as represented by the area under a curve such as this, may be much higher with these arches than with a heavier arch. Such differences in force pattern and continuity must be carefully considered in adjusting initial force levels.

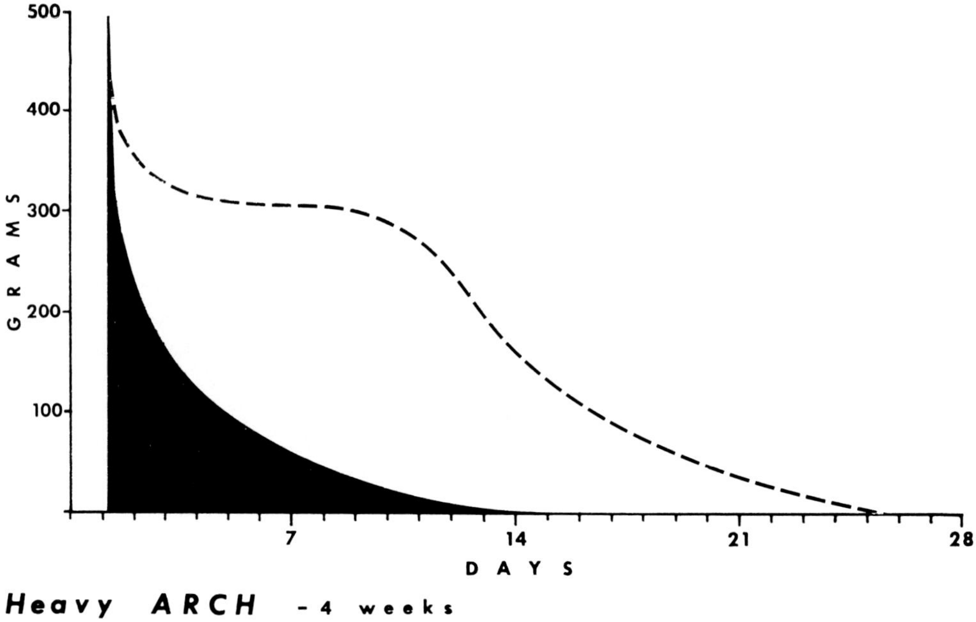

Fig. 11-18. Schematic representation of force application for four weeks with a heavy archwire. Force values shown are arbitrary; this illustration is intended to show trends only. Note that with these very stiff wires there is a rapid drop in force levels with the small movements that take place soon after insertion of the archwire. Later changes are slower, following a course somewhere between the solid black area and the dotted line that represents the refractory period described by Reitan. Actual force application to the tissues in "gram-days" is represented by the total area under the curve.

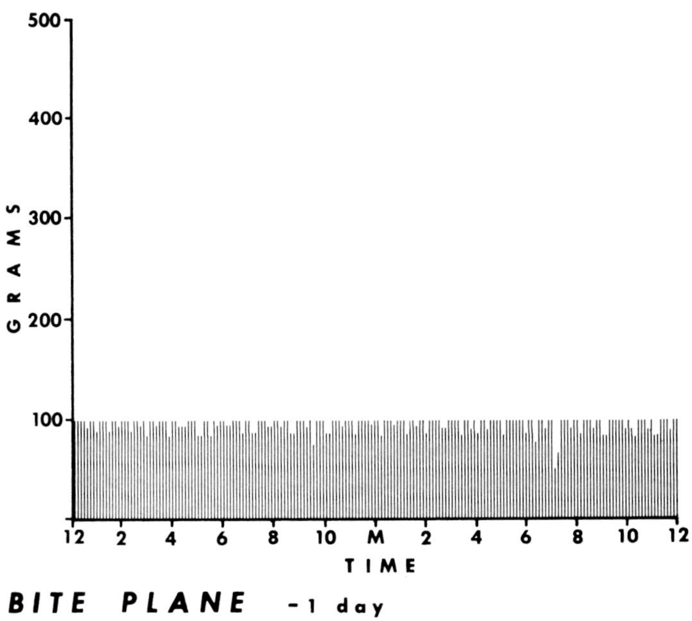

Fig. 11-19. Schematic representation of daily force cycles for a bite plane or similar appliance. Occlusal force is applied for many very brief periods, probably much more numerous and more variable than shown here.

ally so elastic that interruptions actually reverse the force direction instead of merely dropping the level to zero (Fig. 11-16). This can lead to a steady-state level of irritation with no movement at all.

Figs. 11-14, 11-17, and 11-18 show similar rhythms over a four-week period. Here the extraoral appliance continues with essentially identical forces day after day. Archwires, on the other hand, operate with diminishing forces as the teeth move. This is true of all forms of wires and springs, but the rate of the drop can vary widely, as Figs. 11-17 and 11-18 show, for heavy and light wires.

A "heavy" wire (Fig. 11-18) is, by definition, a very stiff wire. This means that it has a steep load-deflection curve with a high initial force that decays rapidly even with small tooth movements. The immediate nonorthodontic tooth movement within the alveolus will produce a sharp initial drop followed by a slower drop as suggested by the two curves in Fig. 11-18. The shape of the curve will depend on the rate of orthodontic tooth movement. The dotted curve illustrates the lag in orthodontic response described by Reitan[18]; the lower curve represents a more uniform response.

Total energy storage in these wires is small in spite of the high force levels. They require frequent adjustments because of the small increment of movement attainable with each. The high initial forces of short duration are soon followed by periods of little or no force, providing time for the tissues to return toward a normal unloaded state.

A "light" wire (Fig. 11-17) may be adjusted to exert a much lighter initial force, but that force will diminish very little with time. Total energy storage is high, and the low stiffness of this type of archwire provides relatively little force decay with large adjustments.

A comparison of Figs. 11-17 and 11-18 shows the fallacy of comparing archwires on the basis of initial force alone. The black areas under these curves represent the actual total force application in "gram-days," and on this basis the light-wire arch actually loads the tissues far more than the heavy-wire arch, while providing no rest or recovery period. It is this change in the rhythm of force application that is responsible for many of the effects often attributed to force levels alone.

These graphs are not intended to demonstrate superiority of one type of arch over another; even accurate measurements of actual forces would do no such thing. The intention is to demonstrate significant differences that must be considered in clinical application.

When stiff wires and heavy forces are used, they must be activated more frequently but still at sufficiently long intervals to provide a rest or recovery period. When light forces are used, they *must* be sufficiently light to permit tissue activity without the intervening rest period. In either case the tissues must be provided with an opportunity to respond with the necessary bone changes. Halfway attempts with "light wires" can apply brutally heavy forces without the benefit of cyclic interruptions.

Many combinations of force levels and rhythms of application will move teeth very effectively if they are properly adjusted in relation to each other. It is this interrelationship of the individual factors, rather than their individual properties, that is most important.

Edgewise practitioners routinely use all types of force, even though the heavy rectangular wires exert a relatively limited range of forces on the teeth. Lighter archwires, extraoral appliances, elastics, tooth positioners, and acrylic and other removable appliances may all be a part of a complete orthodontic armamentarium. It is the skill and understanding that go into the application that are the critical components of success with any pattern of therapeutic forces, and these can be most severely taxed in applying extremely light flexible wires with long working ranges.

12

Orthodontic goals and their clinical attainment

Orthodontic needs cover a broad spectrum from simple tooth displacements to complex facial deformities. This makes a clear definition of objectives an essential part of any individual treatment plan. It is fortunate that more often than not the various possible objectives are complementary so that they can be attained together; but the other side of this coin is the disquieting fact that limited goals may be unattainable without disproportionately intensive efforts and sacrifice. Many times these added efforts must be directed toward problems and goals in which the patient has little or no interest or understanding. For example, satisfactory and permanent correction of a crowded incisor may not be possible without also correcting a mild and otherwise tolerable Class II relationship.

Detailed consideration of orthodontic diagnosis is beyond the scope of this book, but it must be considered in sufficient depth to at least provide a basis for considering the goals of treatment and planning for its successful prosecution.

This chapter is essentially an outline, a brief overview of orthodontic diagnosis and related problems, to provide such a frame of reference for the discussion of therapeutic methods. For treatment purposes, malocclusions can be divided into basic groups, but it must be recognized that these cover broad spectra that can exist either singly or in combination.

ANTEROPOSTERIOR INTERMAXILLARY DISCREPANCIES

Anteroposterior intermaxillary discrepancies are readily identified and often conspicuous, so they often attract a disproportionate amount of attention. Nevertheless, they do provide a useful starting point for the description of a malocclusion.

The Angle classification of malocclusion[19] is still a most workable basis for the gross identification of anteroposterior intermaxillary discrepancies, dividing them into the following four groups based on first molar relationships:

Class I: Normal mesiodistal relationship with the mesiobuccal cusp of each upper first molar seated at or slightly distal to the buccal groove of the lower first molar

Class II, Division 1 (II_1): Maxillary teeth mesial or mandibular teeth distal as determined by first molar relationship, with comparable incisor displacement

Class II, Division 2 (II_2): Same molar relationship as Division 1 without labial displacement of upper central incisors.

Class III: Mandibular teeth mesial or maxillary teeth distal as determined by first molar relationship

Unilateral Class II or Class III: Unilateral Class II or Class III relationships are identified as *subdivisions* of those classes.

Discrepancies in the vertical dimension, arch form, buccolingual relationships, space, and individual tooth position are not described in this classification. These and many other deviations may occur in combination with any class of malocclusion. Nor does the Angle classification consider the skeletal support of the dentition, which may or may not present malrelationships comparable to those of the teeth.

Arch form disharmonies disrupt occlusal relationships, most commonly in the form of crossbite. This is an occlusal relationship in which one or more upper teeth occlude lingual to the lower antagonists. Lower teeth may also occlude completely lingual to the upper arch, taking them out of occlusion in normal jaw positions; and on rare occasions the opposite problem may be present.

Excessive overbite (deep bite) and inadequate overbite (open bite) relationships may also occur in combination with any class of malocclusion as well as in an otherwise normal dentition. These are usually related to functional problems, which can often be a major consideration in therapy.

ANTEROPOSTERIOR CORRECTIONS

Intermaxillary disparities present an extensive variety of problems, both in diagnosis and in treatment. Root movements can be especially deceiving in the absence of comparable crown movement.

"Reciprocal anchorage," "stationary anchorage," and similar terms are actually descriptions of objectives, not precise descriptions of resultant tooth movements. All anchorage is reciprocal, with variations in actual movement depending on a multitude of factors that require continual monitoring.

The most common classes of these tooth movements that can affect intermaxillary relationships are shown in Fig. 12-1. These are the clinical expressions of the tissue responses discussed in Chapter 11. Possible combinations are almost endless, especially when different timings, force levels, and functional factors enter the picture.

There are actually few alternatives for correcting intermaxillary relationships, but the finesse with which they are selected and combined can make a tremendous difference in results. This is an area filled with claims and counterclaims for different methods, offering great things in many different packages. Differences do most certainly exist, but they fall within the same basic framework regardless of the form, material, or name of devices used.

Anchorage

In orthodontic language *anchorage* refers to the resistance of a tooth or teeth to orthodontic movement, and unless otherwise indicated it refers specifically to resistance to mesial movement. As in its nautical usage, anchorage resistance is not absolute; the anchor may drag. One apparent orthodontic exception is extraoral anchorage (p. 280), which provides a base from which to activate distal tooth movement with no reactive mesial force on other teeth.

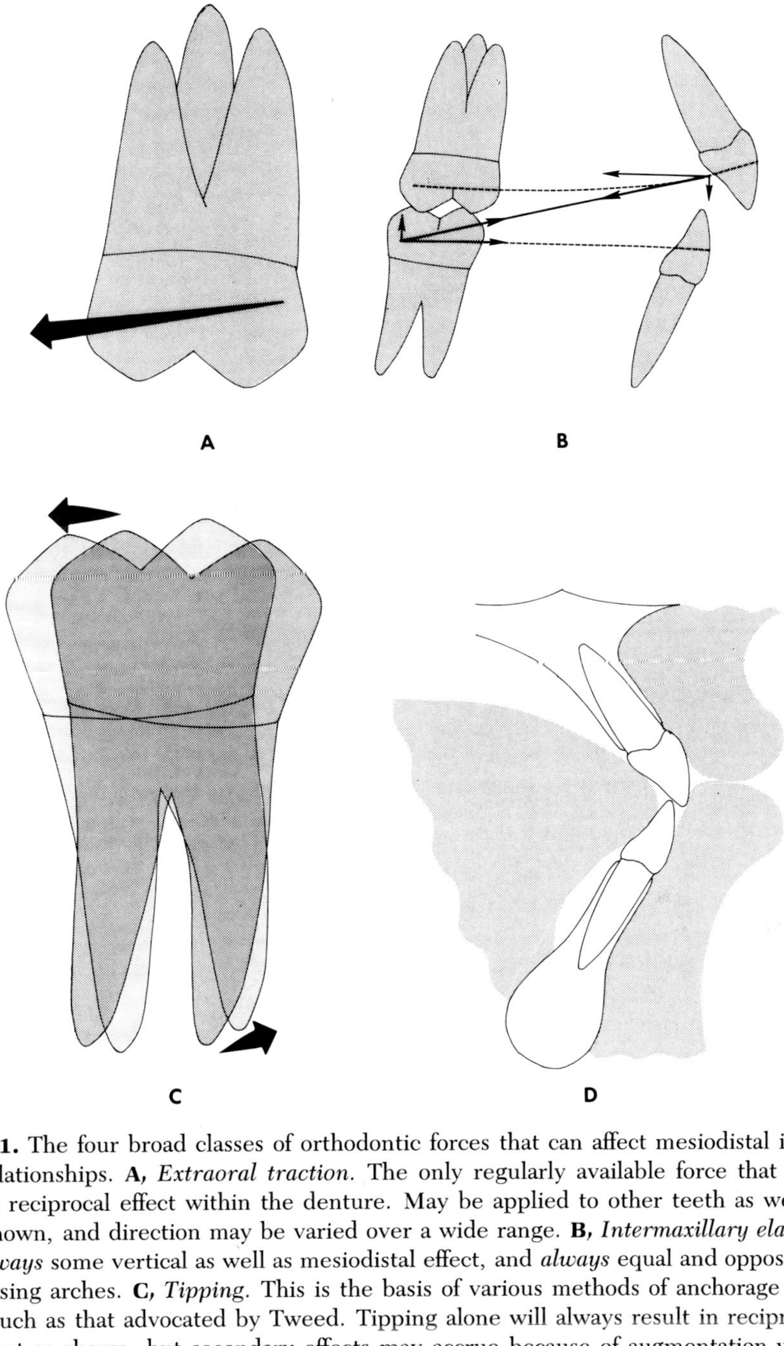

Fig. 12-1. The four broad classes of orthodontic forces that can affect mesiodistal intermaxillary relationships. **A,** *Extraoral traction.* The only regularly available force that does not exert its reciprocal effect within the denture. May be applied to other teeth as well as the molar shown, and direction may be varied over a wide range. **B,** *Intermaxillary elastic traction. Always* some vertical as well as mesiodistal effect, and *always* equal and opposite forces on opposing arches. **C,** *Tipping.* This is the basis of various methods of anchorage augmentation, such as that advocated by Tweed. Tipping alone will always result in reciprocal root movement as shown, but secondary effects may accrue because of augmentation with elastics, elevation such as shown with the tipping molar, and relationships to the functional stroke of the mandible as shown in Fig. 21-1. **D,** *Musculature* can affect mesiodistal movements, often in a negative way. This may sometimes be used to advantage, but most such attempts entail diversion of these forces such as removing lip force from incisors as it is applied to posterior teeth. In such a case there will often be "favorable" incisor changes that will later relapse when the appliance is discontinued and labial forces return to their original pattern.

Anchorage is a factor in most tooth movements, but its most important effects are those that influence intermaxillary relationships. This is true even in movements such as space closure in one arch, where anchorage management can greatly influence relationships of the affected teeth with the opposing arch.

Paradoxes appear to be the rule in this area, most of them resolving into problems in semantics. All claims to the contrary notwithstanding, *a tooth subjected to orthodontic force will move in response to that force.* This is not to say that such movement cannot be controlled, augmented, or retarded, but we must never lose sight of the fact that there will be movement. Most cases of supposed lack of reciprocal movement are merely failures to recognize and identify that movement.

Overbite and arch leveling

Intermaxillary discrepancies may be vertical as well as horizontal, and the two can interact in often inscrutable ways. Such interactions can lead to some of the most vexing of orthodontic problems.

Teeth will normally erupt until they contact an occlusal antagonist in the opposite arch or *some other obstruction.* That other obstruction may be the lower lip, which helps to maintain upper incisors in a normal overbite relationship. It may also be a displaced or malfunctioning lower lip, tongue, or cheek or some external object like a thumb, which can cause and perpetuate a wide variety of abnormal overbite relationships.

Normal resting position of the tongue is within the upper arch, lightly contacting the lingual surfaces of the buccal teeth but not touching the upper incisors. The tip or inferior surface may touch the lingual surfaces of the lower incisors.

If the tongue rests between the incisors, an anterior open bite will result. If it rests over the occlusal surfaces of the buccal teeth, a posterior open bite will result. A posterior open bite in the absence of a comparable anterior condition can be manifested as an extreme incisor overbite on closure, often with accompanying trauma to the palatal tissues. Active tongue thrust may also cause such conditions.

In some individuals, the correction of the malocclusion can lead to a readaptation of the tongue with restoration of normal function. Without this readaptation, posttreatment relapse is likely. Tongue training, while it may be helpful, appears to be of limited value in many of these cases because of the round-the-clock actions and their well-established neural basis.

Mechanical correction of overbite with a fully engaged orthodontic archwire is commonly accomplished by altering the curve of Spee to produce a combination of slight apical movement of the lower incisors with occlusal movement in the bicuspid areas. In this procedure an overbite may be rapidly eliminated, and the lower arch will give the superficial impression that the incisors have been intruded. Actually, these rapid changes are due mostly to the extrusion of buccal teeth.

The mandible at this stage is held open from its original closed-bite position, and normally the muscles of mastication will place increased intrusive forces on all teeth in occlusal function. This can rapidly return the overbite to its original level if positive preventive measures are not applied. For this reason these movements are also among those that should be carried out early in treatment and maintained for a long period of time.

Prolonged retention of such leveling action allows the gradual intrusion of the entire dentition as the mandible returns to its normal closed-bite relationship with the skull. Growth during this readjustment period is a tremendous aid in attaining a more rapid and stable result. Relapse of overbite is still possible if the original functional imbalance has not been eliminated, but controlling the teeth during the return of the mandible to its orginal position prevents new relapse tendencies from being built into the treated occlusion.

Some cases, especially those with steep mandibular planes and weak masticatory musculature, may not return to the original mandibular posture as just described. These facial types can least afford such an opening of the mandible because of the esthetic and functional changes associated with downward and posterior rotation of the chin. Careful differential diagnosis is required in selecting a treatment plan for bite opening in such cases to avoid these undesirable changes. Selective apical movements with interrupted arches and vertical extraoral traction are two very useful approaches under these conditions.

The leveling of the lower arch may also be accompanied by a *tipping depression* of the lower incisors, which may give the outward appearance of actual apical movement. Placing an apical force on the lower incisors without a concurrent retrusive action will cause them to tip downward and forward (Fig. 12-2). Even a force directed straight down from the occlusal plane will have this effect, because of the angulation of the incisor and the labial location of the attachment. These movements produce a depression of the edges of the teeth without actual apical movement of the root.

Flaring the incisors forward in this combination of tipping and depression will level the lower arch, but it will do so at the cost of placing the incisors in a much less desirable relationship to the alveolar process. The gingival ends of the roots are displaced labially, reducing the amount of overlying bone and subjecting the gingival tissues to increased labial pressure. Eruptive potential that could increase overbite is oriented more directly toward the lingual surface of the upper incisor, and a tipped tooth is at an increased mechanical disadvantage in its functional re-

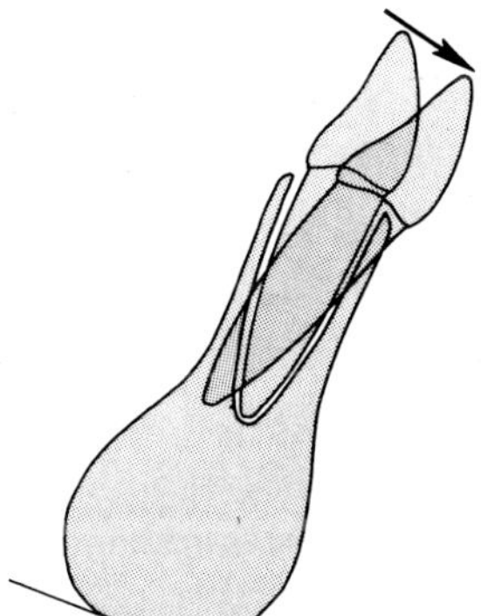

Fig. 12-2. A downward force on lower incisors will tip these teeth forward as the crowns are depressed, but the apex of the root may not be moved downward.

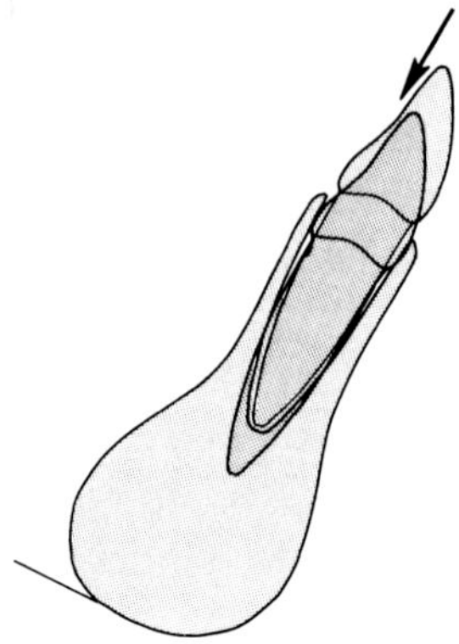

Fig. 12-3. True apical movement of lower incisors is actually downward *and* lingual.

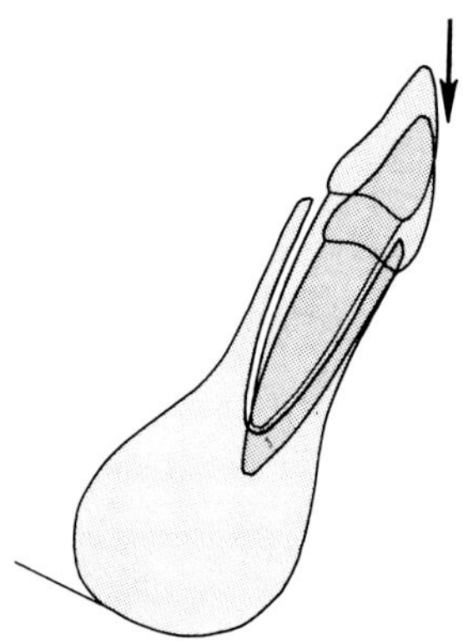

Fig. 12-4. A lower incisor moved downward without change in arch length must undergo translatory labial movement as well as apical movement.

lationship to the upper teeth. This is usually undesirable even though the increased mechanical disadvantage may help to maintain the overbite reduction through the inability of the overloaded periodontal tissues to sustain the tooth in the face of occlusal forces.

In most cases true apical movement of the lower incisors requires a downward *and lingual* force application because of the inclination of the roots of these teeth. This will place the lower incisors in their optimum position in the mandible, but it is much more difficult to accomplish and requires additional arch length because of the lingual repositioning of the incisal edges (Fig. 12-3). Such a force can be applied by a properly adjusted round wire or by a rectangular wire with suitable torqueing adjustments.

A third possibility, translatory anterior movement combined with the apical movement, is a desirable alternative in cases in which some forward movement of the lower teeth is required (Fig. 12-4). This requires a rectangular wire.

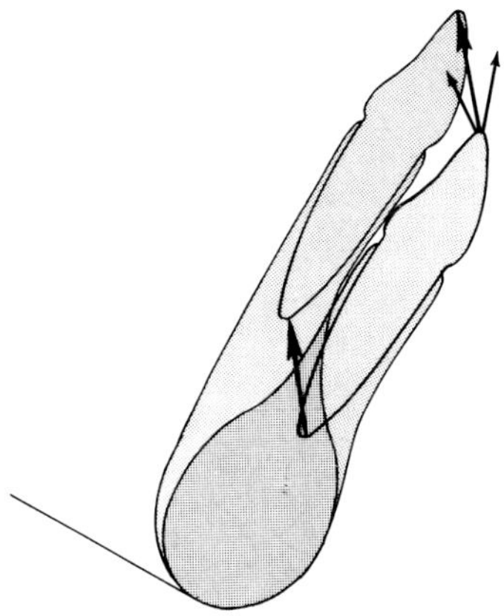

Fig. 12-5. Normal growth pattern in the lower incisor area. Incisors move essentially in a vertical and somewhat lingual direction with little change in axial inclination. The net result is lingual movement in relation to the symphysis.

The only remaining possibility is growth, which can make it possible to level the lower arch without any anterior depression by adding to the vertical height of the face while the lower anterior teeth are held in position. Even in this case, arch length can still be a critical factor and the mechanics must involve some combination of the preceding approaches. Only a careful analysis of all aspects of the problem will provide an adequate basis for action.

Cephalometric evidence, implant studies by Björk,[23] and the work of Enlow[24] indicate an upward *and lingual* migration of the lower dentition on the mandible with growth, as shown in Fig. 12-5. This too can place additional demands on lower arch length.

CROWDING

The disturbances of arch form brought about by crowding are some of the most conspicuous of orthodontic deformities, especially in the anterior region. These space deficiencies may cause a wide variety of rotation and overlapping of adjacent teeth, which in turn may result in a localized crossbite relationship with the opposing arch.

Relief of a crowded condition requires some form of space adjustment, and only two possible courses are available:

1. The arch may be expanded to accommodate the teeth.
2. Teeth may be removed to provide the needed space.

Expansion presents an attractive solution, if for no other reason than that it averts the need for the difficult decision to remove permanent teeth. But this reasoning ignores the fact that the negative decision may prove to be just as problem-laden and irreversible as a decision to extract.

The obvious advantages of nonextraction are that it eliminates all the sequelae of extraction plus the traumatic surgical procedure itself. There is no question that this is the method of choice in cases in which the supporting and surrounding

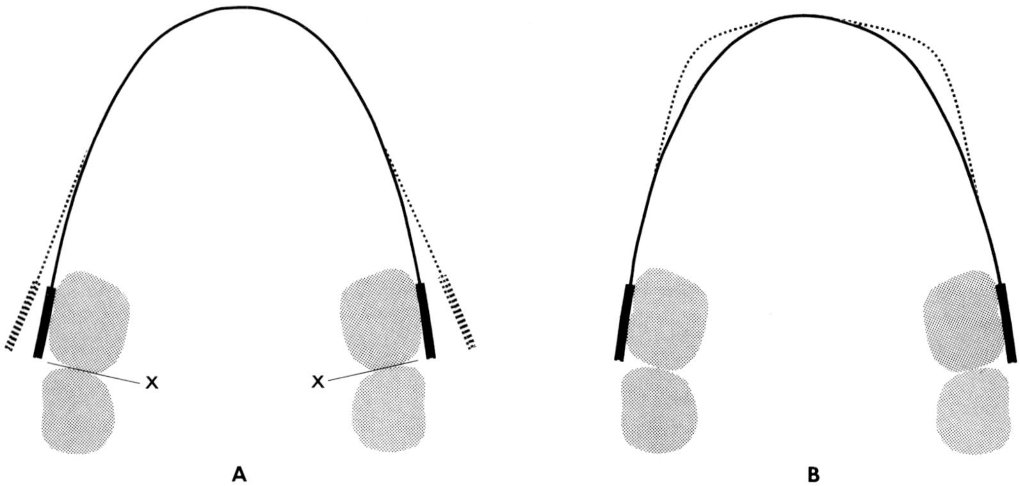

Fig. 12-6. A, Expansion in the molar area offers little increase in arch length. The angulation of the molar contact areas, *x* and *x*, adds to this problem by deflecting the expanding molars in a mesial direction; even unerupted molars lie in this relationship to the roots of the preceding teeth. **B,** Cuspid expansion will increase arch length, but not without risk (see text).

structures can adapt to the necessary changes. The problem is to recognize such cases before treatment.

Extraoral anchorage and other techniques for distal movement of buccal segments without reciprocal mesial movement of other teeth can be a great aid in the nonextraction treatment of truly marginal cases, provided that their other effects are compatible with the total treatment objective.

Effective increase in arch length through expansion requires that a significant part of the expansion be carried out in the anterior part of the arch, which presents a strong possibility of relapse to its original form. Posttreatment studies have repeatedly shown this to be the tendency in a majority of cases.[20-22] Molar expansion is of limited value for this purpose (Fig. 12-6), especially in nongrowing patients, so expansion requires exceptional care in diagnosis, treatment, and retention.

A special warning against expansion in the extraction case is also in order. Teeth are usually removed to obviate the need for excessive expansion of the arch, but *extraction does not prevent expansion or its sequelae.* If extraction is followed by expansion, as in the flattening of the incisor segment with widening at the cuspids, it is entirely possible to produce a result that combines many of the disadvantages of both extraction and nonextraction therapy.

Some techniques may reduce the demands on anchorage by the expedient of tipping cuspids laterally instead of moving them distally along the line of the arch. Such a course solves one problem at the cost of introducing another, and the consequences may be either later demands on anchorage, increased relapse tendency, or unphysiologic tooth positions.

Extraction has the obvious advantage of providing a measurable amount of space for the rearrangement of the remaining teeth within the original arch form. Obtaining space with minimum change in arch form can be a major contributor to long-term periodontal health while also making it possible to avoid distortion of the labial musculature and profile by increased dental protrusion.

Extraction can present problems of a different nature. Maintenance of symmetry requires that most therapeutic extractions be carried out bilaterally, even when this provides more space than may otherwise be needed or desired. Asymmetrical crowding is frequently related to a shift of anterior teeth toward the crowded side, and this will be aggravated even further by unilateral extraction and subsequent space closure on the affected side.

Excess space derived from extraction can sometimes present difficult closure problems. This is especially true in a lower arch that requires considerable mesial molar movement, and in those patients with tooth size discrepancies or overbite problems. Space closure requires careful control over the inclinations of all affected teeth, especially incisors and those adjacent to the spaces. Excessive lingual tipping of incisors with space closure can produce an "extracted look" as undesirable as the "protrusive look" of injudicious nonextraction.

All of these problems must be considered in the initial extraction decision and, just as important, in planning the exact treatment procedures that are to follow. The mere fact of extraction should not automatically establish all succeeding procedures.

Extraction is the most obvious of treatment procedures. Even years after all treatment has been completed, only a casual count of the teeth is required to establish the fact of therapeutic extraction. There may be no other way of even detecting past orthodontic treatment, much less knowing what appliances were used or how they were used. It is even more difficult to determine pretreatment or posttreatment problems unrelated to the orthodontic therapy, but the tendency all too often is to attribute all findings (good or bad) to the extractions or the lack thereof.

Extraction is only one small part of treatment. The decision on extraction will not treat the patient, but it will have a tremendous effect on the course of all of the treatment procedures that follow. This makes it a basic decision that must be resolved before any further plans can be established.

It is fortunate that this is no longer the highly charged subject that it was a few years ago. Nevertheless, it is still one of the most difficult decisions faced by the orthodontist, and it is still obscured by many objective and subjective smoke screens ranging from impersonal statistics to highly personal emotions. Prejudice is not an adequate justification for following a particular course of action, and neither is some combination of measurements, no matter how "scientific" they appear. Even with the most sophisticated aids available, this decision must ultimately depend on carefully considered professional judgment.

SPACING

Spacing of teeth can be just as great an esthetic and functional handicap as crowding.

The key factor in space closure is the *total* space in the arch. Closing and maintaining a small space in an otherwise intact arch presents few problems compared to those in the arch with generalized spacing.

Space closure presents two histological problems that can be especially important in retention:

1. The spaced teeth are separated by excessive soft tissue that will behave elastically for an extended period of time after being compressed in closure. This redundancy is most marked in the labial frenum, which is largely made up of dense fibrous tissue, but it is present to some degree in all spaces.
2. Transseptal fibers that normally maintain contact integrity by literally tying the teeth together with elastic fibers are either absent or rendered ineffective by the negative tension induced by space closure.

The combined effect of those two conditions is a strong tendency for orthodontically closed spaces to partially reopen for a long time after treatment.

Measures for controlling this problem include the following:

1. Surgical excision of redundant tissue
2. In extraction cases, removing teeth where possible *before* adjacent teeth erupt so that they will erupt with minimum intervening tissue and more normal interdental tissue (extractions after eruption leave *two* interdental papillae plus healed gingival tissue at the extraction site)
3. Planning treatment for early closure so that adaptation of proximal tissues begins as soon as possible
4. Treating to secure occlusal and proximal relationships that will favor maintenance of the space closure by hindering any tendency of the teeth to drift apart.

The last of these measures is the most important of all, and often the only one available to the orthodontist. Excision of redundant tissue will not restore transsep-

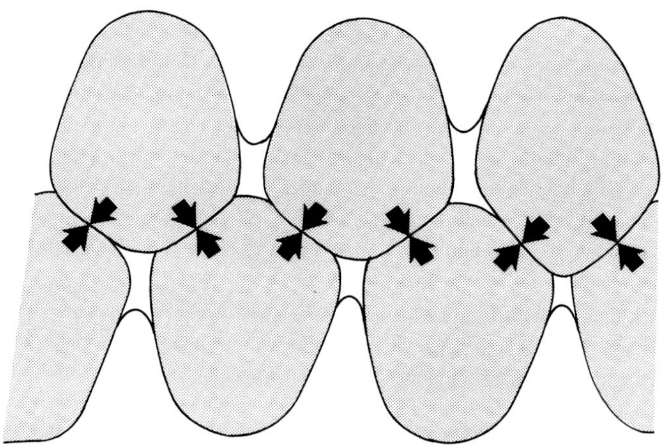

Fig. 12-7. Spaces in the bicuspid region are often maintained by the wedging action of opposing teeth. This presents an increasing problem with larger spaces because of the need to intrude opposing teeth to effect space closure.

tal fibers, and scheduling of extractions or other treatment measures must be based on many considerations in addition to this one.

Special care must be taken to close nearby spaces in the course of any space closure. Residual spaces in the arch present a possibility for relapse in direct proportion to their proximity to the original space.

Occlusal forces from the opposing arch may resist space closure in any part of the arch. In the incisor segment, occlusion can keep upper teeth from moving far enough lingually to close spaces, especially when discrepancies in tooth size exist. In bicuspid areas, the action of an opposing tooth wedging into a space can have a powerful effect, requiring bite opening or intrusion of these teeth for successful closure (Fig. 12-7).

Most (but not all) spaces larger than 1 or 2 mm should be closed with a fixed appliance to control axial inclinations, but finishing frequently requires a removable appliance. With multiple spaces the elastic positioner, augmented with extraoral traction where not contraindicated, is excellent for this purpose, but simpler appliances are more suitable for single spaces. These are discussed in more detail in Chapter 20, "Coordinating treatment procedures," and Chapter 21, "Finishing or 'retention.' "

SPEED OF TREATMENT

Time is always a factor in any orthodontic correction. How fast can or should teeth be moved? Speed has great attraction for several reasons, not the least of which is patient satisfaction. The caries hazard can also be reduced by a short treatment time, but this is related more to the time with fixed attachments on individual teeth than to overall elapsed time.

Rapid treatment is not new. The four cases shown by Angle[31] in his original presentation of the edgewise appliance were completed in less than eleven, five, and eight months, respectively. Those are certainly minimal treatment times even today. It should not be unusual for some cases to require two years or more for completion of the active phase of treatment.

Speed in treatment is a legitimate goal, and it will receive considerable attention in later chapters; but it must be kept in perspective. One problem in discussing speed lies in relating it to the overall treatment situation. Rapid movement and short treatment time are not necessarily synonymous. Initial movements can and should be accomplished rapidly, but this is often the point where the real work begins. Careful finishing into a good occlusion can take time, and rapid initial movements with unwanted secondary effects can have a net negative effect.

Nor are elapsed treatment time and total chair time always proportional. Finishing a case requires certain clinical movements, and a shorter treatment time may require more intensive effort at the chair, telescoping the total expenditure of time and effort into a shorter period.

Physiological considerations also influence the time factor. Some movements such as anterior alignment can and should be accomplished in a matter of weeks. At the other extreme, extraoral therapy aimed at the orthopedic modification of overall maxillomandibular relationships is most effective when it is acting concurrently with growth. Sufficient growth seldom occurs in one year or even two, so unless treatment coincides perfectly with a very active growth period, this type of therapy must operate over an extended period of time for optimum results.

ESTHETICS

Esthetics is an important consideration for many patients, but it cannot be isolated from other treatment effects.

Physical appearance is often a major incentive for seeking orthodontic help, and the correction of disfiguring deformities can be one of the most important services provided by the orthodontist. Orthodontics is basically a health service, and its contributions to mental health and personal effectiveness in the socioeconomic environment can sometimes far outweigh any local benefits ensuing from occlusal relationships. Few will disagree on this point, but the widely divergent means of defining and attaining subjective goals such as esthetic improvement can lead to many different clinical approaches.

Esthetic needs and benefits must be evaluated with due consideration for the patient's total health and well-being. Obvious deformities may cry out for correction, but excessive preoccupation with a minor dental irregularity may be a symptom, rather than a cause of other emotional problems. Correcting such a defect can leave the patient still unsatisfied and perhaps more disturbed than before because the underlying nonorthodontic problem goes on unabated.

While the patient's wants cannot be ignored, they should be tempered by sufficient knowledge to recognize how the best long-term satisfaction can be attained. Nor should professional criteria be ignored, with appropriate recognition of their proper place as one part of the total picture.

If *all* criteria are considered, we will not lose sight of the fact that *the look of beauty is the look of health,* and to be truly beautiful *for a lifetime, if possible,* teeth must be placed in a sound, healthy relationship to one another and to their supporting tissues. Sacrificing dental function or health for a transitory esthetic gain can lead to the premature loss of all three.

DIAGNOSIS

Planning orthodontic correction, even in "simple" cases, requires a careful evaluation of the dentition and its total functional environment. Any orthodontic intervention will have lasting effects on dentofacial relationships, and the total mechanism is too thoroughly integrated for casual interference.

Minimum diagnostic records for most problems consist of accurate plaster casts of the dentition, cephalometric radiographs and panoramic or intraoral radiographs as may be required. Facial and dental photographs are also very useful. These records together with observations from direct examination and an adequate history provide the basis for consideration of the immediate problem and a projection of anticipated future conditions with and without all possible courses of treatment.

As noted earlier, the personal preferences or prejudices of the orthodontist are not an adequate justification for following a particular course of action; *neither is some combination of measurements,* no matter how "scientific" they may appear. Masking our prejudices or replacing our minds with the trappings of science is not enough.

Cephalometric evaluations are an invaluable starting point in orthodontic diagnosis. They indicate where the patient's problems and general skeletal configuration fit into the overall range of humanity as a whole, giving meaningful direction to the clinical evaluation. Computer techniques have now been adapted to facilitate this task of orientation to the general population and when judiciously used as a supplement (not a substitute) for professional evaluation they can be very helpful.[25,26]

This orientation, by whatever means, merely sets the stage for the final steps in diagnosis that still must be subjective. As the techniques of evaluation progress they continue to add to our knowledge of orthodontics and of the individual, but even the most sophisticated are still nothing more than *descriptive techniques* that should in no way be confused with decision-making techniques. Description forms an important basis for decision, but the ultimate decision must still be a function of the clinical judgment of the orthodontist. It is the skilled human mind that must provide the final analog integration and output stage of the analysis, and the real contribution of any mechanical preliminary analysis lies in freeing the mind from becoming bogged down in the minutiae of the preliminary routine information-gathering stages so that is can concentrate on the vital final phase.

Beginning with a cephalometric evaluation, we must then consider *why* we found the cephalometric measurements as we did. We must go back to the radiographs, photographs, and dental casts and look again at the actual flesh and bones that make up the dentofacial complex.

We must look at the size and form of the alveolar processes (Figs. 12-8 and 12-9) on which all orthodontics depends. Is the mandibular symphysis thin or thick? Are the upper central incisors located in a central position in the alveolar process, or are they situated near or at the labial surface? These relationships are often reflected indirectly in cephalometric measurements, but that is a roundabout and less reliable approach to information that is more clearly seen directly on the radiographs.

Direct inspection of the investing tissues in the mouth and on casts and photo-

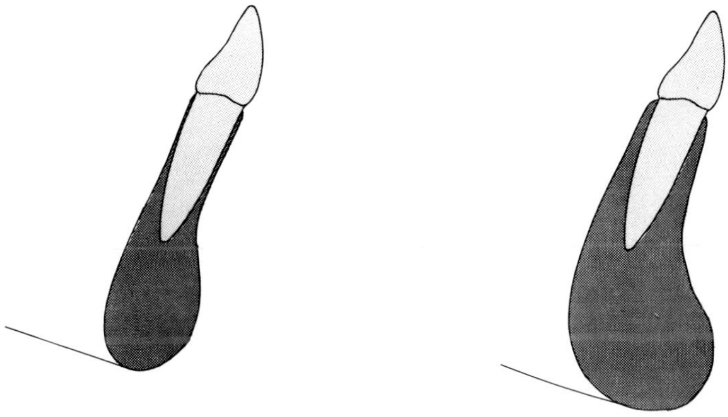

Fig. 12-8. Alveolar process may be either thin or thick, presenting considerable differences in root support and periodontal nutrition.

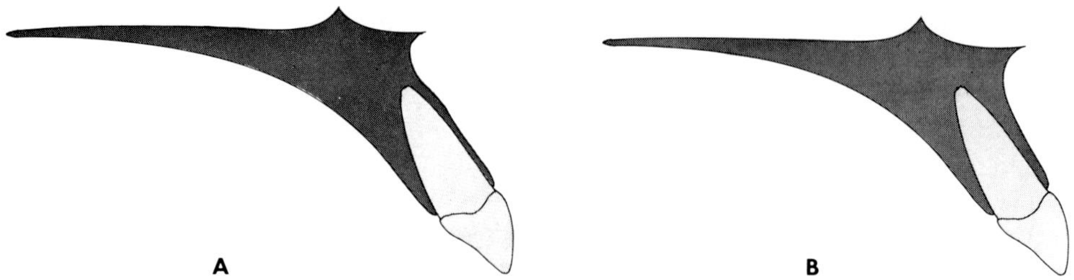

Fig. 12-9. Relationships of incisors to the alveolar process are not fully described by angulation, which is the same in the two cases shown. Linear measurements and relationships of cephalometric points describe these differences more fully, but the actual picture of roots and bone as seen above provides the most reliable and sometimes critical information.

graphs will also give clues to their general state of health as well as the abundance of circulatory nutrition.

The tongue, lips, and cheeks also make vital contributions to present and future dental relationships. These should also be evaluated both in the lateral radiograph and by direct clinical examination.

The important point is *not* which cephalometric or other analytical procedure is used or its level of sophistication or automation. It is whether or not these aids are applied with understanding. The routine formal analysis delineates and describes the problem to a point; then it is up to the clinician to complete the evaluation and develop a workable plan for correction. Mere blind treatment of a number, by the numbers, or for the numbers is as unfair to the patient as it is unworthy of a professional person.

DENTOFACIAL ORTHOPEDIC RESPONSIBILITY

Most other dental procedures do not upset the original balance of the denture as the dentofacial orthopedic changes of orthodontics do, so they are usually planned and executed on the assumption that the denture and its interrelationships are static. When a dental procedure does alter the original balance, whether it is orthodontic therapy, an occlusal adjustment, or a restoration that changes contact or occlusal relationships, the dentist initiates certain ongoing changes. No such procedure can be considered successful or complete until the teeth have had time to adjust to their changed environment and reach a new balanced relationship.

It is certainly true that no professional can be responsible for all of the changes that follow treatment. The mere act of placing an appliance or a restoration must cause minor changes in tooth relationships as an integral part of such treatment, and many additional changes take place as a result of the patient's conduct and the continual changes that are a part of life. In orthodontics the patient is not anesthetized or immobilized during treatment. Daily routines go on almost unchanged, using and abusing teeth and appliances alike in many ways. The patient must take proper care of the appliances, maintain good oral hygiene, and follow instructions for wearing removable auxiliary devices. And added to all of this are the predictable and unpredictable effects of growth.

All of these factors are out of the orthodontist's control throughout treatment, and to the extent that they are beyond professional control, they are beyond professional responsibility. On the other hand, many basic factors in diagnosis and treatment planning are under the orthodontist's control, and for these there is a responsibility both during and for some time after treatment. Removal of the appliance cannot mark the end of that responsibility, and arrangments for treatment should take this into account. Posttreatment changes, to the extent that they have been influenced by the appliances, are just as much a part of therapy as if the appliances were still on the teeth.

In the case of dentofacial orthopedics, the extent of professional responsibility is further complicated by growth and development. The occlusion is an especially changing mechanism through the entire period of growth, and the orthodontist must continually keep this in mind. A patient who seeks orthodontic care places *all* dentofacial orthopedic problems in the professional's hands, not just those that are immediately apparent or that may require the installation of a certain appliance.

The period of active appliance therapy is only one phase in a patient's developing occlusal problem, and we must take care not to ignore the pretreatment and posttreatment periods, which may be equally important. Many patients, especially those with intermaxillary malrelationships, will show continuing changes long after growth stops, requiring periodic supervision at least until sometime after the third molars are either "in" or "out". An unfortunate aspect of the mobility of today's population is that these changes are so unique and our service so personal that it is difficult if not impossible for any orthodontist other than the one who originally rendered the service to bring equal insight and familiarity to bear on later changes. Follow-up care can be provided with a high level of knowledge and skill, but can be seriously limited by the lack of long-term personal observation.

LIFELONG CHANGE

Continuing change of a usually minor nature is to be expected as a normal part of maturation and aging. Life is change. Teeth retain their responsiveness to environmental forces throughout life, maintaining a balanced condition through all of the changes wrought by wear and tear and alterations in facial muscle function.

Such changes are seldom related to treatment, even though they may obviously affect teeth that were previously moved. Orthodontic therapy offers valuable developmental guidance and recovery from nature's mistakes, but it cannot confer unnatural stability because the dentition is by its very nature a dynamic changing mechanism that will continue to adapt to functional and environmental influences as long as a person lives. Our responsibility is to place teeth in balanced relationships that will optimize those later ongoing natural adjustments as much as possible.

PART III

Clinical procedures

■ Clinical correction of dentofacial orthopedic deformities with an orthodontic appliance requires practical application of the principles presented in Parts I and II.

Fixed appliances capable of three-axis control offer a wide latitude for variations in design details, as is attested by the plethora of components on the market. Each has its own minor differences from the others, but all function in essentially the same way and all must be used with an understanding of the underlying mechanics.

The clinical principles that follow apply to any appliance with comparable control capabilities regardless of its heritage. Specific procedures are shown to illustrate specific points, not as specific recommendations. The objective is to provide a basis for informed judgment without promoting any specific appliance or therapeutic approach.

Orthodontics has long been overblessed with personal cults and cure-all therapies, and they continue to proliferate. The following material is intended to provide a basis for evaluating and using available options without adding yet another.

13

There are exceptions to every rule, including this one.

Orthodontic appliance selection

Moving teeth is one of the most easily accomplished procedures in all of dentistry. Even a child can do it with no outside instructions whatever and with no equipment other than a thumb. Any pressure, from a few grams to several pounds from any source, is capable of causing teeth to move and even to alter the underlying supporting structures.

Moving teeth well—directing them into healthful, esthetic, and functionally stable positions with a minimum of discomfort or other undesirable effects—is one of the most difficult and exacting procedures in all of dentistry. Those who have devoted their lives to the problem find new challenges around every corner, with the ultimate panacea always seeming to move farther out of reach.

The facts behind the preceding two paragraphs have been responsible for nearly a century of confusion and misunderstanding, with all the problems and unpleasantness that such conditions can evoke. The confusion continues unabated; only the names have changed. Some orthodontic appliances look so complex that it appears that some form of sorcery must be required to make them work, so finding that teeth can actually be moved with ease is a heady draft indeed. Add to this a few broad claims of "new, quick, and easy" methods and devices, and we have the beginnings of a new cycle of confusion and frustration.

The exhilaration of finding that teeth are so easy to move is something like the first experience in applying a bur to a tooth. All that was necessary was to hold the bur against the tooth and guide it. Nothing could have been simpler. The entire field of restorative dentistry dissolved into the simple process of steering a bur.

The apparent simplicity gave no hint of the many problems and pitfalls that are a regular part of accumulating experience with dental procedures. Orthodontics is no exception, but it has the added problem of a very insidious time lag. It does not take long to find out whether or not a bridge is going to fit, but the dentofacial orthopedic correction of an orthodontic problem can go on for years to an apparently successful conclusion, only to collapse later because of factors not recognized or anticipated in the original diagnosis.

The really difficult problems in orthodontics lie not in making teeth move, but in making them move to the right places. This means, first, knowing the right places, where the teeth will be healthy and stable. It also means moving the teeth to these places without simultaneously moving other teeth into less desirable positions. In addition, all of this *must* be accomplished with reasonable comfort for the patient and with minimum risk for the teeth and supporting tissues.

The evolution of orthodontic therapy is essentially a story of increasing diagnostic understanding combined with improved control over tooth movements. The earliest appliances depended on simple tipping as teeth were nudged into more acceptable positions. Successive developments brought control over vertical movement and rotation around the various axes. Rotations around the long axis, mesiodistal tipping, and labiolingual tipping have all come under orthodontic control.

These increases in the range of feasible movements made it possible to raise diagnostic sights toward increased benefits and in turn opened the way to even more therapeutic techniques. An important case in point is extraction, a powerful therapeutic tool that can prove disastrous without adequate control over tooth levels and tipping.

The edgewise appliance was the first to offer complete three-axis control, opening the door to modern orthodontics. By providing at least the theoretical feasibility of any conceivable tooth movement the edgewise appliance set the stage for the present phase of technical refinement.

Emphasis gradually shifted from feasibility to facility, a search that is responsible for today's plethora of orthodontic gadgetry. These are all variations on a few basic themes, each offering some unique combination of advantages and disadvantages that vary with the patient, the problem, and the orthodontist.

An insidious factor that moves through this picture almost unseen at times is the many reciprocal and collateral effects. An attachment capable of moving a tooth in a given direction is only part of the picture. Much of the continuing advancement in orthodontics revolves around increasingly sophisticated control over the secondary effects that often occur in areas far removed from the primary action site.

This submerged part of the iceberg goes far beyond simple reciprocal movement of nearby teeth. All of the other teeth, mandibular position, lip posture, tongue function, and breathing are some of the other important factors that can be influenced by the movement of even a single tooth.

There is no clear-cut universal superiority in any one appliance because of the many interrelated variables in clinical application. It is only through an understanding of underlying principles that a clinician can evaluate, compare, and selectively apply appropriate mechanical procedures for each patient's problem.

ORTHODONTICS TODAY

Most appliances introduced in the fifty years since the original introduction of the edgewise principle are capable of inducing all types of tooth movements. It would be gross presumption to attempt a detailed comparison of the relative merits of these various methods here, but neither can the present profusion of appliances be ignored.

As noted earlier, modern orthodontics has much more to offer than the mere installation of an appliance. Orthodontic problems cover a broad spectrum, and any dentist who undertakes their treatment must be prepared to do each of the following:

1. Choose the time for the most effective intervention, considering the *total* dentition and face.
2. Choose the most effective appliances for the patient's situation.
3. Anticipate, recognize, and cope with new problems as they arise.

No one appliance, no single age for treatment, and certainly no rote procedure can meet all requirements. The orthodontist of today must work with a varied armamentarium of diagnostic techniques and appliances to provide an optimum of service with the mechanical intervention carefully tailored to individual needs.

The edgewise appliance does not represent minimum mechanical intervention, and this fact alone makes it clear that it cannot be the method of choice in *every* situation. Many cases are better served by a partial or modified application of the edgewise mechanism, sometimes in conjunction with other devices. Still others may be served equally well or even better with a completely different therapeutic approach.

THE COMPLEAT ORTHODONTIST

The selection of an adequate armamentarium is an essential part of every orthodontic practice. There is obviously no need for everyone to be prepared to use every appliance; in fact, any such effort would certainly lead to a dilution of skills. What is needed is a selection of methods with varied potentials, so that all demands of treatment may be met with maximum efficiency and minimum duplication.

The following tabulation includes most of the commonly used devices, going from relatively simple to complex, with brief comments on the applications for each. In comparing these appliances one must not overlook the fact that *mechanical simplicity bears no relation to diagnostic or therapeutic simplicity.* This basic fact can easily deceive those with a restricted viewpoint who may still regard orthodontics as a purely mechanical exercise, when in fact some of the greatest challenges lie in the effective selection and application of seemingly simple therapeutic measures such as the following:

1. Space maintainers and simple removable appliances can guide an *otherwise normal* occlusion into good relationships. Their use for a local problem where other problems may need later attention can be wasteful duplication.
2. Bite plates and guide planes can temporarily remove occlusal interferences. This can make it possible for teeth blocked by such interferences to erupt into better positions, or allow the mandible to regain its normal posture. More elaborate functional appliances can also serve to redirect functional forces and growth patterns as part of an overall treatment program.
3. Extraoral anchorage can correct intermaxillary discrepancies through distal or apical movement of upper (and sometimes lower) teeth, as well as alter relationships of deeper facial structures.

   ADVANTAGES

   a. Early resolution of these problems restores normal lip function before growth is completed, resulting in optimum improvement.
   b. Minimal appliance mechanism is required.
   c. Guidance of upper molars can provide some gain in anterior arch length and improved vertical relationships.

DISADVANTAGES

a. Additional correction is usually required.
b. Space may be inadequate in the upper molar region, limiting the correction that can be achieved without compounding later problems there.
c. The wide variations in individual response to these powerful effects on growth patterns can result in unfavorable as well as favorable effects, making continuous cephalometric monitoring an essential part of this treatment.

4. Nonbanded or minimum-banded appliances can align teeth within the arch and may be used to adjust some intermaxillary relationships with supplementary elastics.

ADVANTAGES

a. Minimum appliance mechanism is required and is most useful where limited control is adequate.
b. Hygiene may be easier.

DISADVANTAGES

a. Lack of a positive attachment provides limited control over individual teeth.
b. Horizontal movements are essentially tipping, so they must be limited to short distances. This can be extremely critical in intermaxillary corrections.
c. Closure of extraction spaces requires more tooth movement than may be safely accomplished by tipping, so extraction should not be considered without the availability of full-control appliance therapy.
d. Treatment of many cases without extraction creates a temptation to use expansion as the alternative. This carries potential risks of relapse and loss of alveolar bone when inappropriately applied.
e. Vertical control is often limited.
f. Removability adds to problems of loss and damage.

5. Multiple-attachment appliances such as Edgewise, Universal, Twin-wire, and "light-wire" provide maximum control over individual teeth. The various appliances in this group differ in mode of operation, but they are generally capable of controlling rotations and tipping in most directions.

ADVANTAGES

a. Full control enables the operator to place most teeth in optimum positions in relation to function and supporting bone.
b. Space closure can be carried out with adequate control over tipping.
c. Roots of anterior teeth can be moved labially or lingually as required.

DISADVANTAGES

a. Reciprocal effects are more complex.
b. Archwires need careful adjustment even in areas requiring no movements.
c. Arch movement is restricted by multiple attachments, requiring many adjustments or selective banding for some situations.
d. Hygiene is complicated by fixed attachments and arches.

The preceding descriptions are simply orientation sketches, representing the general ranges of application. Variations in the appliances and their use can impair or augment these factors in many ways, so the mere presence of a particular appliance tells virtually nothing about the treatment being applied.

TREATMENT TIMING

Appliance selection depends both on the occlusal problem and on the age of the patient or, more specifically, the stage of development. Some problems that may be treated most effectively at one stage with one appliance may require an entirely different approach at another time. We may or may not have a choice in these situations, depending on when the patient first appears for evaluation.

The accompanying charts (Figs. 13-1 to 13-8) are intended to give an overall view of the types of therapy that *might* be considered at different ages for the broad major classes of orthodontic problems listed. These charts are obviously gross generalizations and should be interpreted accordingly. It should also be noted that many patients may present problems appearing on more than one chart (such as a Class II relationship with crowding), which will require judicious integration and coordination of treatment.

Classes of orthodontic problems

ARCH LENGTH	
Space deficiency	Fig. 13 1
Space excess	Fig. 13-2
SKELETAL ABERRATIONS	
Convex profile	Fig. 13-3
Concave profile	Fig. 13-4
Width	Fig. 13-5
OCCLUSAL ABERRATIONS	
Class II	Fig. 13-6
Class III	Fig. 13-7
Crossbites	Fig. 13-8

SPACE CONTROL IN THE MIXED DENTITION

Space deficiencies in the mixed dentition may sometimes be alleviated by intervention at this stage. The overriding consideration here is the provision of maximum service with minimum intervention.

The course of action selected often depends more on coexisting problems than on the obvious space deficiency. It is wasteful and sometimes even counter-productive to carry out an early local corrective program where other problems will require later treatment that could accomplish the same result as a part of the comprehensive therapy.

Serial extraction

Removal of deciduous teeth for the temporary relief of crowding initiates a complex chain of events usually culminating in the removal of permanent teeth and the need for comprehensive orthodontic therapy. Many of these situations also require some form of intermediate space control following the extractions to avoid negative long-term effects.

Text continued on p. 140.

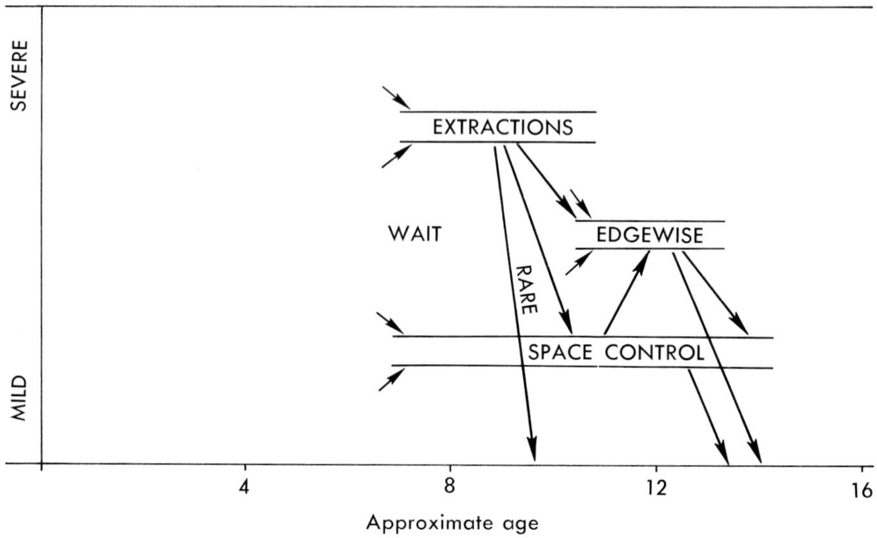

SPACE DEFICIENCY

Fig. 13-1. Space deficiency must be corrected either by extractions or by control of existing space as with space maintainers or extraoral anchorage. The choice depends primarily on the severity of the problem. These measures are usually begun earlier than comprehensive correction with an appliance such as the edgewise. As indicated by the arrows, all of these may require comprehensive (edgewise) therapy for full correction.

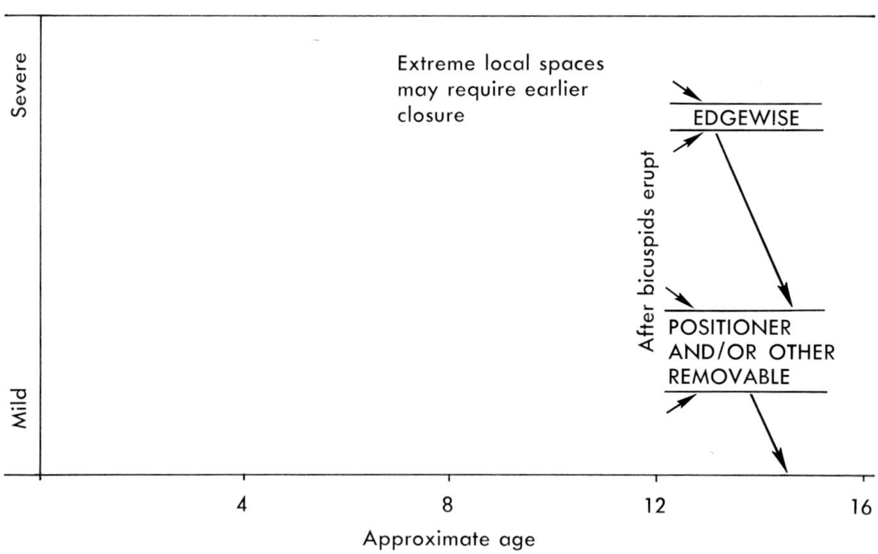

SPACE EXCESS

Fig. 13-2. Excess space can seldom be corrected before the deciduous teeth have been replaced. Severe local problems may be corrected earlier, with due regard for the stage of root development. Small spaces may be closed with removable appliances, but large discrepancies require the control of fixed attachments.

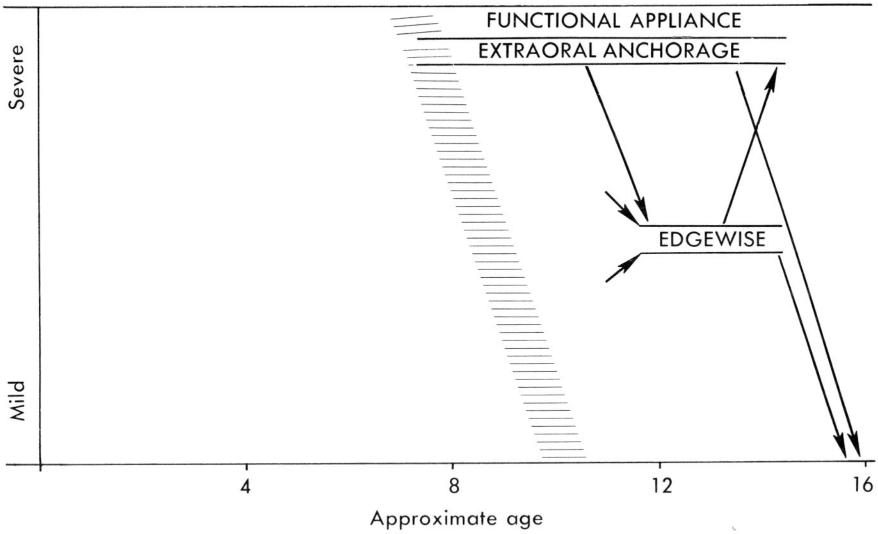

FACIAL CONVEXITY

Fig. 13-3. Facial convexity may be corrected with extraoral anchorage, functional appliance, edgewise, or a combination depending on severity and the time that the patient comes in for treatment. Edgewise therapy in these cases often includes intermaxillary elastic traction or other auxiliary forces.

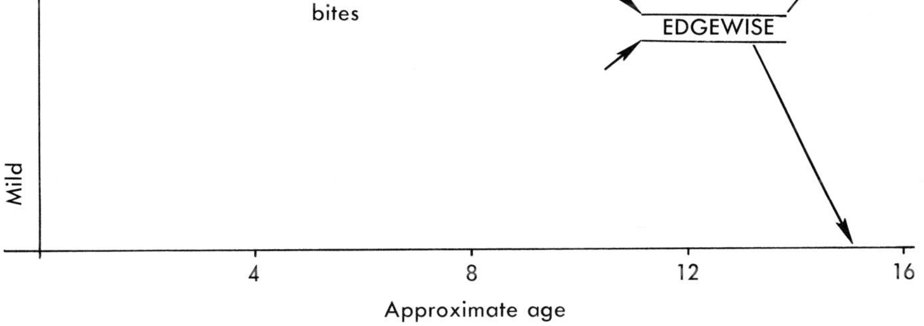

FACIAL CONCAVITY

Fig. 13-4. Class III skeletal relationships cannot be fully corrected until growth is complete, requiring mandibular surgery in extreme cases. Earlier treatment is aimed at minimizing the problem by controlling crossbites. Chin cap traction is of dubious value but may be considered in some cases.

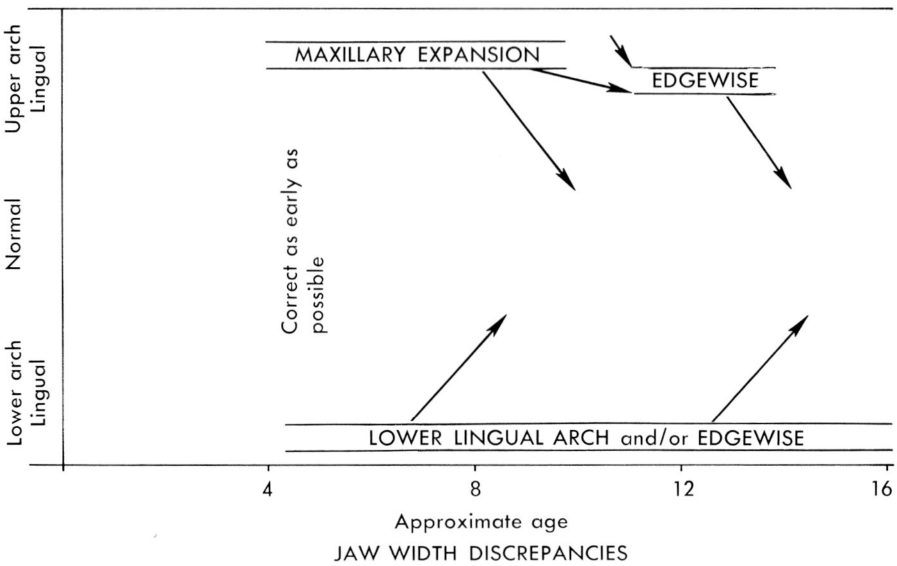

Fig. 13-5. Discrepancies in jaw width (various forms of buccal crossbites) are usually corrected as early as possible because of their potential for creating progressive disruption of the occlusion and growth. Early intervention may be all that is needed, or additional help may be required as the dentition matures.

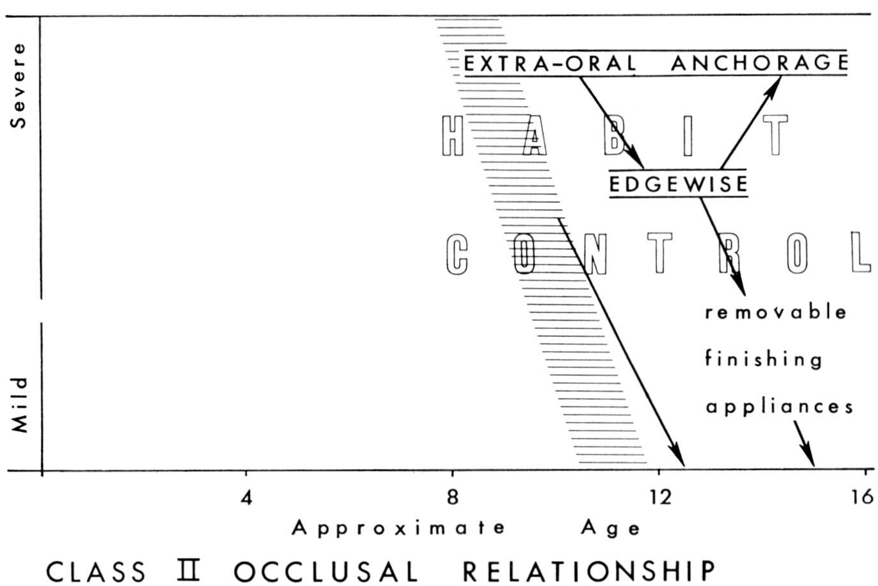

Fig. 13-6. Class II occlusal relationships, in the absence of comparable skeletal discrepancies, may be related to oral habits or space problems. Correction may be initiated early with extraoral anchorage or later with edgewise, with finishing depending on remaining habits or muscular dysfunctions.

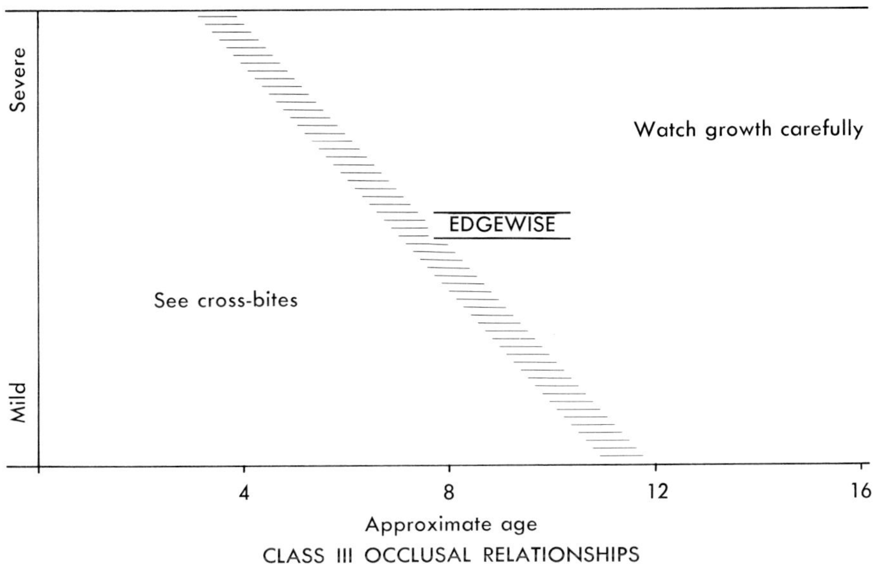

Fig. 13-7. Class III occlusal relationships usually require comprehensive banded therapy, with the final course dependent on growth. Early measures may be limited to crossbite control.

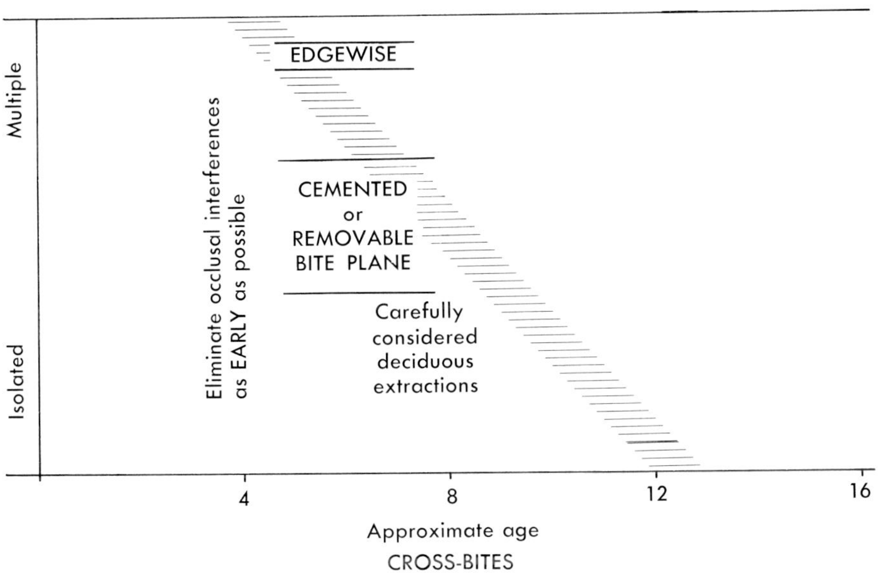

Fig. 13-8. Crossbites should usually be corrected early to avoid secondary effects. Deciduous extractions may be considered in some situations, but not without careful consideration of the effects on succeeding teeth. Only the more severe multiple crossbites require edgewise therapy in the mixed dentition, but in older patients comprehensive therapy becomes increasingly necessary.

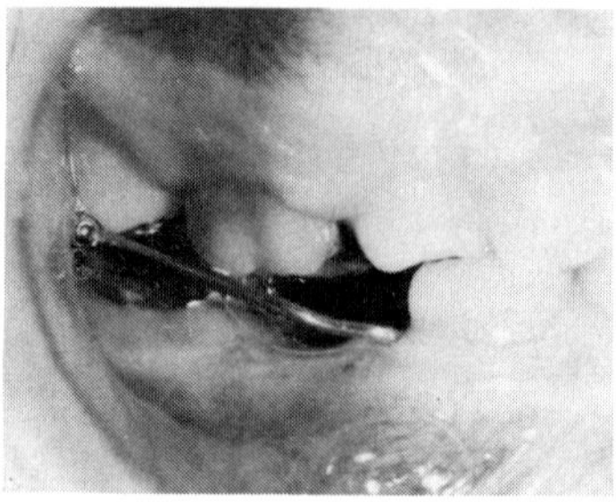

Fig. 13-9. Upper second deciduous molar erupting into lower space maintained without an adequate occlusal stop. The succeeding bicuspids will erupt into the same occlusal relationship if this condition is allowed to persist. This illustration also shows the tipping described in Fig. 13-13.

Diagnosis and case selection for this procedure must go far beyond the gratifying initial improvement of incisor alignment. Such extractions can seriously complicate a developing malocclusion if they are not followed by close supervision throughout the mixed and early permanent dentition periods.

Space preservation

Space preservation, as the term is used here, refers to the preservation of space following the early loss of deciduous teeth. Such space can be lost in both *horizontal* and *vertical* directions; it is of little avail to maintain a mesiodistal space for a lower second bicuspid while the upper bicuspid drops down into the space from above (Fig. 13-9).

All concurrent problems must be considered in any effort directed toward space preservation. For example, the patient shown in Fig. 13-10 is obviously suffering a severe space deficiency far beyond that which threatens as a result of the loss of the upper left first deciduous molar. The space maintainer shown is clearly helpful in preventing further space loss in an already deficient situation. On the other hand, it is also maintaining the anterior malocclusion, and its effectiveness depends on a deciduous tooth that can be expected to shed before the need for space maintenance has passed. In such a situation the patient is better served by measures coordinated with the final resolution of the total orthodontic problem rather than piecemeal local efforts.

For example, in this case the space between molars and central incisors is more important than the space between molars and the deciduous cuspid, which will shed soon. This could be controlled either with an acrylic space maintainer, a lingual arch, by banding molars and incisors, or by extraoral traction—any of which would be more effective. The individual choice should be based on a detailed evaluation of the total problem.

Acrylic space maintainers. A simple acrylic space maintainer is often the most effective means for replacing deciduous molars. For the upper arch it may be constructed entirely of self-curing or vacuum-formed acrylic. Lower appliances should be reinforced and stabilized by a lingual wire with the ends formed into occlusal rests in the central fossae of the first molars (Fig. 13-11). The same type of appliance can also serve as a posttreatment retainer in some situations.

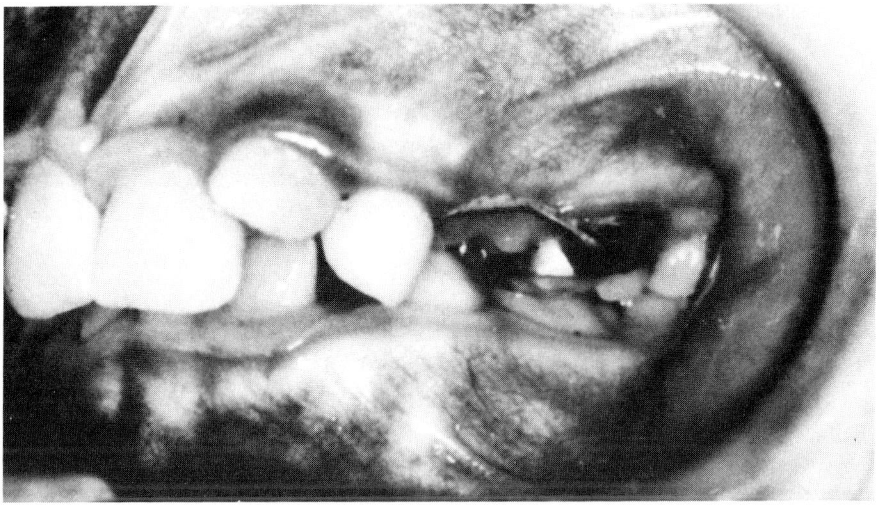

Fig. 13-10. Space maintainer holding space for the upper first bicuspid, with crowding already a serious problem anterior to the space. This is a futile gesture. Space conservation measures with preexisting malocclusion should be based on the long-range total problem.

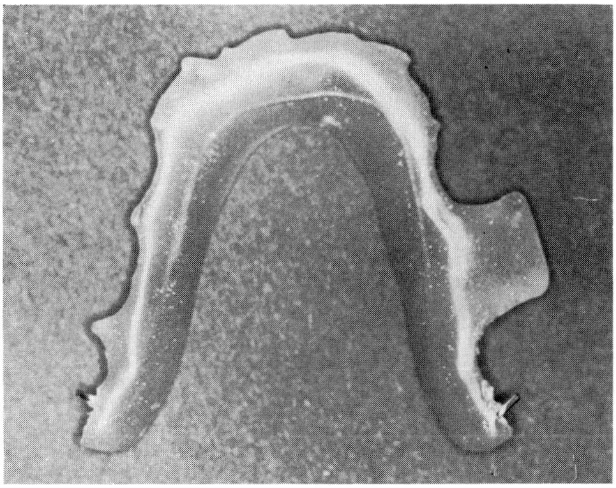

Fig. 13-11. Lower removable acrylic space maintainer replacing a missing second deciduous molar. The acrylic block that fills the space prevents elongation of the opposing tooth. Remaining teeth enjoy maximum freedom of movement in growth and in eruption, since the material may be selectively relieved wherever indicated. Note the reinforcing wire that ends in small occlusal rests on the first molars.

ADVANTAGES

1. Dental hygiene is not unduly complicated with these removable appliances, and experience shows that there is virtually no risk of increasing caries when they are made without clasps.
2. Minimum supervision is required. Because there is no increase in caries hazard and there are no parts that may be bent, patients using these space maintainers do not require the frequent examinations that are necessary when using cemented or removable wire appliances.
3. Vertical spaces are maintained. The plastic fills the space formerly occupied by any missing teeth, effectively preventing overeruption of opposing teeth.
4. The acrylic in the space may be relieved as required to permit eruption of succeeding teeth into the spaces being held.

DISADVANTAGES

1. Loss and breakage can be problems. The risk of loss is obviously increased with removable appliances. Breakage is comparable to that experienced with other appliances.
2. Cooperation is required. The patient must wear the appliance if it is to be effective. This is rarely a problem in practice because it it not uncomfortable when worn continuously, and full-time wear is not essential to holding space.
3. Growth may require replacement, especially with palatal appliances. Over a period of time, alveolar growth can carry the dentition away from the appliance and so negate its effectiveness (Fig. 13-12).

Cemented unilateral space maintainers. Many forms of space maintainers may be constructed using cemented bands or crowns on adjacent teeth as a support. Construction details can be varied in many ways but, with the exception of those mentioned below, these variations are generally unimportant.

Occlusal level must be maintained. Where there is no occlusal stop for the opposing tooth, some form of rigid metal or plastic occlusal surface must be provided to prevent overeruption. If wire is used, it must be adequately smoothed and reinforced for the occlusal function.

Cantilever cautiously. The tipping moment of a cantilever can easily tip the abutment tooth far enough to destroy the effectiveness of the space maintainer (Fig. 13-13). An occlusal rest will prevent this tipping, as will banding teeth on both sides of the space. Possible early loss of deciduous teeth must always be considered in the overall plan. If additional therapy is contemplated, space maintainers can be fitted with suitable attachments for later incorporation into the complete appliance.

ADVANTAGES

1. Minimum demands are made on patient cooperation.
2. Alveolar growth will not reduce effectiveness.

DISADVANTAGES

1. Hygiene problems and caries hazard increase. Cleaning is more difficult because the appliance is not removable. Undetected partial or complete loosening of an anchor band can lead to caries in that tooth. This consideration is especially important when the first permanent molar is used for this purpose over an extended period.
2. Frequent examinations are required. The possibilities of bending, breaking,

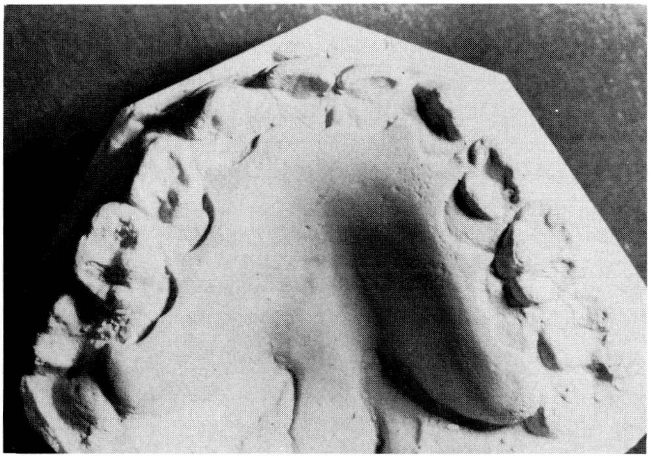

Fig. 13-12. Growth pattern in upper arch as shown by relationship of teeth to a cleft palate prosthesis worn for a long period of time. Similar changes can occur with removable space maintainers, requiring regular adjustment or replacement.

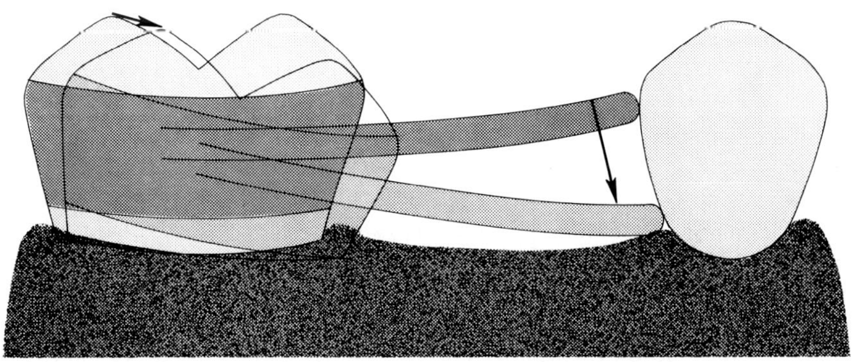

Fig. 13-13. Cantilevered space maintainer can easily tip and lose space. Occlusal forces can accelerate this action (Fig. 13-9). Resting the wire on soft tissue is not an adequate safeguard; only a secure rest or a band on the other abutment will provide adequate stability.

or loosening without detection by the patient make regular professional supervision a necessity.

3. Removal must be carefully and precisely timed. A cemented space maintainer may deflect the erupting tooth for which it was holding the space, yet space must be held until the new tooth is in place.
4. Shedding of a tooth adjacent to the space may necessitate construction of a new space maintainer. This is a common occurrence because the mesial teeth usually shed first. This is a very critical time, when the missing tooth should still be maintaining distal arch integrity.

Cemented bilateral space maintainers (usually a form of lingual arch). Lingual arches, either fixed or removable, may be used as space maintainers. These are especially effective in the lower arch where several deciduous teeth have been lost or there is a possibility of later loss of additional teeth. Space is held without interruption throughout the period of bicuspid eruption unless the arch interferes with the eruption of a lingually inclined bicuspid.

ADVANTAGES

1. No large demands are made on patient cooperation.
2. Little or no change is required through the transition to permanent dentition.

DISADVANTAGES

1. The hygiene and caries problems are the same as with other banded devices.
2. The need for supervision is the same as with all banded appliances.
3. A lingual arch does not maintain vertical dimension, so its use for an extended period is often contraindicated. This appliance is best suited for the transitional period when bicuspids are erupting or when teeth opposing the spaces are also missing.

Extraoral anchorage. The appliances for extraoral anchorage are discussed in more detail in Chapter 19. These are ideal upper space maintainers for multiple spaces, or where their retracting action is required for concurrent problems. Initiating Class II correction with this appliance in the mixed dentition obviates the need for any other upper space maintainers.

Split palate. Narrow maxillary arches may be widened with fixed banded appliances, removable wire or acrylic appliances, or cemented acrylic appliances. Of these, the acrylic appliances differ in that they apply force to the palatal tissues, as well as to the teeth.

The construction and application of the cemented acrylic appliance has been described in detail by Haas.[27] The rationale of the cemented jackscrew type of appliance is based on the premise that heavy forces will separate the maxillas before much tooth movement can take place. This effect has been demonstrated clearly, but similar though less spectacular results may also be obtained with removable appliances. Either can be extremely beneficial in the correction of crossbites. Most unilateral crossbites are actually mild bilateral problems in which the mandible is displaced on closure to facilitate chewing, so bilateral expansion is often indicated for unilateral as well as bilateral crossbites.

Expansion of this type can provide some additional arch length, but not nearly as much as the overall expansion. All but the simplest cases treated in this way will still require additional measures to provide an adequate occlusion.

Edgewise appliance. Space management in cases that will require later treatment with the edgewise appliance can sometimes be provided by placing part of that appliance as a space maintainer. Most frequently this will mean banding molars and placing a lingual arch, or also banding incisors for a space-holding arch similar to that shown in Fig. 18-20.

Bands used with other space maintainers may also be equipped with edgewise attachments to facilitate later incorporation of these teeth into the appliance.

HABIT CONTROL

Oral habits of every description can influence tooth positions. The most common include thumb sucking, finger sucking, tongue thrust in all its variations, lip biting or sucking, and bruxism.

When we have said that these habits can influence tooth position, we have about covered the area of agreement on this subject. Corrective measures range from the strictly psychologic approach to the crudely mechanical, and the entire field is much too broad and complex to permit any adequate treatment here.

It is usually considered unnecessary, if not undesirable, to initiate corrective measures before 4 to 6 years of age, and many of these problems will not be amenable to treatment until much later.

Some habits are at least partially dependent on the accompanying malocclusion, making orthodontic treatment a logical first step in correction. This improvement of the oral environment can be an essential first step in normalizing parafunctional habits. Any such treatment should be presented to the *child* patient as a purely orthodontic measure, with *no* mention of its relation to the habit. Not "making an issue" of the habit will solve the problem for many patients without jeopardizing their orthodontic cooperation by associating it with the habit-breaking effort.

Correcting an incisor overjet with extraoral or functional therapy can alter the relationships in this area enough to discourage many sucking habits at the same time that it brings lips into a more natural posture. This in itself can be enough to solve many problems, but the really dedicated practitioner of one of these habits will not be discouraged by such simple measures.

Direct mechanical "habit breakers" are seldom effective in the refractory case, and these devices must be used with great caution to avoid increasing patient resistance to later treatment.

OTHER TREATMENT

Other treatments referred to in Figs. 13-1 to 13-8 are covered elsewhere, mostly as part of the overall edgewise therapy or as finishing procedures. Of course this does not exhaust the list of orthodontic approaches to malocclusion, but it does provide a framework into which other variations may be fitted as desired.

14

Edgewise appliance

During the first thirty years of this century, Dr. Edward H. Angle brought orthodontics from the simple E arch through the ribbon arch to the edgewise mechanism. In the edgewise mechanism Angle gave his specialty an appliance that was perfected in principle and fully adaptable to later progress in related scientific and technologic fields. The problem for the present generation is to maintain perspective and to identify, adopt, and adapt those changes that are most beneficial. This is possible only with a good understanding of the basic mechanism and its function.

The objective of this chapter is to present that basic edgewise mechanism as a base on which to build and consider the newer modifications so that they can be selected and used to best advantage. In this description liberal use will be made of Angle's original work since no such description could be complete without either direct or indirect quotation of these orthodontic classics.[28–31]

Our technology may have advanced in the last fifty years, but the underlying design and function of the edgewise mechanism remain essentially unchanged. They are based on immutable physical laws and biologic principles. We may gloss over the outward appearance with superficial refinements, new names, and countless variations, but skilled application still requires the ability to see past the surface to the level where the real action takes place.

In applying mechanical devices to the teeth an orthodontist steps in for a rather brief period in the patient's life, alters the relationships of the teeth to each other and to the surrounding structures, and then steps out again. The untreated occlusion is in a sort of disordered balance. If the teeth of the treated occlusion are not carefully ordered, or if they are not in balance, the ultimate result will be unstable, unsatisfactory, or both. Angle addressed this important point in 1928, when he said:

> Orthodontists [must] fully realize that in treating malocclusion of the teeth such corrections must be made as will reestablish the denture as a self-sustaining, self-maintaining unit or organism; in other words, that all parts of the denture which exert force and all those which sustain and distribute force must be perfectly balanced, in pairs, in groups, and as a whole; for BALANCE is the greatest word in orthodontia. [Balance] is the law of the successful maintenance of that denture which reaches normal development naturally, and it is the law which must be observed in detail if treatment of an unbalanced denture—malocclusion—is to be successful. These details are as follows:
>
> First, there must be established fully normal proximal contact relations of teeth arranged in arches of normal individual typal form and size;

Second, there must be established fully normal cusp and inclined plane interrelationships; and

Third, and quite as important as the other two, though seeming as yet to be little appreciated, there must be established fully normal upright axial positions and relations of the teeth. [This is essential] if the teeth are to balance with the muscles and sustain and normally maintain the great [force] of occlusion.*

Those objectives of orthodontic correction are no less important today, but their attainment has been expanded immeasurably since Angle's time. Improvements in appliances and materials have been helpful, but ironically the full achievement of the balance to which Angle referred was not possible until the profession reevaluated the therapeutic extraction of teeth, which he abhorred, in light of cephalometric radiography and the full three-dimensional control afforded by today's edgewise armamentarium.

The turning point came with the searching studies of Dr. Charles H. Tweed and his carefully considered report to the profession in 1941.[32] Downs' introduction of cephalometrics as a diagnostic tool in 1947[33] closed a large remaining gap by providing the diagnostic means for a more complete evaluation of dentofacial relationships. These have been followed by a continuous stream of clinical studies that have undoubtedly changed the nature and potential of orthodontic therapy as much as the edgewise concept itself.

Extraction is far from a cure-all, and it is no less subject to misapplication than any other therapeutic modality. Enthusiasm may fluctuate excessively in one direction or another from time to time, but this broadened approach to treatment has certainly enlarged the capability of orthodontic therapy to attain the objectives described by Angle as essential to a healthy, balanced occlusion.

The unique contribution of the edgewise appliance toward attaining these objectives is *complete control* over axial inclination of *all teeth* in *all directions*. This is essential for root control in horizontal tooth movements as well as for correcting teeth that have an abnormal inclination. The classical mechanical means for exercising this control is the engagement of the archwire in the slot of the bracket on the tooth (Figs. 14-1 and 14-2). Tipping the archwire as it is engaged in the brackets will cause the seated arch to tip the root mesially or distally. A rectangular archwire or suitable auxiliaries can accomplish the engagement that is necessary to tip roots buccally or lingually as desired.

Using this potential for control with discretion and finesse is essential to effective application of this appliance. It is unnecessary and often undesirable to control root tipping in all directions at all times in all cases. This is frequently true in the case of buccolingual root movement with a rectangular wire. If no buccolingual root control is needed, the use of a rectangular wire merely adds unnecessary complication to the adjustments and increases the stiffness of the wire. Those complications are not eliminated by angulated slots, which still retain the potential for undesirable actions.

The name of the edgewise appliance has created some confusion on this particular point, since the appliance is obviously named for the edgewise rectangular

*From Angle, E.H.: The latest and best in orthodontic mechanism, Dental Cosmos **70**:1143-1144, 1928.

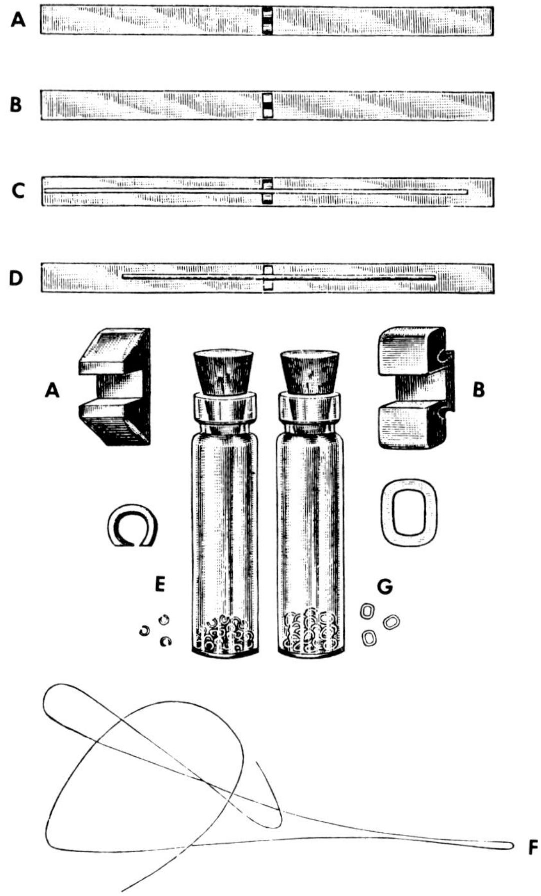

Fig. 14-1. *Top: A-D,* The original edgewise attachments; brackets soldered to band strips, ready to be formed into bands. Sections of archwire are shown in the slots at *C* and *D*. *Below: A,* The obsolete wingless anterior bracket; *B,* the prototype of the present edgewise brackets; *E,* staples, enlarged and actual size; *F,* a ligature wire for tying the arch to the bracket; *G,* washers that can be threaded on the arch to control space. (From Angle, E.H.: Dental Cosmos **70:**1146, 1928.)

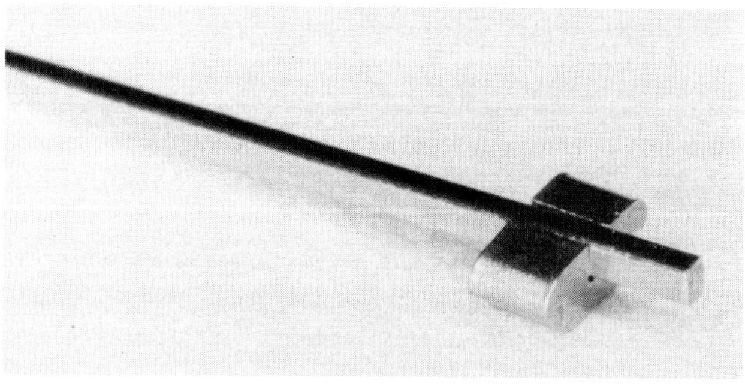

Fig. 14-2. The basic edgewise bracket and rectangular wire. Engagement of this wire in the slot prevents rotation of the wire and so provides positive control in all planes of space when securely tied into the slot.

wire. This does *not* mean that use of the edgewise wire itself is an essential element of the appliance.

In his original presentation of this mechanism, Angle did not call it the edgewise mechanism; in fact, he did not give any name to the complete appliance. He recommended that *both round and rectangular wires* be used in treatment, according to the dictates of the case, much as is done by most orthodontists today. To differentiate between the round and the rectangular arches that he used, Angle called the rectangular one the edgewise arch. This was done to avoid confusion with the earlier ribbon arch, which was also rectangular but was seated in the bracket with the widest surface facing the tooth (flatwise). Angle's ribbon arch bracket has since been adapted as the attachment for the Begg technique and in a more modified form for the Universal technique.

ATTACHMENTS

Brackets or tubes are attached to the teeth to serve as handles—a means for attaching the working arch to the tooth. In most cases all teeth from the first molars forward require such fixed attachments for adequate control. They may be left free only when the plan of treatment does not require that they be moved or controlled by the arch. Where anchorage considerations, positions of second molars, or severity of the curve of Spee make control of second molars desirable, these teeth may also be controlled through part or all of treatment. Fig. 14-3 shows some of the variations of the edgewise bracket. These brackets are typically used on the labial or buccal surface of every tooth, with the exception of the last molar on each side. They may vary in dimensions and in certain details, but all have the horizontal slot for the arch across the face, with upper and lower wings for ligation. The archwire is tied to the bracket by means of a soft ligature wire or elastic ligature with the wings used as shown in Fig. 14-4. Brackets are also available with various latching devices to replace the ligature. Selection of optimum bracket and archwire dimensions is discussed in detail in later chapters.

The last molar on each side is usually fitted with a rectangular tube or sheath that serves the same function as the bracket—holding the archwire to the tooth. The use of tubes on these teeth makes it unnecessary to use ligatures in this difficult posterior position and, more importantly, the tubes hold the ends of the arch in place as soon as it is inserted. This stabilization greatly simplifies the problem of holding the arch in position while ligatures are tied to the other teeth. During the interval between adjustments, the complete enclosure provided by the tube protects the patient from the sharp end of the arch and also provides a smooth guide for movement of the archwire in response to tooth movement.

Fig. 14-5 shows arches in place in the mouth. The cuspids and bicuspids are fitted with the original type of narrow (.05-inch or 1.25-mm) bracket shown in Figs. 14-2 and 14-3, *A*. Double-width brackets (.10-inch or 2.5-mm), also called molar-width brackets, are shown on the incisors. The upper arch is fitted with a rectangular wire and the lower arch with a round wire. This case is shown for illustration only; these are not the brackets in general use today.

In the original edgewise appliance bracket slots and openings in molar tubes were .022 inch (.56 mm) wide by .028 inch (.71 mm) deep. There has been a strong

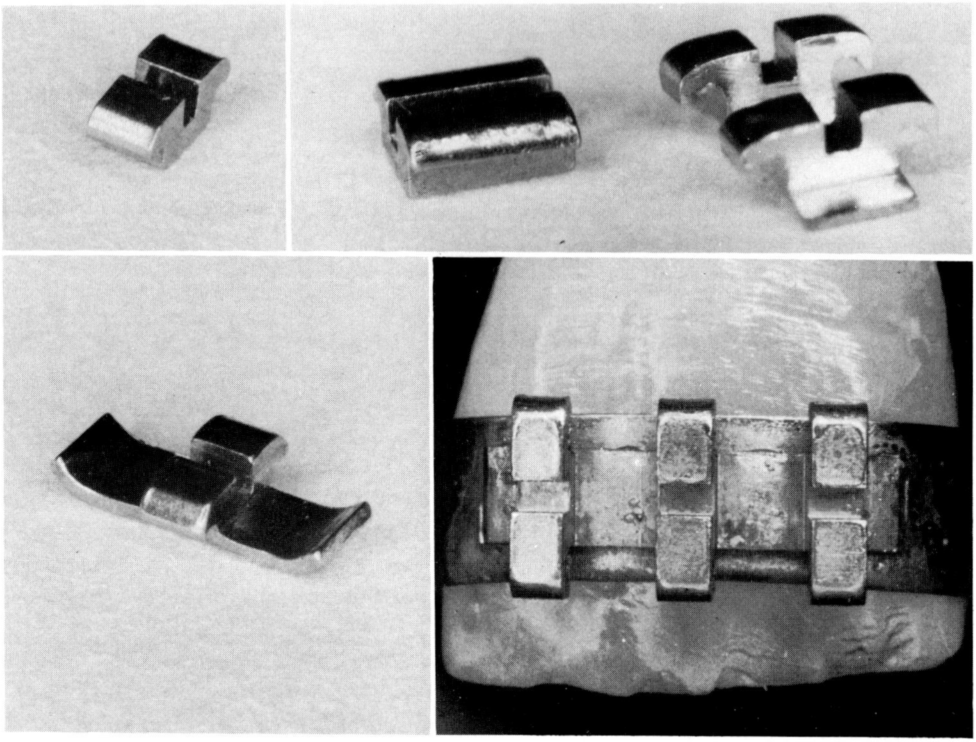

Fig. 14-3. A, Original narrow-width edgewise bracket, .05 inch (1.25 mm) wide. **B,** Left, double (molar)-width gold edgewise bracket, .1 inch (2.5 mm) wide. Right, wide twin stainless steel edgewise bracket, .14 inch (3.5 mm) wide, with welding flanges. **C,** Single-width bracket with rotating wings that contact the archwire and so control axial rotation of the tooth. These brackets are available with either rigid or flexible wings. **D,** Triple brackets on a central incisor. May also be used on molars. These brackets provide an additional mechanical advantage for rotation and tipping adjustments with light wires, plus a ready fine control over rotation by selective tying of only one or two of the brackets.

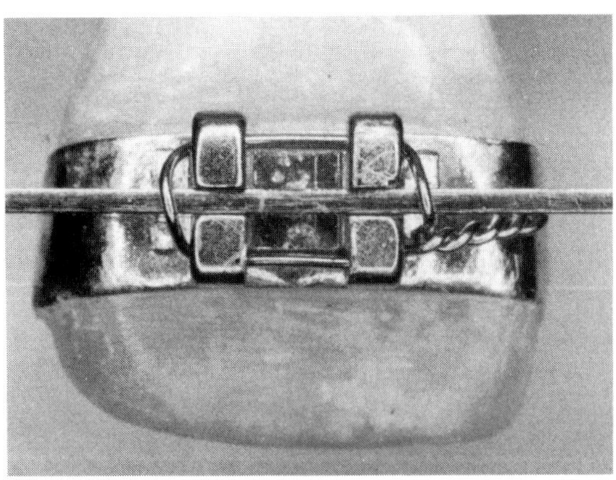

Fig. 14-4. Ligation of the arch to the bracket with stainless steel ligature wire.

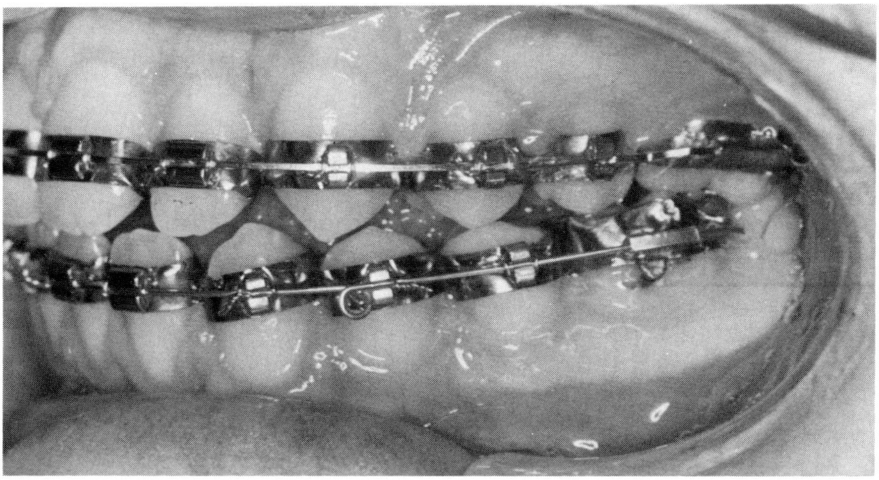

Fig. 14-5. Arches in place in the mouth, showing the original narrow form of bracket on buccal teeth and wide (molar) brackets on incisors.

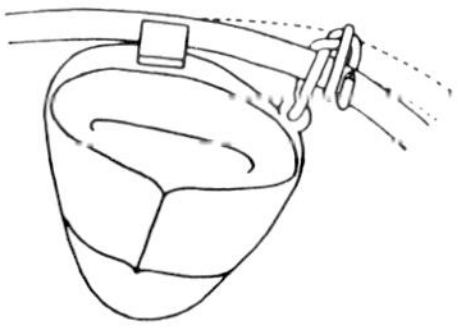

Fig. 14-6. The use of a staple in rotation. Arch movement and the resulting rotation are greatly exaggerated in this illustration. (From Angle, E.H.: Dental Cosmos **71**:170, 1929.)

trend in recent years toward a narrower slot, now standardizing at .018 inch (.48 mm) wide and from .025 to .030 inch (.63 to .78 mm) deep. Each size has its advantages and limitations, and comparable force levels and control are attainable with either. The choice depends largely on personal preference in the use of wires and auxiliaries. Some of the considerations related to these dimensions are discussed in detail in Chapters 17 and 18.

Staples and other rotating attachments

An important auxiliary attachment in the original edgewise appliance that is still useful in some situations is the staple or eyelet (Fig. 14-1, *E*). This tiny eyelet, just large enough for a ligature wire to pass through, is attached to the band at any point where a pull might be required. The original location was mesial or distal to the bracket, where tying it to the arch placed a rotating action on the tooth. This action is illustrated in Fig. 14-6, where Angle has positioned the bracket off-center to give a more effective rotating action. In current practice this application of the staple has been largely replaced by a second bracket in the double-bracket arrangement. In rotations this second bracket replaces the staple in Fig. 14-6 and functions in the same way. This provides a bonus feature in providing a similar mechanical advantage for mesiodistal tipping actions. Other rotation devices, such as the winged bracket (Fig. 14-3, *C*) and the rotating spring wedge, are also available, but these offer no advantage over the second bracket when arches are formed to take full advantage of their rotation potential.

In current practice the staple principle is still widely used with lingual eyelets, buttons, or hooks for rotation control. These are more often activated with elastic ligatures than with wires, but either may be used as the dictates of movement require.

ARCHES

All banded teeth are normally under the influence of the archwire, whether they are being moved actively, held immobile, or used as relatively stable anchorage or resistance units. The formation of the archwire and the coordination of its often subtle actions is a critical factor in successful treatment.

Some of the arches in current use are a far cry from Angle's ideal edgewise arch, but their underlying form and function are still the same even though the resemblance may not always be obvious. Mechanical devices may change from time to time, but normal occlusion does not!

The metal orthodontic arch is the form that molds the dental arch, with every bend in the wire reflected in the positions of the teeth. If the teeth are finally to be positioned in their best esthetic and functional relationships, this wire arch must be carefully formed in every detail.

With a heavy archwire the teeth are eventually moved into position on that arch, so that the dental arch and the wire arch will have the same form. With more flexible wires, the force levels are so low that the force required to deflect the arch may be in the same range as physiologic and functional forces acting on the teeth. This means that the dental arch will never attain a form duplicating that of the wire arch, so the process of arch formation must include a visualization of final form and deflecting forces as they relate to the passive wire form. *This is of critical importance*, because forming a "light-wire" arch to ideal form *cannot* be expected to induce that form in the dental arch. This holds true even more in vertical relationships than in the horizontal plane.

Normal arch form

The form of the dental arch and the form that the wire arch must have to produce it have been carefully described by Angle, who began with an important description of what the arch form is not:

> If asked to demonstrate the form of a normal upper dental arch, nearly all will give a semi-ellipse, or a horseshoe pattern, with the central and lateral incisors and the cuspids all of the same height and in the same alignment, and nearly always with the bicuspids buccally to normal. . . .
>
> Teeth without artificial support could never possibly remain in such positions, for there could not be mechanical balance mesiodistally between the normal proximal contacts of the teeth, nor between the inclined occlusal planes of opposing teeth, nor balance of the muscles, nor of teeth and muscles with the [temporomandibular joint]. . . .
>
> Now how is the proper shape of the metal arch to be determined? There are in

> dentures five points or 'landmarks,' so to speak, from which the ideal—the typal—form of both dental and metal arches may be quite accurately determined, regardless of the irregularity of position in which the teeth may be found. . . . These landmarks are indicated at *A, D, D', E,* and *E'* in Fig. 14-7, which is a drawing representing the ideal arrangement of the teeth in a fairly average normal upper dental arch, with a metal arch lying in juxtaposition to the teeth. . . .
>
> It will be noted that there is a straight line from the center of the labial ridges of the cuspids, *D, D'*, to the center of the mesiolabial ridges of the first molars, *E, E'*. This line is always straight, regardless of the degree or form of the curve of the anterior part of the dental arch or of the lateral width between either the cuspids or the molars.*

Angle goes on to describe the unique alignment of the upper lateral incisor. This tooth is thinner, labiolingually, than the central incisor and much thinner than the cuspid. The *lingual* surfaces of these teeth should form a smooth curve for occlusion with the lower teeth; thus, the *labial* surfaces must be adjusted to compensate for the differences in thickness. This requires close observation of the peculiarities of the individual teeth, which in most cases will require that the lateral incisor be placed slightly lingual to the adjacent teeth, as shown in Fig. 14-7. The lateral incisor should also be slightly shorter than the adjacent teeth, as shown in Fig. 14-8. This position compensates for the difference in crown length and thickness, so that the incisal edges can function smoothly with the lower teeth.

Note in Fig. 14-7 that the contact points *do* lie on an ellipsoid curve; the deviations noted by Angle are in the buccal contours, due to differences in tooth anat-

*From Angle, E.H.: The latest and best in orthodontic mechanism, Dental Cosmos **70**:1153-1154, 1928.

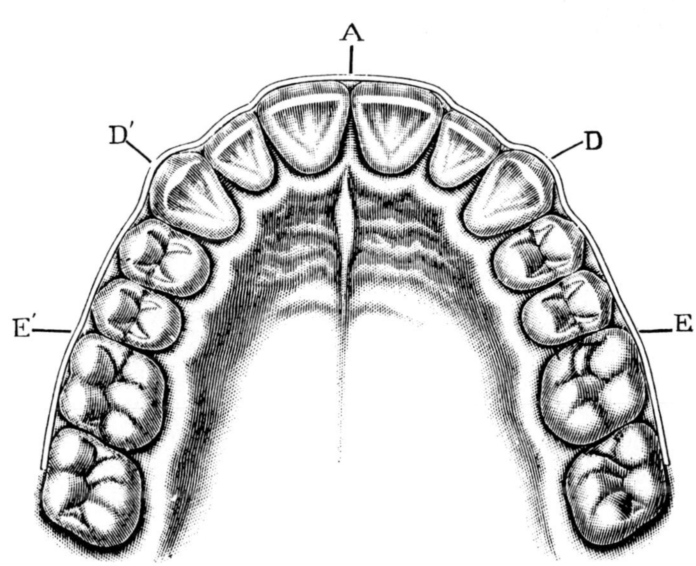

Fig. 14-7. The upper dental arch with a wire contoured to the buccal surfaces. (From Angle, E.H.: Dental Cosmos **70**:1154,1928.)

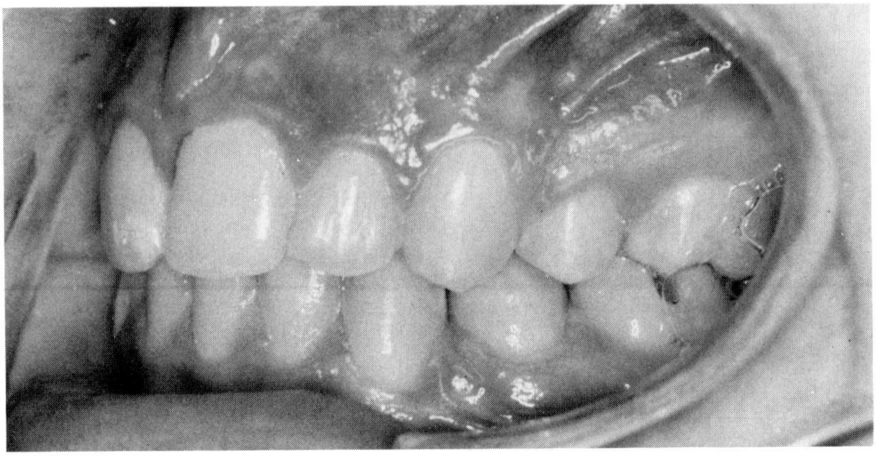

Fig. 14-8. The normal position of the lateral incisor is slightly lingual and gingival to the adjacent teeth. This is essential to compensate for the thinner, shorter crown of this tooth.

omy. The form of this curve also changes as we proceed from occlusal to gingival, especially in the lower arch, because of differences in inclination of the buccal surfaces. Modern bracket and tube configurations and positions require smaller adjustments in the form of the wire arch.

In the buccal segments the arch continues to follow an ellipsoid curve as it arcs progressively inward. Angle described a straight buccal line from the cuspid to the mesiobuccal cusp of the first molar, but *the arch does not continue in a straight line beyond that point.*

This takes on added significance with the popularity of appliances that attempt to build all adjustments into the attachments; such attempts beyond the first molar can lead to an excessively buccal position of the second molar.

The mesiobuccal cusp of the first molar is the inflection point. The arch curves progressively inward from there, often much more than shown in Angle's illustration in Fig. 14-7. This can be critical in the second molar area because of the position of the developing third molar, which lies in close proximity to the distobuccal surface of the second molar root.

Each molar erupts with a distobuccal inclination, dropping lingually and distally into function under the guidance of buccal musculature and the distal surface of the preceding molar. The distal crown surfaces of the upper molars are angulated distolingually, and this angulation is increased by mesial rotation. Excessive buccal tipping of upper molars is usually the result of inhibition of normal functional adjustment by some combination of distal space deficiency in the tuberosity and excessive mesial rotation of the preceding molar.

Shaping the arch

Many different instruments can be used for bending round wires. Large-radius bends are most easily made with the fingers, but small, sharp bends require the use of pliers or special loop-forming instruments. Four very useful types of wire-bending pliers are shown in Fig. 14-9.

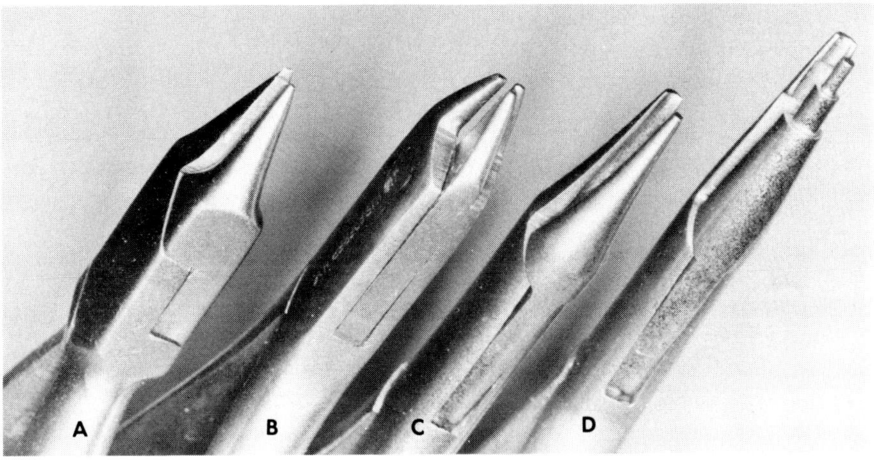

Fig. 14-9. Pliers for bending round wires. *A*, Angle wire-bending pliers No. 139. *B*, Triple-beak clasp-adjusting pliers. *C* and *D*, Pliers for bending and forming loops, especially in small-diameter wires. *A* is used to hold the wire while it is bent around one beak with the fingers. *B*, *C*, and *D* will also produce a bend by merely closing on the wire; greater bends are made by continuing the bend with the fingers or by successive small bends.

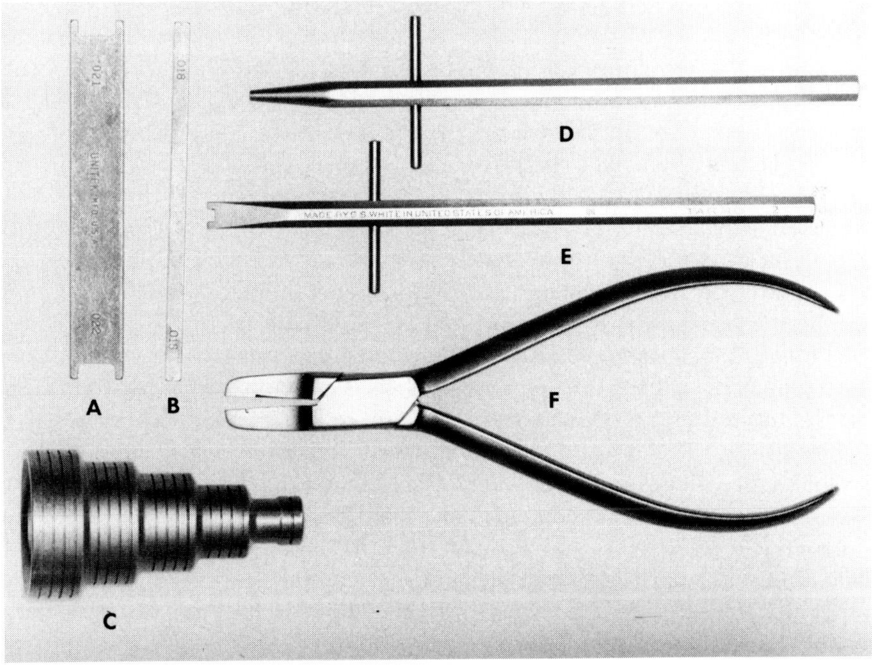

Fig. 14-10. Instruments for bending rectangular wires. *A*, *B*, *D*, and *E*, Torque keys with slotted ends machined to engage the flat sides of the wire securely. *C*, Arch former with slots machined around the circumference to fit different thicknesses of rectangular wire. *F*, Angle pliers No. 142, with a precision groove in the lower beak for the wire.

The bending of rectangular wires requires instruments designed to keep the wires from twisting as they are bent, as well as to introduce torquing adjustments (Fig. 14-10). The arch former has slots of several widths on each of the four large turrets. The wire is placed in the narrowest slot that it will fit and is then bent around the slot with the fingers. There is a great deal of spring-back from these large-radius bends, so the wire must always be bent on a turret that is smaller in diameter than the desired bend. This is especially true in the case of stainless steel wires. The best procedure is to overbend the wire slightly and then return it to the desired curvature with the fingers. The slots of the various torque keys and the No. 142 pliers are used in many combinations with each other and with the fingers for small, simple bends.

For torquing (twisting) of the wire, two slotted instruments must be used in combination with each other, one holding the wire at either end of the section that is being twisted. An exception is made when a large segment, such as the incisor region, is being twisted in relation to a segment that lies almost perpendicular to it. In this case much of the twisting adjustment can be made by holding the anterior segment with a slotted instrument and bending the buccal segment up or down with the fingers. This type of admustment may also be reversed by holding the buccal segment with the slotted instrument and bending the anterior segment up or down as required. In the first case the torque will be changed mesial to the cuspid, and in the second case it will be changed distal to the cuspid.

Torquing adjustments usually distort the plane of the arch, so they must be followed by a gentle reshaping with the fingers and verification of the final net torque adjustment.

Shaping of the metal arch is illustrated in Fig. 14-11. The original procedure, with gold wire, was to scribe the arch at each of the points shown in Fig. 14-11, according to measurements taken from plaster casts of the teeth. This is not suitable for steel archwires, especially in the smaller sizes, because of the weakening effect that such marking has on these harder metals. Marks on hard archwires should be made either with a pencil or with a special marker, or the arch can be formed by repeated fitting in the mouth without any marking. Arches may also be partially formed on the casts, with final adjustments made as they are fitted in the mouth.

The first bend shown (Fig. 14-11, *I*) determines the labial curvature of the incisor segment, and in many ways this is the most important bend of all. Curvature of this segment *must* be based on the individual patient's optimum arch form and *not* on the natural curve of the wire as it is placed in the mouth, or on any other stereotyped form. This anterior curve controls intercuspid width, one of the most important single dimensions in the arch. The bend is made with the fingers on the arch former if the wire is rectangular and with or without the arch former if the wire is round.

The second bends (Fig. 14-11, *II* and *III*) are the sharp bends at the cuspid prominences. These are made with the small end of the arch former, with the fingers, or with a pair of pliers. The degree of offset in this bend must be based on the individual dentition and exact bracket positions. With double brackets, which do not lie on the most prominent part of the cuspid, this bend will be less severe than that shown in this illustration.

The last bends (Fig. 14-11, *IV* and *V*) are the subtle adjustments at the lateral incisor and molar. These are made with the No. 142 or three-point clasp-adjusting pliers, and once again must be individualized for each case. Tooth anatomy and bracket levels can dictate a much smaller offset for many patients.

Careful attention should be given to the molar bend, for the previously mentioned straight line from cuspid to molar ends at the mesiobuccal ridge of the molar. If the buccal surface of the molar were to follow the same straight line, the tooth would be rotated mesially. Molars are often found rotated in this way before treatment, so the very first arch should be carefully formed to correct or prevent such a rotation.

The bend in the arch mesial to the first molar can be deceiving. If the mesial end of the molar tube is placed at the center of the mesiobuccal cusp, and if the bend is made exactly at this point, only a simple bend will be required. If the same simple bend is positioned mesial to this point, it will position the bicuspid too far buccally or the molar too far lingually. In this situation a double bend is required to correctly offset molar and bicuspid.

The offset of the two bends mesial to the molar depends on their position between molar and bicuspid and on the amount that the molar must be rotated in relation to the straight bicuspid section of the arch (Fig. 14-12). Whenever an angled arch moves distally through the molar tube, it will move the molar buccally and the bicuspid lingually in relation to each other; therefore the adjustment of this bend must be watched carefully throughout treatment.

Angulated molar tubes will minimize the need for this bend, but they cause more cheek discomfort. Either means can accomplish correct molar rotation.

The actual procedure for bending arches may be modified in many ways, at the operator's discretion. The important consideration is the final form and function of the arch rather than which bends are made first. Small round arch wires are most easily formed if the operator starts with a slight anterior curve to establish the plane of the arch and then begins detailed adjustments at the left molar. Bends are then made tooth-by-tooth, around the arch from left to right. Measurements can be made with dividers as required, or the partially completed arch may be tried directly in the mouth. The arch can often be positioned and partly bent at a bracket to mark the location of the next bend. Working in this way with a long piece of stock wire is especially useful when incorporating loops into the arch.

The arch just described is the ideal as it should be at the end of treatment. Earlier arches may have to be modified to partially adapt to the malocclusion, but any such modifications must always be made with the final form in mind. This requires that *more, not less*, attention be given to arch form in these early stages.

The lower arch is similar to the upper, but without the lateral incisor offsets.

The inclination of the buccal surfaces of teeth makes the vertical position of the bracket or tube an important factor in arch form. If the attachment of one tooth lies more gingival than that of an adjacent tooth, the compensating bend should be accompanied by an offset to avoid moving that tooth buccally or lingually (Fig. 14-13).

Torque adjustments are placed in rectangular wires after the arch form has been completed. This must always be done by first adjusting the wire so that torque is

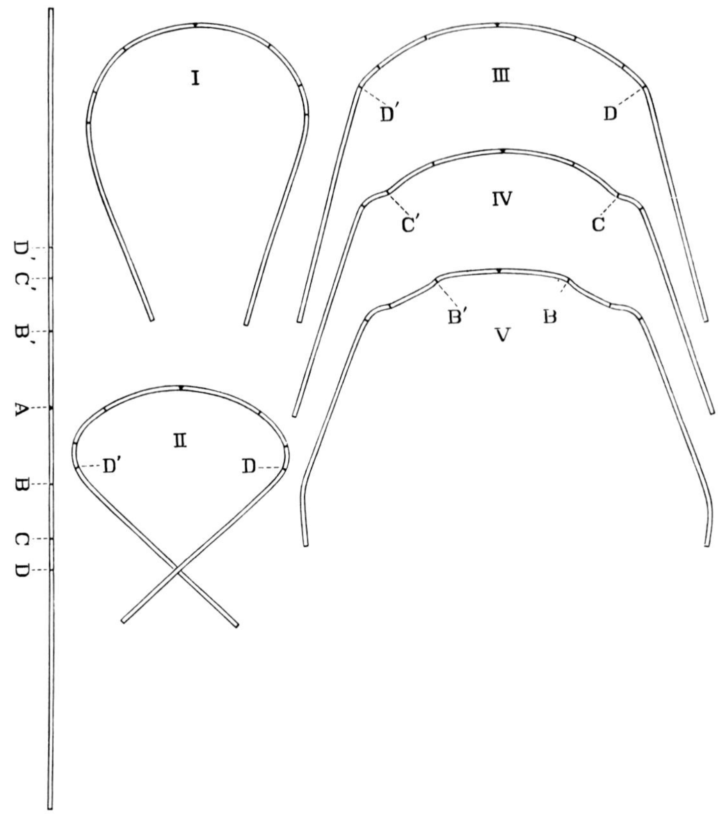

Fig. 14-11. Forming the upper arch, as originally described by Angle. Bends are somewhat exaggerated for purposes of illustration, and the arch form is more "square" than would be suitable for many cases. (From Angle, E.H.: Dental Cosmos **70:**1155, 1928.)

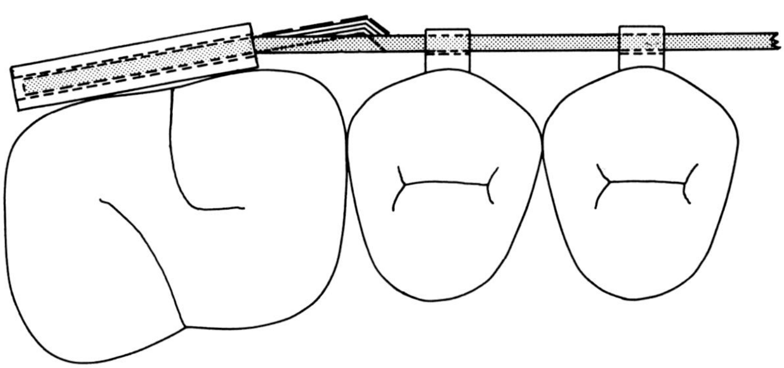

Fig. 14-12. The bend in the arch at the upper first molar. A simple bend is correct over the mesiobuccal molar cusp, but a double bend is required if the bend is positioned more mesially. Angulation of the molar tube may be used to obviate the need for this bend.

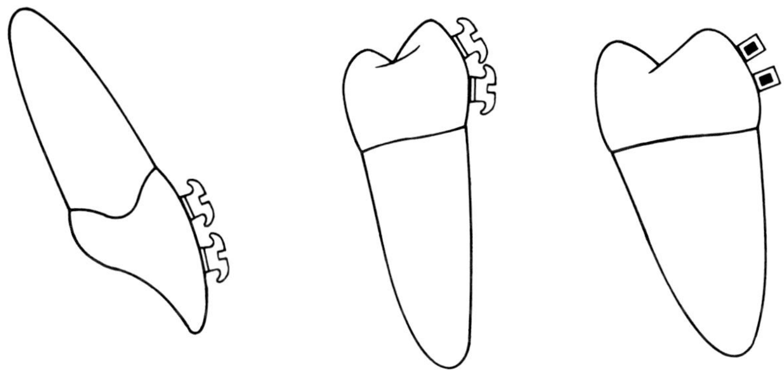

Fig. 14-13. The level of the attachment on the tooth affects the buccolingual position and the torque effect of the archwire, requiring compensating adjustments. Individual tooth anatomy introduces another variable.

essentially passive in the mouth. Slight activating adjustments can then be added as required. Active torque with rectangular wires must be used with great care, as is noted in more detail in the discussion of slot dimensions on pp. 168-172.

Initial arches

Careful design and formation of arches from the very beginning can save much time later. The most rapid tooth movement is accomplished with the small-diameter wires and sectional or interrupted arches that are usually used first. Details that are not attended to in the early stages can easily prolong treatment with the added attention that they require later. This is clearly reflected by Angle in the following comments on arch formation:

> [The] mechanism employed for orthodontic treatment should be such that from the first, in each case, its operation [will] result in the continuous and physiologically rapid movement of each tooth . . . into its own individual position in the line of occlusion, the ideal and the means of gaining the ideal thus closely coordinating from the beginning to the end of active treatment.
>
> . . . This is now possible . . . by shaping the metal arches so accurately that from the very beginning of treatment they have *ideal typal* forms, or forms that closely correspond to the desired ultimate forms of the dental arches in each individual case. Thus shaped, sprung into, and secured in their attachments, they must immediately begin to exert force automatically on the malposed teeth, in directions and amounts most favorable for the direct movement of these teeth into their correct positions in the individual, typal line of occlusion. The relation between the activity of the mechanism and the typal positions of the teeth is, therefore, not vague and problematical, but closely correlated from the beginning of treatment to its completion. But it will be realized that the shaping of the metal arches must be done *carefully*, and that in size and form they must [conform to] the required (normal) sizes and forms of the dental arches in each case, indicated by the sizes and typal pattern of the teeth, the type of the face and skull and the general type of the individual.
>
> Owing to the delicacy and great elasticity of the two forms of metal arches (round and edgewise) and to the . . . form of the bracket-slot attachments of the new mecha-

> nism, the full, free, maximum elasticity of the ideally formed metal arches is accessible from the first for direct distribution to the teeth individually and collectively for their direct movement from their abnormal into their normal positions. These arches will thus naturally be operative over much longer periods before changes in their attachment relations become necessary than will those of the usual types of mechanism. *This is especially true in the use of the delicate round arch, and its use is often preferable,* particularly in beginning treatment.*

That description sounds almost as though it might have been written to describe some of the current "light-wire" techniques. Today's light resilient wires far surpass the materials available to Angle in their orthodontic potential, and they are an important part of modern edgewise therapy.

These wires appear to bring us close to the ideal to which Angle alluded when he said:

> Ideally, of course, the force would be positive and uninterrupted from the beginning to the completion of the required movement of each individual tooth, and the movement would be as rapid as fully normal stimulation of bone cells warrants.
>
> If force could be thus ideally applied, the requirements of physiology and dynamics would be fully met. However, no mechanism has yet been devised that admits of the exertion of the proper amount of force in all required directions to complete in all cases all necessary movements of all teeth from a single, initial adjustment.†

A casual look at some of the capabilities of wires now available might suggest that we are close to the ideal sought by Angle, but closer scrutiny shows a different picture.

It is entirely possible to achieve rapid movements with highly flexible archwire mechanics, but rarely is a gain achieved without a price. That price can be especially high when it goes unnoticed.

In these cases the price is excessive movement of adjoining teeth. Excessive movement is always undesirable, and in some of these situations it can be irreversible as well.

When wire flexibility is increased, there is a comparable change in its force management capabilities. Some of the superflexible wires that are available to the orthodontist of the eighties so far surpass the elastic range of more conventional materials that they require a complete reassessment of the force and distribution system. These effects are a direct function of the high range/stiffness ratio, so the multistranded wires of conventional materials and the solid wires of such materials as Nitinol and other titanium alloys produce the most extreme effects.

Such wires almost inevitably function as primary energy storage units, with severely limited distribution capabilities. This is a complete role reversal from conventional wire arches. Physical properties of these wires are characterized by *low stiffness and strength* combined with *high working range.* The low stiffness means that forces cannot be transferred by these wires in a distribution function without

---

*From Angle, E.H.: The latest and best in orthodontic mechanism, Dental Cosmos **70:**1152-1153, 1928; italics added.

†From Angle, E.H.: The latest and best in orthodontic mechanism, Dental Cosmos **71:**260-270, 1929.

the large deflections that result in inevitable storage of a significant part of the applied force.

Their high flexibility makes these wires most effective over short spans, so they are widely used for their effects on individual teeth rather than overall arch form. Less flexible wires accomplish such changes in small, controllable increments, but the superflexible wires can work through long, sweeping movements.

Such movements use the adjoining teeth for reciprocal anchorage, taking them along for the ride as they provide backup for the low stiffness of the wire. These secondary effects require even more attention than the intended action when these wires are used.

While seeming to bring us closer to the goals described by Angle, these wires fall far short in exerting the proper amount of force in *all required directions.* They can be a valuable addition to the orthodontic armamentarium, but only when they are used with care in carefully selected situations that may benefit from their unique capabilities.

15

Attachments

Bracket and tube attachments are the most distinguishing features among the different fixed appliances. Within the edgewise group the various forms of these attachments differ from one another almost as much as they do from those of other appliance systems. Slot dimensions and angulations, overall dimensions, numerous auxiliary functions, and design details all contribute to the range of available choices.

The different attachments form the basis for many of the variations in technique. Each of these will perform well, but with its own unique advantages and problems, so selection is a matter of weighing all factors and choosing the most agreeable compromise. *Understanding all of the unique characteristics of the ultimate choice, both favorable and unfavorable, is far more important than the choice itself.*

BRACKET WIDTH

The original edgewise bracket, 1.25 mm wide, has now come to be known as the "narrow" bracket. The first new size, introduced a few years after the narrow bracket, was 2.5 mm wide. This was the first attempt at gaining added mechanical advantage through bracket width, and though it was originally intended for use on the molar teeth as an aid in tipping control, its obvious advantages soon led to its use on other teeth as well. The next step was soldering two narrow brackets in exact alignment on the same band. Those were the precursors of today's multiple brackets that are milled as a single unit on a common base. Keeping the brackets on a single base keeps the slots in alignment and greatly simplifies the attachment of more than one bracket to a single tooth. These brackets, which may be called twin, double, dual, or Siamese brackets, vary from about 2 to 4.5 mm in overall width. Triple brackets, with the same spacing as the 3.5-mm double brackets and an overall width of 5 mm, are preferable to the extra-wide spacing of two brackets for most applications where this added width is required.

The divided form of the multiple brackets makes it possible to bend the base between brackets to fit individual tooth contours. This is especially important in these wider sizes.

Attachment width and arch efficiency

Attachment width is instrumental in root control in both the mesiodistal plane and in axial rotations. Since archwire mechanics is essentially the same for both movements, tipping control will be used as the basis for discussion.

Resistance and response in tooth movement depend on the force that reaches the supporting tissues. In root movement the archwire applies a tipping rotation to the tooth as a moment, rotating the bracket and the attached tooth in a vertical plane (Fig. 15-1).

It can be assumed that there is an optimum moment that must be applied to accomplish this movement; therefore we can consider the moment load imposed on the tooth merely as some definite moment that must be attained without considering absolute values. The objective in treatment is to apply this moment over the greatest possible working distance to reduce the number of necessary adjustments. This requires using the most flexible wire possible to attain the required force level.

The limiting factor is the load on the archwire, so optimum bracket dimensions are those that will deliver a maximum tipping moment to the tooth in proportion to the bending load imposed on the archwire.

The tipping moment is delivered to the tooth through the two points where the arch contacts the bracket or tube at its outer ends (Fig. 15-1). This will be true in tipping actions whether a bracket is single or divided into multiple brackets. For rotations the usual curved contour of the tooth brings the archwire into contact with the inside edge of the bracket, so the working span for most of these actions is actually between the outside of one bracket (where the ligature engages the wire) and the inside of the other (Fig. 15-2). These two points, together with the activating force, form a simple beam arrangement. The load and critical section are at the bracket edge nearest the activating force. For the present we can ignore the fact that the arch continues on to contact additional teeth on either side.

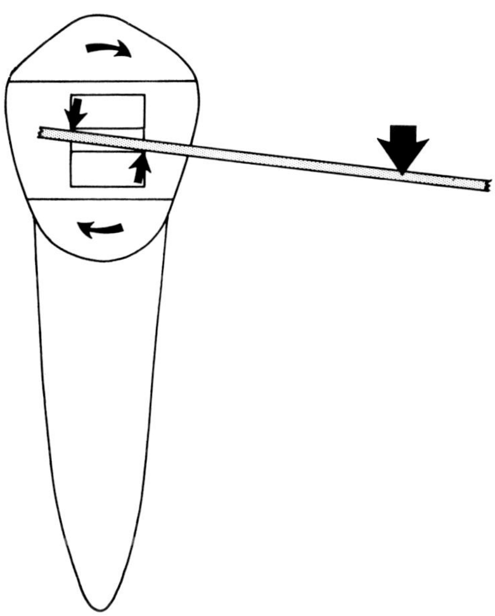

Fig. 15-1. Tipping action on a bicuspid. Arrows at arch show force application to the arch; forces on the tooth at these points will be in opposite directions.

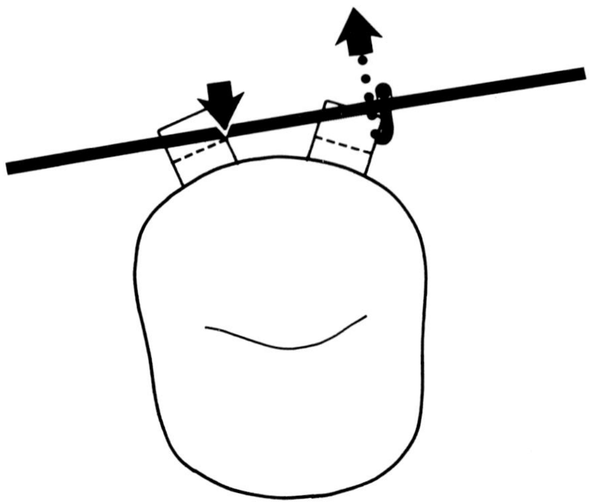

Fig. 15-2. Axial rotations are controlled by two-point arch contact, usually at the inside edge of one bracket and the ligature opposite the outside edge of the other.

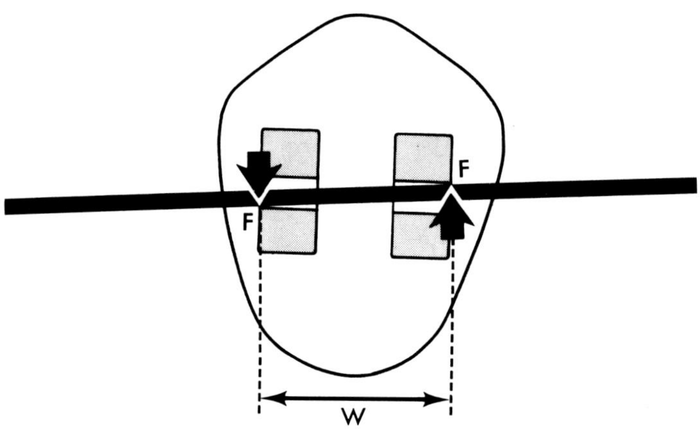

Fig. 15-3. The moment of the couple operating to rotate a tooth in either tipping or axial rotation *(M_t)* is the product of the applied force *(F)* and the distance between points of application *(W)*. $M_t = FW$.

The mechanical effectiveness of the archwire in this situation depends on several interdependent factors.

Required force

First, there is the force that is applied to the tooth to produce the couple acting to tip or rotate it. The moment of this couple on the tooth *(M_t)* will be equal to the force at one end of the attachment *(F)*, multiplied by the attachment width *(W)*, or, $M_t = FW$, as in Fig. 15-3. Any increase in bracket width will proportionately reduce the force required at the bracket ends to produce this tipping moment.

This relationship between force and width is equally important in the use of elastic ligatures to control rotations, because they also operate with a limited available force whose effectiveness will be directly proportional to bracket width.

Bending moment on wire

Second, there is the bending moment produced in the wire by the application of the required force. This is best represented by the third beam illustrated in Fig. 4-4, where the value of the maximum moment in the wire (M_w) is $\frac{Fab}{L}$. The relationship is shown as it applies to a tooth in Fig. 15-4. This is the simplest configuration, such as might be encountered with a tipping or rotating auxiliary. The force levels are higher with a continuous arch rigidly attached to adjacent teeth, but the relative effects of bracket width are essentially the same.

Going back to Fig. 15-3, we can rearrange the formula $M_t = FW$ to the form $F = \frac{M_t}{W}$. Our values for substitution in the formula for maximum bending moment now are:

$$F = \frac{M_t}{W}$$

L = span between tooth centers (about the same as tooth width)
a = W
b = L-W (span minus bracket width)

Substituting these values in the formula $M_w = \frac{Fab}{L}$, we have

$$M_w = \frac{\frac{M_t}{W} W (L - W)}{L}$$

$$= \frac{M_t (L - W)}{L}$$

$$= M_t \frac{L - W}{L}$$

From this we see that bracket width (W) occupies an important position in the numerator, where *any increase will reduce the bending moment on the wire.*

Working range

Third and last is the working range, which will be at its maximum with a bracket width equal to half the span (half the tooth width). In the preceding formula, this is the situation where $a = b$, and $L = 2W$, which is the same configuration as the center-loaded span shown in the second column of Fig. 4-4.

With the bending load on the wire decreasing and working range increasing as this width is approached, it becomes obvious that any narrower width will be less desirable. Even greater widths will reduce the load on the wire more, but the

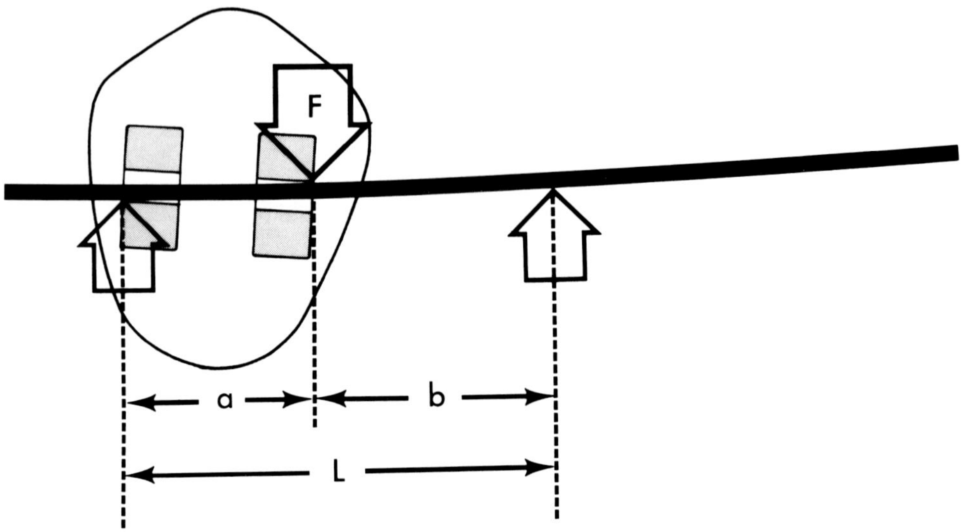

Fig. 15-4. The maximum bending moment applied to the wire (M_w) is at the point of application of the middle force (F). The value of this moment depends on the spacing of the counterforces on either end, as indicated by the dimensions a and b. The formula for this moment is: $M_w = \frac{Fab}{L}$. In this situation F is equal to the sum of the two forces at either end. The smallest force of the two applied to the tooth (left-hand arrow) determines the tipping moment applied to the tooth. The additional force applied at F, which is equivalent to the force of the right-hand arrow, merely adds a translatory effect that in this case will tend to move the tooth occlusally.

simultaneous loss in working range, along with other problems associated with wider brackets, makes any further increase impractical for most applications.

All things considered, optimum bracket width is half the width of the tooth. Differences in effectiveness are small as long as width is close to this size, so that exact width is not critical.

According to this criterion, a bracket 3.5 mm wide will be suitable for bicuspids, cuspids, and upper lateral incisors.

Lower incisors require close control over rotations; therefore brackets of the same width (3.5 mm) may be used on all but the narrowest of these teeth where overlapping contacts do not preclude their use. Severe rotations of lower incisors should be corrected with arch loops or elastic ligatures, and in either of these cases the penalty in working range does not apply as the bracket width increases beyond half the width of the tooth. Loops and elastic ligatures have no practical limits of working range for this application, so every increase in bracket width gives a fully proportional increase in rotation control. Large corrections in mesiodistal tipping, which can be limited when wide brackets of adjacent teeth lie close together, are rarely required for lower anterior teeth, but bracket levels must be controlled carefully because there is little space for compensatory arch adjustments.

Upper central incisors are best managed with *triple* brackets. Individual brackets are spaced the same distance as on the double bracket, so these triple brackets

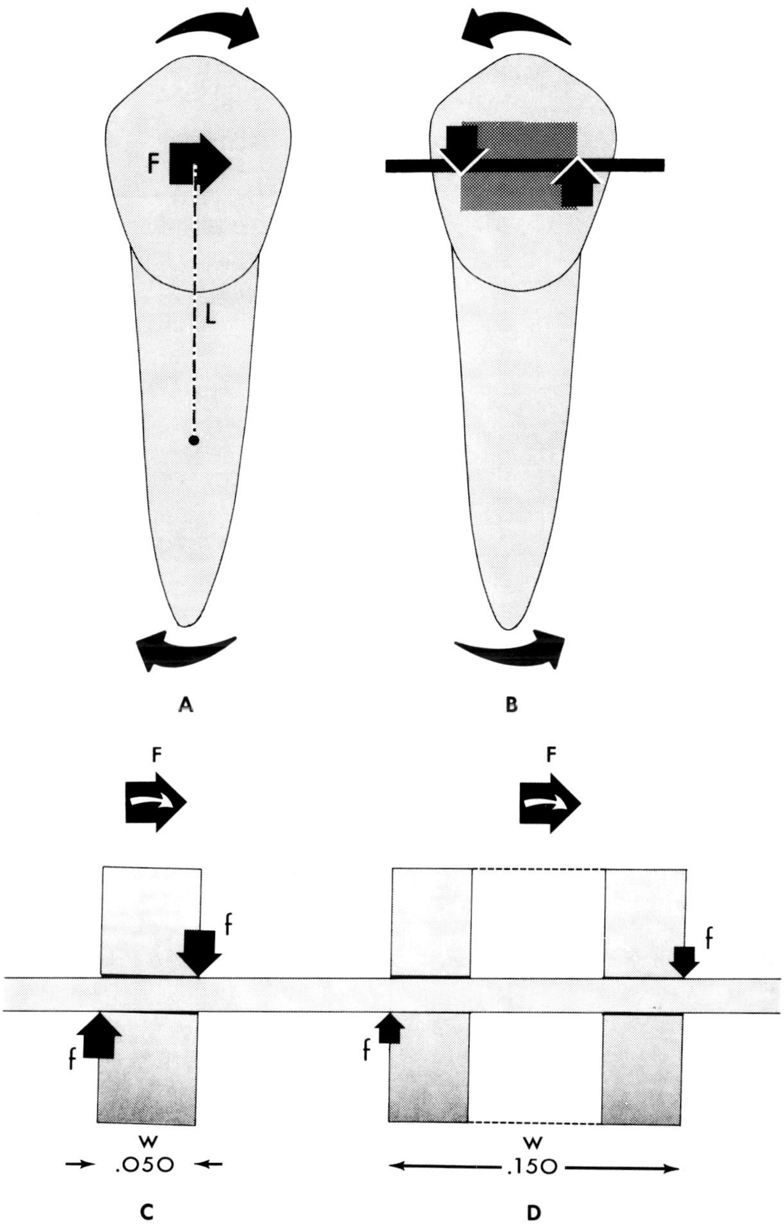

Fig. 15-5. Sliding friction on an archwire is caused by bracket pressure resulting from tipping moments in the tooth. **A,** A tooth being moved laterally will be tipped with a moment, *FL,* equal to the horizontal force, *F,* multiplied by the length of the moment arm, *L.* The moment arm will vary with the nature of the applied force, but it will always terminate somewhere in the root. **B,** The tipping moment is balanced by a couple with an equal moment, formed by the forces exerted by the archwire on the edges of the bracket. The bracket also exerts equal and opposite forces on the archwire at these points. **C** and **D,** The moment of this couple is *fw,* so the actual force on the archwire, *f,* is inversely proportional to the width of the bracket, *w.* Friction is directly proportional to this force, so friction is also inversely proportional to bracket width. In this illustration, the narrow bracket at **C** will generate three times as much frictional resistance as the wide twin bracket at **D.** This difference will become even greater if the narrow bracket allows increased tipping with an accompanying increase in the tipping moment and associated forces.

are less conspicuous than a more widely spaced pair. It is seldom necessary to tie more than two of the three, and selecting the inner or outer pair gives an extra measure of rotation control with minimum arch adjustment. The third (untied) bracket still provides tipping and rotation control as the arch rests in its slot (Fig. 15-15, *A*).

Molars, when they are fitted with brackets instead of tubes, can be well controlled with the same triple brackets used for central incisors.

Bracket width and friction

Friction of bracket on archwire is a consideration whenever a tooth must be moved by sliding it along the wire. Other means are available for horizontal movements, but sliding is often most desirable if friction is not excessive.

Two factors determine friction in any situation: (1) the coefficient of friction of the two surfaces in contact and (2) the force applied between the surfaces. Note especially that *area of contact is not a factor*. Increasing area of contact adds friction-creating surface at exactly the same rate that it reduces force per unit area, so that these effects neutralize each other. Area of contact is important only in the extreme case in which at least one surface becomes so small that it digs into the opposing surface.

In the case of brackets and wires the surfaces are generally smooth and the coefficient of friction is reasonably uniform. The important variable is the force generated between bracket and wire as the collateral tipping tendency of the tooth is resisted by engagement of the wire in the slot. In other words, it is control of collateral tipping and rotation that introduces the friction; so the objective is to achieve that control while still keeping induced friction at a minimum.

The wide bracket also presents a clear advantage in this situation. The same force picture that minimizes distortion of the archwire also results in minimum friction-producing force between bracket and wire.

Fig. 15-5 shows that these frictional forces are inversely proportional to bracket width. A narrow bracket can also increase friction in two other ways; the higher forces with a narrow bracket increase the possibility of indentation, and the increased tipping that it allows can cause a progressive increase in friction-producing force.

A very important point to remember with frictional resistance is that *increasing force will not help* overcome it. The friction-producing force in such toggle locking is derived from the motive force itself. Since frictional resistance is proportional to the force between the surfaces, any force increase will be met with a comparable increase in frictional resistance.

Once frictional locking conditions are encountered in this type of situation, the only hope for restoring movement is to alter the tipping moment that is converting part of the motive force into frictional pressure between the sliding parts.

These principles are readily demonstrated by banding extracted teeth and tying them to a wire or using the arrangement shown in Fig. 18-4 and sliding by hand.

SLOT DIMENSIONS

The original dimensions of the bracket slot and the opening in the molar tube of the edgewise appliance were .022 by .028 inch (.56 by .71 mm). Several bracket slots of smaller dimensions have been introduced since, the most popular being .0185 by .025 or .030 inch (.47 × .63 or .76 mm). While these are manufactured to a .0185-inch standard to provide freedom of fit for full-dimension wires, they are usually referred to as 18-thousandths slots.

Importance of slot and bracket width in tipping actions

Using a wire smaller than the size of the bracket slot will permit a tooth to tip before the ends of the bracket engage the wire. This effect can be seen in Fig. 15-1. Such tipping can be countered by an adjustment in the arch, but making many of these bends routinely is an unnecessary chore. Effective compensation by this method becomes practically impossible in the case of narrow brackets and small wires.

The actual amount of tipping permitted in these situations is presented graphically in Fig. 15-6, which shows, for example, that the narrow 1.25-mm bracket with a .022-inch (.56-mm) slot fitted with a .015-inch (.38-mm) wire will permit nearly 8 degrees of tipping in either direction, a total of 16 degrees. This is excessive. The clinical problem is illustrated in Fig. 15-7, where a .016-inch (.40-mm) wire has permitted considerable tipping in the lower arch. In practice, tipping will usually exceed the values shown in Fig. 15-6, for the graphs are based on precise dimensions. Bracket wear and manufacturing tolerances tend to increase clearances and resultant tipping.

Less than 5 degrees of tipping clearance is not serious, for it is easily controlled. All of the wider brackets stay well within this limit in both slot sizes, so slot size is not an important factor in tipping movements with the recommended wide brackets.

Slot size and freedom of wire movement

Some tooth movements require movement of the wire through the slot. Spaces may sometimes be closed by sliding a tooth along the archwire, and most axial rotations require mesiodistal movement of the bracket along the archwire as the tooth turns. Even very small irregularities in an archwire, such as a straightened bend, can inhibit these movements when the clearance between wire and slot is less than .002 inch (.05 mm).

Slot size and torque control

Torque control with rectangular wires is the *only* movement that requires close engagement of wire and bracket slot. A .001-inch (.025-mm) freedom of the wire in the slot (wire .001 inch or .025 mm thinner than slot) will give from 2 to 4 degrees of freedom in tipping in the direction of torque with common wire widths. A difference of .002 inch (.05 mm) brings this freedom to well over 5 degrees, so for all practical purposes the thickness of any rectangular wire used for torque control should be kept within .002 inch (.05 mm) of the width of the slot. For narrow wires, such as .016 inch (.40 mm) square, even this will provide excessive freedom.

The .018-inch (.45-mm) slot was developed as an adaptation to the higher stiffness of stainless steel. If solid stainless or chrome-cobalt rectangular wires are to be used to apply buccolingual tipping (torque) action, the .018-inch slot is most suit-

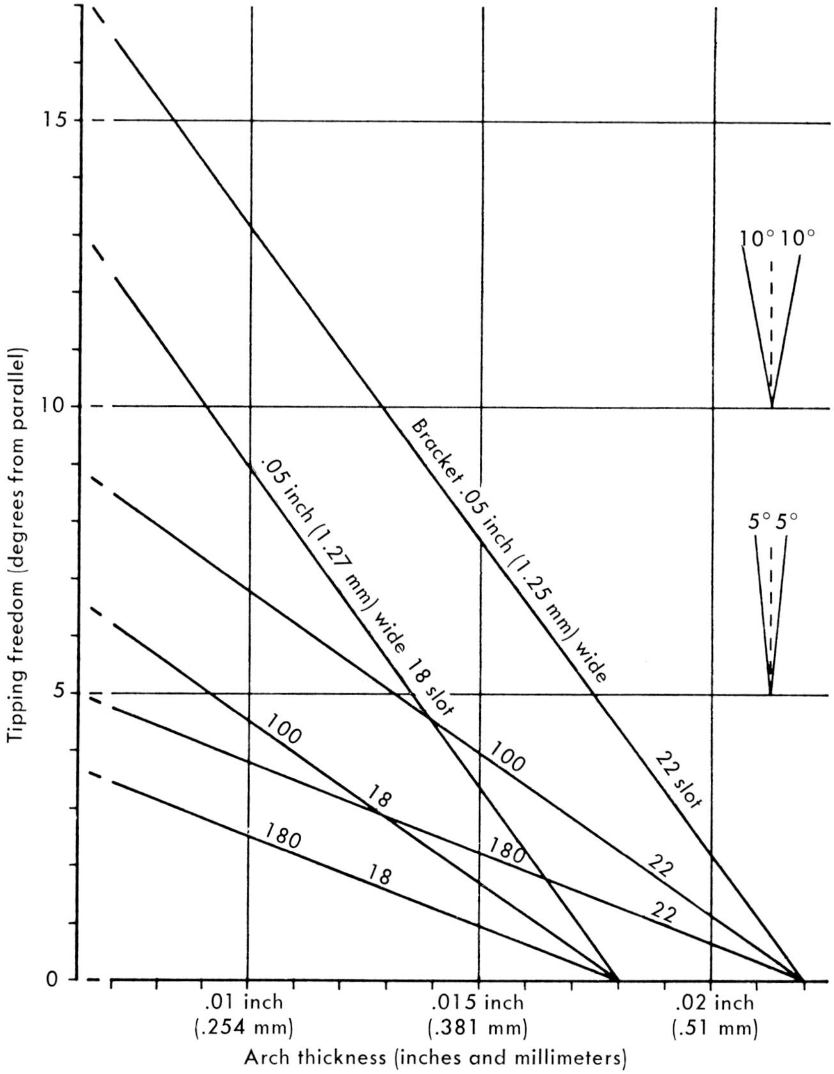

Fig. 15-6. Tipping freedom as it is related to slot width and size of archwire. Graph shows how far tooth can tip in either direction due to "play" of arches from .007 to .022 inches (.18 to .56 mm) in thickness. It shows these effects for brackets .05, .1, and .18 inches (1.25, 2.5, and 4.6 mm) wide, both with .018- and .022-inch (.46- and .56-mm) slots.

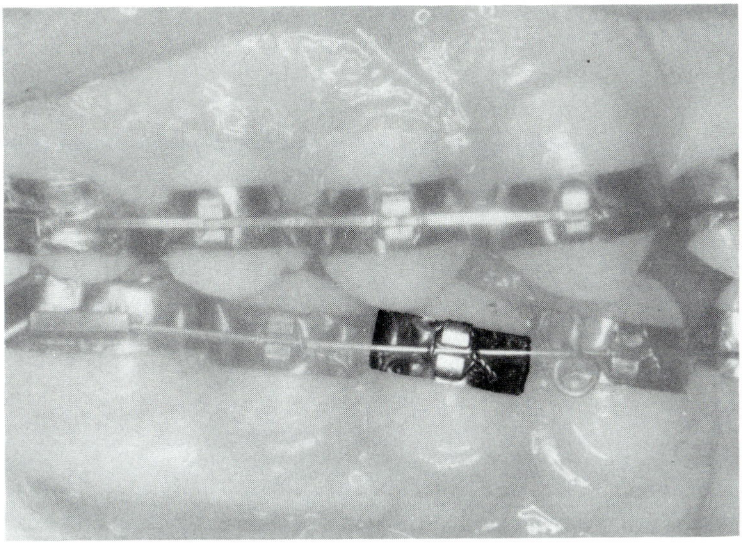

Fig. 15-7. Tipping of buccal teeth with .050-inch (1.25-mm) bracket and .016-inch (.4-mm) lower archwire. Close-fitting rectangular upper archwire shows good control.

able. If gold or laminated stainless steel wires are to be used, the .022-inch (.56-mm) slot may be more effective. The smaller wires cannot be used to apply these actions in a large slot, and the stainless materials in the large size are too stiff for any application other than stabilization.

For all other actions, such as mesiodistal tipping and rotation, the small-diameter wires of any dimension can be used with equal effectiveness in slots of *either* size.

Undersized wires for torque

An important consideration in torque action is the use of undersized wires. Wires that fit the slot too precisely should not be used to torque individual teeth. When a wire with torque action is seated in a bracket, the activation extends over the entire length of the arch. If the passive wire fits passively in the brackets of other teeth, the activation will tip them in the opposite direction. This effect is most pronounced on adjacent teeth, where it will almost equal the intended action in magnitude. The adjacent teeth will not be permanently moved if the arch is left in place long enough to return to a passive state, but in the course of the movement they will have been subjected to an unnecessary back-and-forth action.

Wires adjusted to torque individual teeth should be sufficiently undersized to allow the adjusted wire to rotate in the slot of the adjacent teeth with no transfer of the torque action.

Where all the teeth in an arch need some simultaneous torquing action, a close fit in the slot is not such a problem. In these cases the wire can engage all teeth and move them simultaneously without adverse actions on individual teeth.

The basic rule in this adjustment is that the archwire should be sufficiently undersized to permit free reverse movement equal to any active torque action that is being applied to an adjacent tooth. Freedom of .001 or .002 inches (.025 or .05 mm) will provide this margin with careful adjustment.

Sectional arches or torquing auxiliaries are more suitable for buccolingual root movement in most situations, while a rectangular arch is most effective for maintaining or fine-tuning existing angulations.

Slot depth

Rectangular wires in torque applications must be seated with their outer working edges fully engaged in the slot. Slots should be deep enough to ensure such full engagement. This helps to thwart any tendency for the wires to creep out between adjustments. Even a very small labial movement of a torqued wire can be enough to disengage it from effective activation.

LIGATURE WINGS

Ligature wings on edgewise brackets should be wide and deep, with ample clearance between the wing and the bracket base or band. Each bracket will be tied many times, and any design features that will facilitate this procedure are of distinct value.

Brackets can be situated in very inaccessible spots, and they may become worn or distorted by occlusion. Wide and easily engaged wings can make the difference between a usable and unusable bracket in some of these situations. This is especially true where severe rotation places a bracket deep into an interproximal space.

The improved method of securing ligature ends shown in Fig. 15-15, *B* and *C*, is most easily applied with a relatively wide wing, one that can amply accommodate the twisted pair of wires in addition to the single strand.

Elastic ligatures require more space under the bracket wing than wires do, so they can be much more easily applied when ample space is available.

ANGULATION OF ATTACHMENTS AND SLOTS

Angulation

Angulation of the archwire slot was described by Angle in the series of articles that introduced the edgewise appliance to the profession in 1929. It has been an integral part of the appliance ever since, with ongoing evolution, refinement, and occasional rediscovery over the intervening years.

Like every other detail of appliance design and application, angulation is neither a simple nor an unmixed blessing. Using angulated slots introduces several new considerations that should be evaluated for each application.

It is important to bear in mind that *slot angulation in no way affects the treatment potential of an appliance.* It is a convenience factor and nothing more, so selection decisions should be made on that basis only.

Slots may be angulated in two planes. Occlusogingival angulation, in the plane of the face of the bracket, will influence mesiodistal tipping. Buccolingual angulation of the milled slot, so that a rectangular wire will enter the slot on some angle other than perpendicular to the face, will affect buccolingual tipping in the same way as twisting (torquing) the wire.

Occlusogingival angulation

The objective of occlusogingival angulation of an archwire slot is to reduce or eliminate the need for archwire adjustments for mesiodistal tipping control. Angulating the slot so that it is parallel to the occlusal plane instead of perpendicular to the root of the tooth accomplishes the objective of optimizing the mesiodistal tipping angulation of the tooth without the need for corresponding bends in the archwire. This was the objective of the angulation described by Angle in his classic 1929 article (Fig. 15-8).

The slot angulation may be accomplished in either of two ways: angulating the bracket on the tooth, as in Fig. 15-8, or angulating the slot in the bracket. The effects are identical. Convenience in bracket and archwire placement is the only consideration in the choice between the two.

Angulating the bracket is the simplest and most controllable approach; angulation is under direct control as the bracket or band is applied, so it can be adjusted as required for the anatomy of the individual dentition.

Angulating the slot in the bracket is a manufacturing process in which the angle must be based on average values; it is controllable by the doctor only by compensatory angulation of the bracket on the tooth at the time of application.

Two parameters can be affected by mesiodistal angulation of the arch slot: arch adjustment and effective bracket width.

Arch adjustment. Built-in preangulation of the bracket slot can eliminate the need for basic arch adjustment in the affected plane, but the necessity for compensatory adjustments to adapt to the requirements imposed by collateral tipping, individual anatomy, wire size, and stiffness will still remain. Ignoring these needs on the assumption that a standardized bracket angulation will meet them can be disastrous.

Special attention is required to prevent excessive tipping when overcompensations are built into the preangulation, as in those sometimes referred to as "extrac-

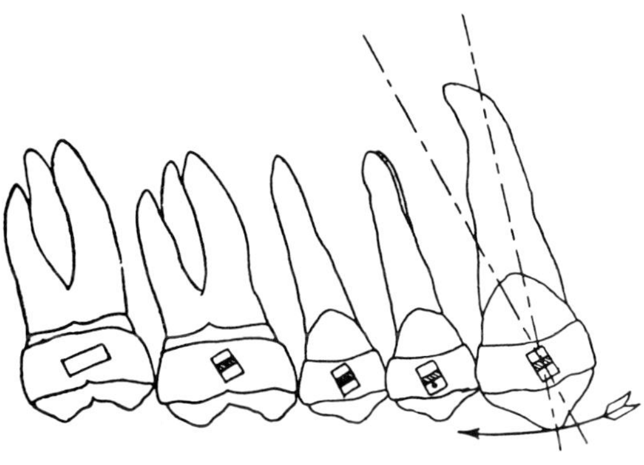

Fig. 15-8. Angulating brackets, as recommended by Angle, to induce distal tipping in the buccal segment. Inserting a straight arch into such angulated brackets has the same effect as multiple tipping bends in the arch. These angulations are the opposite of those in current use to control distal tipping. (From Angle, E.H.: Dental Cosmos **71**:262, 1929.)

tion" brackets. Optimum angulation of the teeth is not related to whether or not other teeth were removed in the course of treatment.

Effective bracket width. Brackets control tipping by contact with the archwire at the top on one end of the slot and at the bottom on the other end. The critical mesial and distal working contacts between archwire and bracket are usually on the side of the slot that is shortened by angulation of the slot within the bracket. The result is a bracket that appears to be much wider than its actual effective working width (Fig. 15-9). The geometry of these brackets also increases the span of the ligature across the wire, reducing its effectiveness proportionately.

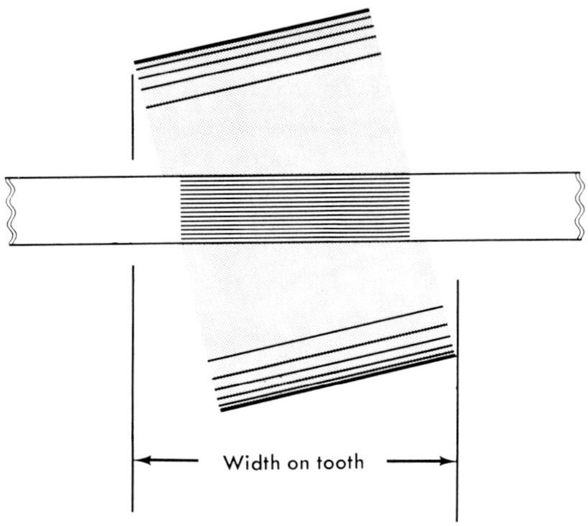

Fig. 15-9. Effective working length of angulated slots is less than the slot length and much less than the mesiodistal width of the bracket on the tooth. Bracket engagement to accomplish the tipping control for which the slot is angulated is on the short side of the slot at each end, as shown by the shaded section of wire.

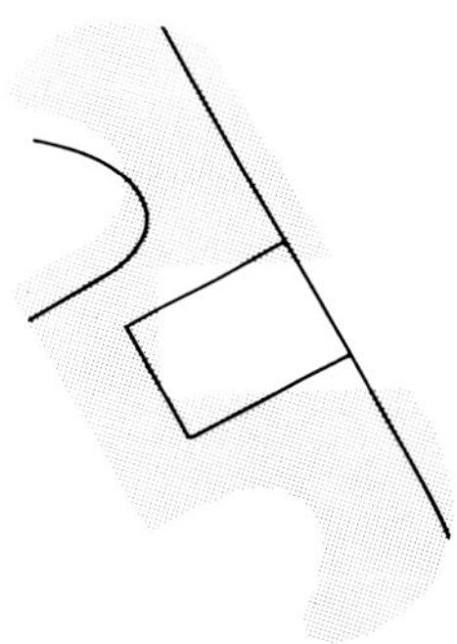

Fig. 15-10. Buccolingual (torque) slot angulation requires increased bracket dimensions to maintain thickness and strength. The lines show the more compact dimensions for comparable strength with a perpendicular slot.

Buccolingual angulation (torque)

Angulating slots for buccolingual tipping control follows the same rationale as other built-in angulations, but the side effects are more subtle and numerous. Accomplishing the angulation without compromising slot depth requires either a reduction in bracket strength or an increase in bracket thickness (Fig. 15-10).

The side of the critical working contact between archwire and bracket slot for torquing action is usually the shallowest side, making full slot depth and full seating absolutely essential for control.

No torque adjustments are required if the angulation of the slot is ideal for the patient's needs, but additional tipping or compensatory relief of excessive tipping is often desirable in individual cases.

Vertical effects (for both round and rectangular wires). Built-in torque control introduces a subtle vertical effect that can have a significant negative influence. A slot oriented to the occlusal plane instead of to the tooth is actually inclined occlusally in relation to the root of the tooth (Fig. 15-11).

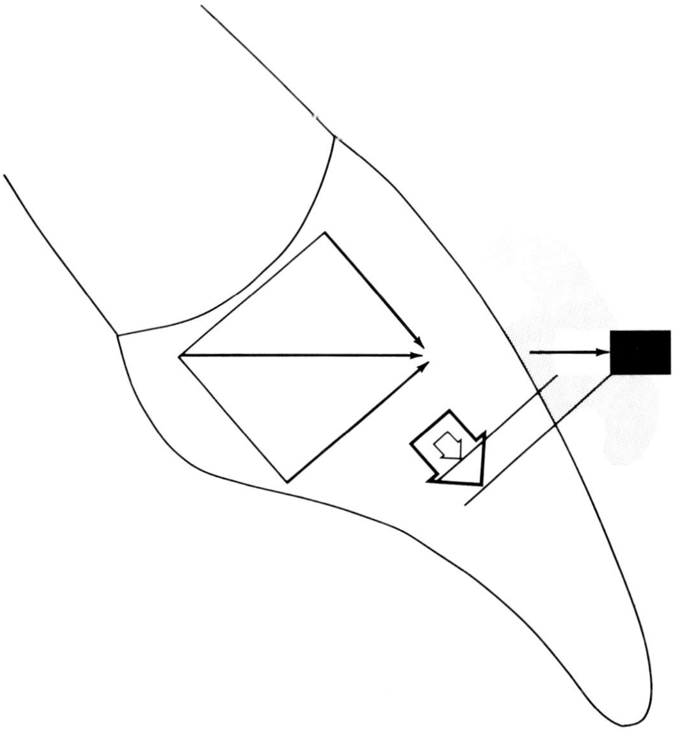

Fig. 15-11. Buccolingual (torque) angulation introduces a subtle elongating effect whenever the passive archwire does not seat completely in the slot. Slot angulation includes a significant incisally directed component, as shown by the vector diagram. The short lines mark the distance that the tooth will be extruded in its socket when ligated to the archwire shown. Each archwire change can impose this effect on at least some teeth, so the cumulative effect over a complete treatment program can be significant.

Ligating an archwire toward a fully seated position in the slot when it does not seat passively in the bottom of the slot will cause the tooth to move in a direction guided by the walls of the slot. The occlusal component in the orientation of angulated slots will cause the tooth to move occlusally (extrusion) in relation to the alveolar socket. Such extrusion is usually unwanted.

A single movement of this kind may be small, but repeated ligation of successive archwires as treatment progresses can have a large cumulative effect. This makes it especially important to very carefully adjust archwires for full bracket slot engagement in the passive condition when they are being used with torque-angulated bracket slots.

Visual cues in archwire adjustment

Ambiguity and loss of important visual cues for archwire formation and adjustment with angulated bracket slots can have an insidious effect on treatment quality, efficiency, and convenience.

Archwires are typically adjusted by introducing bends deviating from the level arch in the direction of the desired tooth movement. Angulation of bracket slots to accomplish some of these same ends without archwire adjustment will have one of the following three effects, depending on the needs of the individual patient:

1. It will eliminate the need for an adjustment.
2. It will reduce the amount of adjustment required.
3. It will overcompensate, requiring a negative compensating adjustment in the archwire.

It is the third of these situations that can add to the difficulty of fine control over tooth movement. With the bracket slot oriented for too much of a good thing, the archwire must be adjusted in what would ordinarily be an unwanted direction. That kind of adjustment is ordinarily made only in the early stages of treatment to partially adapt to a malocclusion. Succeeding adjustments gradually eliminate or even reverse them.

When such atypical adjustments must be incorporated into the finishing arches, unusually close attention is required to make them correctly and to avoid inadvertently removing them at later visits.

Conservative slot angulations unlikely to require such reverse compensation will minimize this type of problem. It is much easier to finish a case with small adjustments acting in concert in similar directions than with a mixture of positive and negative adjustments.

The problems of visual cues are especially difficult to deal with in the buccolingual (torque) adjustments, where no good visual references are available for monitoring adjustments with angulated slots. In the mesiodistal direction the long slot provides a good visual reference for arch adjustments in this plane, even when angulation of the slot in the bracket makes the other bracket surfaces useless for this purpose. No comparable reference remains when a slot is angulated buccolingually for torque control purposes.

When the slot has been milled perpendicular to the face of the bracket, applying a torquing key to the wire and observing its relationship to the bracket face gives a quick and accurate visualization of the activation of the wire even before it is inserted into the slot. With an angulated slot there is no surface available for such use as a visual reference. The wire must be actually inserted into the slot, observing the movement of the seating instrument as the arch is seated to determine its effective activation. This can be especially difficult to accomplish with adjustments that involve closely adjoining teeth.

Other considerations in slot angulation

One of the major advantages of slot angulation, especially buccolingual angulation, accrues as a result of the reduction in bends in the archwire between teeth. This leaves the arch smooth for attachments to slide along the wire as teeth move, without the need for careful positioning of bends in anticipation of such movements.

On the negative side, inventory requirements are greatly increased with right and left versions required in most situations. This carries with it an increase in the probability of misfiled attachments and resultant placement of attachments in the wrong position.

The benefits of added convenience are gained only with consistent use of a specific type of slot angulation for a specific tooth in the arch, such as cuspid or central incisor. This is true whether the angulation is the basic perpendicular or some other type. Using one type of angulation only in selected cases can complicate rather than simplify overall appliance management.

On the other hand, angulating the attachment on one tooth in a specific way does not necessarily create a need to use a similar angulation elsewhere in the arch.

With the foregoing considerations in mind, the following suggestions are offered for specific teeth. The simple governing rule is to orient the attachment to a level arch rather than square it to some arbitrary part of the tooth that lies at a different angle to the plane of the arch.

Bicuspids and lower incisors

Bicuspids and lower incisors can be adequately controlled by means of wide brackets and arch adjustments, with no angulation of either bracket or slot. When the narrow .050-inch (1.25-mm) brackets were used, it was necessary to angulate bicuspid brackets to *prevent* tipping due to freedom of fit in the bracket, but the control afforded by wide double brackets makes this unnecessary.

Cuspids

Cuspids should be fitted with brackets attached at an angle of about 5 degrees. These brackets are angulated for mesial crown angulation, so different attachments will be required for right and left sides when angulated slots or brackets prewelded to bands are used. (This angulation is the opposite of that shown in Fig. 15-8.)

Bracket slots on cuspids need not be angulated for torque, but these teeth do require torque control when rectangular wires are used, to keep roots tipped lingually. This can be done by arch adjustment with any slot angulation.

Upper central incisors

Upper central incisors are managed most effectively with triple brackets. All three may be tied, or selective tying of the mesial or distal pair will provide fine rotation control with minimum arch adjustment. These brackets harmonize well esthetically with double brackets on lateral incisors because the spacing between individual brackets is the same.

If torque slots are used on these teeth, the angulation should be 20 or 25 degrees. No bracket angulation is required.

Upper lateral incisors

Upper lateral incisors are the only teeth that can benefit from angulation of both bracket and slot. Because of the shape of these teeth, the best-fitted band will usually be inclined so that the mesial side of the band is in a more gingival position than the distal side (Fig. 15-12). Angulating the bracket 4 to 8 degrees will offset this effect and make it easier to keep the correct axial inclination of the tooth. Bonded brackets are not affected by this band-related angulation.

These teeth also need some torque action, but not so much as the central incisors. Angulating the slots of the brackets about 5 degrees less than the central incisors will maintain an approximately correct relationship between lateral and central incisors.

Molars

The wide variations in molar anatomy make individualization very desirable in many cases. This can be achieved fully by welding attachments at the time that bands are fitted, or partially by prewelded attachments specially oriented for each right and left position.

The last molar to be under archwire control is normally fitted with a buccal tube. Angulation for a slight distal tipping action is desirable in most cases (Fig. 15-23). A double tube in this position adds great versatility, providing two alternatives for archwire level as well as a means for attaching a broad variety of auxiliaries.

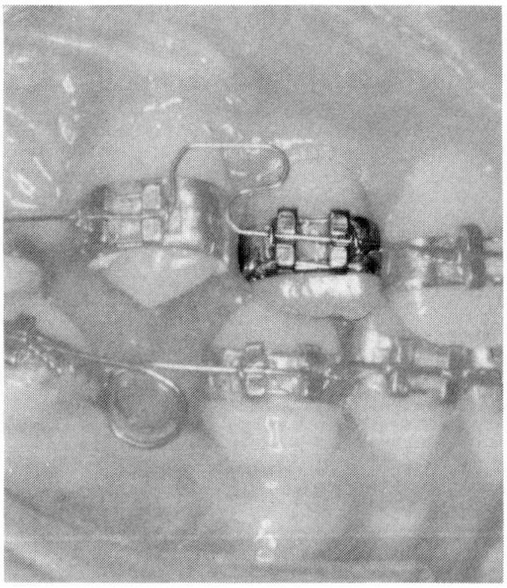

Fig. 15-12. Angulation of the bracket on a lateral incisor will compensate for the natural angulation of a band on the tooth, but this large compensation is not a factor with direct bonding.

When the first molar is not the last controlled molar, it is usually fitted with a wide bracket instead of a tube. A tube may be used, provided that first and second molar tubes are aligned with sufficient precision so that no archwire adjustments will be needed between the two teeth, but this can be difficult to achieve.

Numerous bracket variations are used in this position. Bracket width is a great advantage in controlling these large teeth, so this is the primary consideration. Triple brackets or very wide double brackets are recommended. A removable cap on the bracket may be used to convert it into two short tubes and so eliminate the need for ligation, but threading an archwire through both brackets can often be as difficult as ligation.

Auxiliary attachments cover a broad range of options. Hooks may be attached buccally or lingually, especially when a tube is not available for adding one later. A lingual arch provides exceptionally effective molar control, and its lingual tube can also provide attachment for an auxiliary hook when the arch is not being used.

LIGATURES

Arches are held in place in the bracket slots by fully annealed stainless steel ligatures .008 to .012 inch (.20 to .30 mm) in diameter, or by elastic ligatures. These may be applied in many ways, depending on requirements. My preference in nearly all situations is hand tying with .009-inch (.23-mm) wire. Smaller wires may break, and heavier wires do not adapt as well to the bracket and archwire without mechanical aid. The added stiffness of heavy wires results in a looser ligation with hand tying, so these wires are often placed with a ligature locking and tying pliers that provides the mechanical advantage necessary to pull them snugly into position. Whenever a ligature must sustain a heavy load, the larger wires applied with the pliers are most effective.

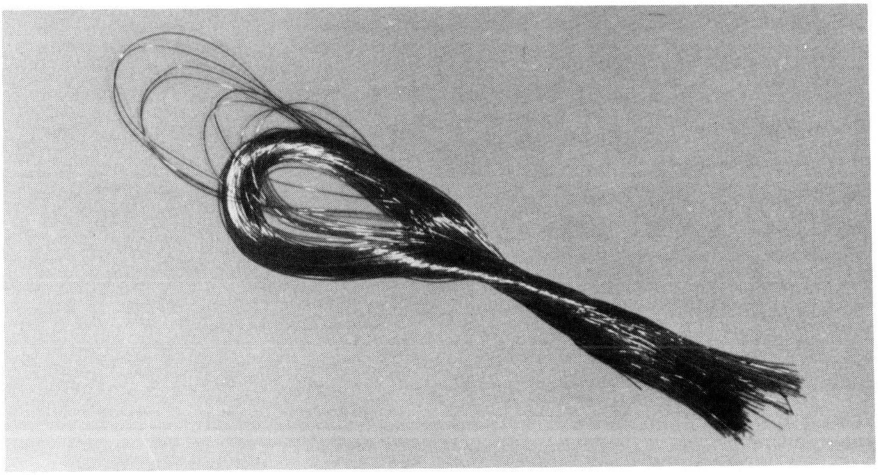

Fig. 15-13. Hank of ligature wires cut in individual lengths.

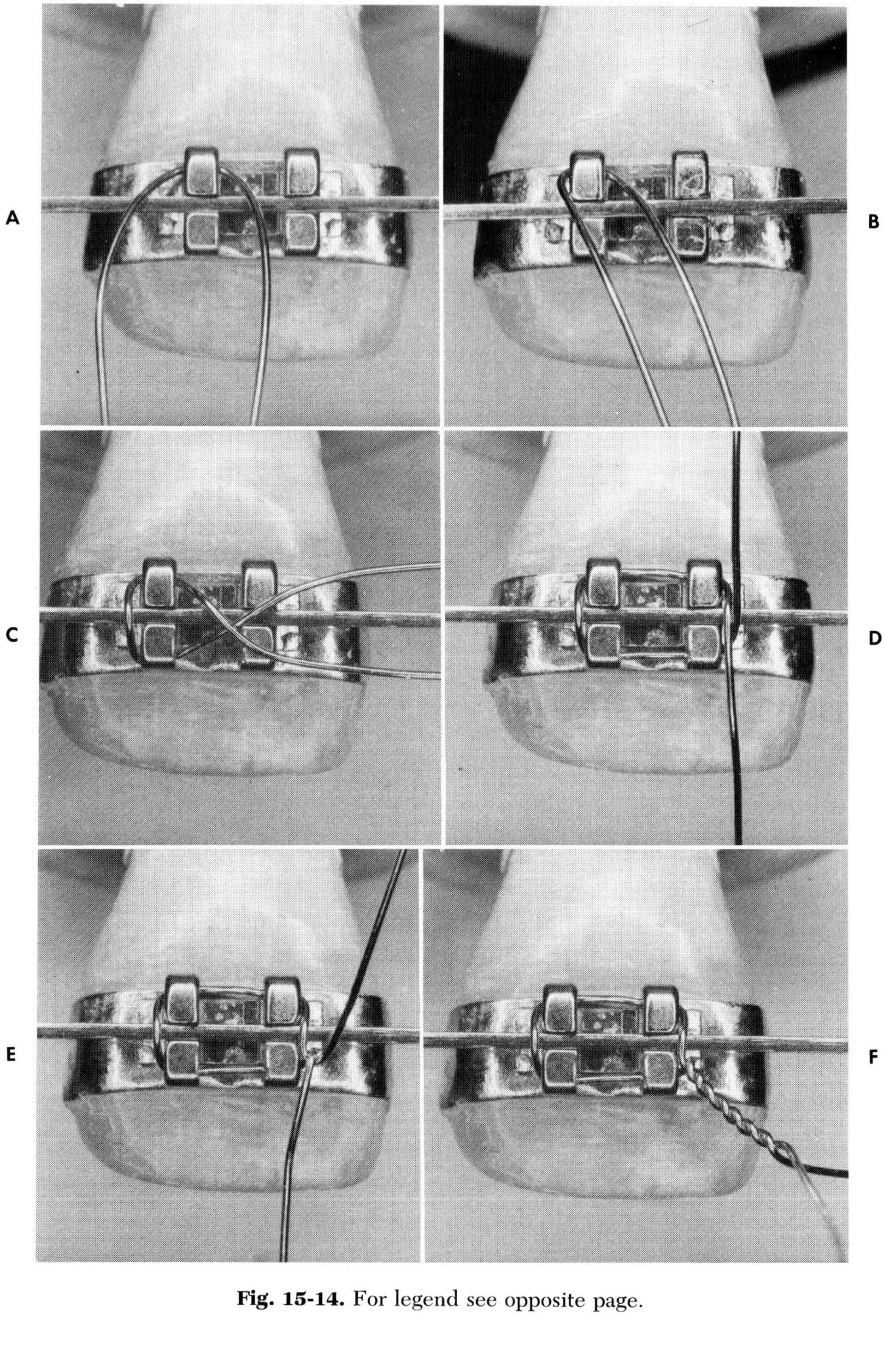

Fig. 15-14. For legend see opposite page.

G 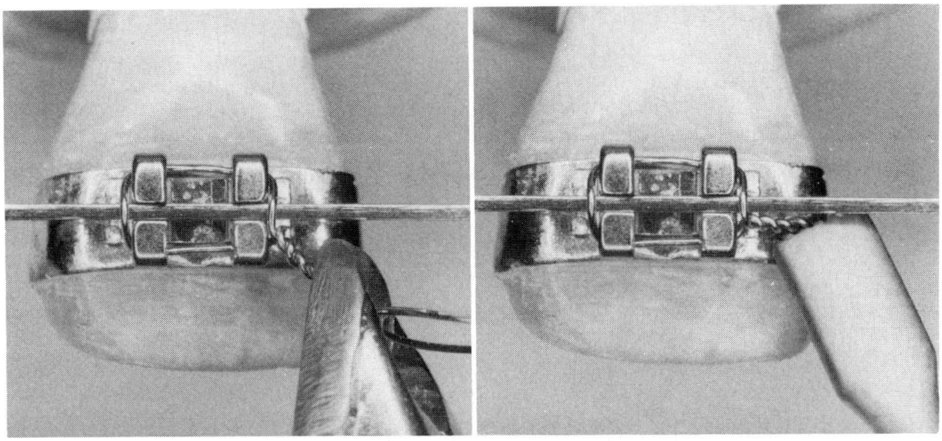 H

Fig. 15-14. Wire is looped over gingival wing, **A,** pulled tight to conform to the bracket, **B,** brought over incisal wing, lightly crossed, **C,** and pulled tight again for shaping. The wire is then brought under the wings of the other bracket and pulled tight across the archwire, **D.** The first twist, **E,** must be made tightly. This locking twist establishes the tightness of the ligature; it cannot be effectively tightened by later twists. The strand that crosses the archwire should lie against the bracket. Twisting is continued, **F,** to form an ample "pigtail." In conventional tying, the wires are cut, **G,** and the end is tucked under the arch wire, **H.**

Breakage of ligature wires in service is hardly ever a tension failure; it is fatigue failure due to localized work hardening. Tying technique should be so controlled that the wire is never bent more than once at any one place, because repeated bending will rapidly harden and embrittle it enough to cause breakage. Care should be taken to avoid applying excessive loads with the ligature locking and tying pliers. Breakage between appointments is usually brought about by the patient's finding a loose end and either playing with it or bending it repeatedly in an attempt to tuck it out of the way.

Another common cause of breakage is attempting to tighten a ligature by tightening the twist with pliers. Tightness should be established with the first half-twist, with additional twists serving to keep this load-bearing twist from unwinding. Further twisting with pliers subjects the sharply bent wire to loads more than a hundred times the force applied at the pliers handle.

Ligature wire is stocked in hanks of individual 12-inch (30-cm) lengths (Fig. 15-13) from which single wires may be pulled as needed.

Basic ligation

The basic procedure for ligation with a double or twin bracket is shown in Fig. 15-14. The looped ligature wire is caught under one wing of the bracket (Fig. 15-14, *A*), pulled tight to give it a bend at the bracket edge (Fig. 15-14, *B*), and then caught under the other wing and pulled tight (Fig. 15-14, *C*). It is next brought under the two wings of the other bracket, and the ends are pulled across the arch to shape it at these bracket edges (Fig. 15-14,*D*). One end is kept across the arch, and the two ends are kept under light tension as they are twisted on one side of

A

B

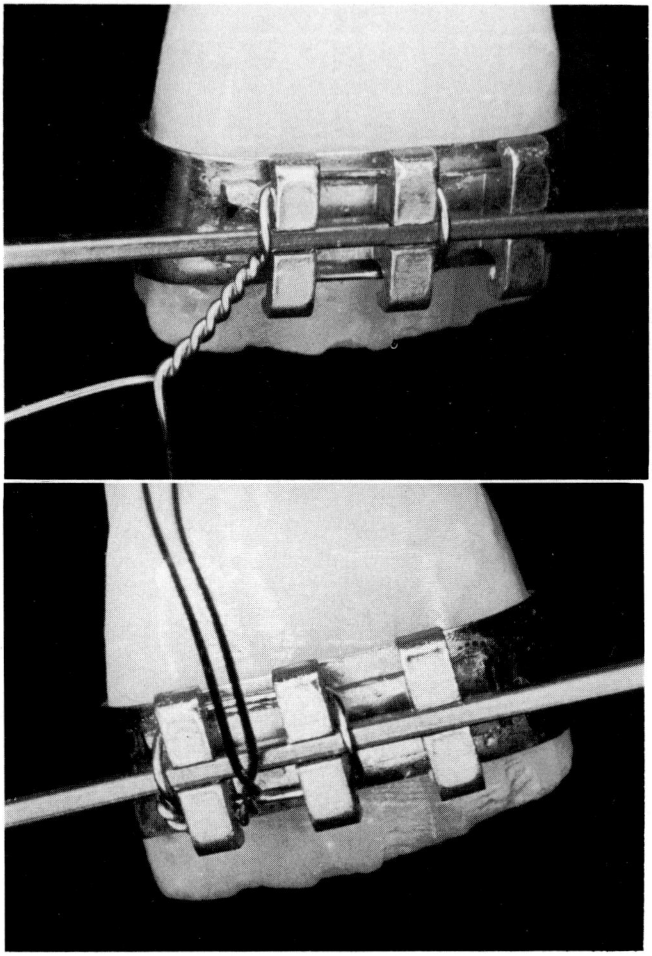

Fig. 15-15. A to **C,** Wide-wing brackets permit an improved method of securing the end by twisting the ends as usual, pulling the twisted pair under the bracket wing, grasping lightly with the cutters and pulling tight with a rotating action against the bracket, then cutting the end flush with the bracket edge.

the arch (Fig. 15-14, *E* and *F*). The end that crossed the archwire should be closest to the bracket as the twist is begun.

It makes no difference whether the two ends of the wire are twisted on the occlusal or the gingival side of the arch, but they must not be twisted directly over the arch.

In the classical edgewise ligation the twisted ends are cut with ligature-cutting pliers (Fig. 15-14, *G*), and the end is tucked under the archwire (Fig. 15-14, *H*). The end must be tucked under from the side on which the twist was begun, not across the arch and then under. This helps to keep the ligature tight and the surface smooth.

An improved method of completing the ligation is made possible by the wide

C

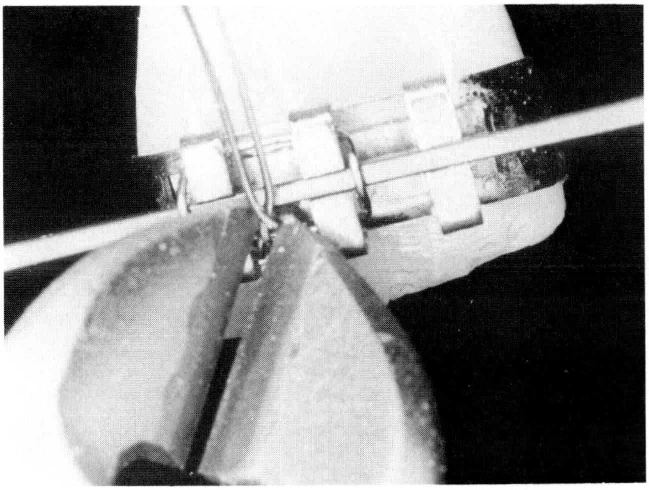

Fig. 15-15, cont'd. For legend see opposite page.

bracket wings that will easily accommodate the twisted "pigtail." In this method the twisted end is pulled under the bracket wing as soon as the twisting is completed (Fig. 15-15, *A* and *B*). It is then grasped lightly with the ligature-cutting pliers (Fig. 15-15, *C*), and, with a twisting action against the bracket, pulled snugly under the wing. The ligature cutter is then shifted to lie closely against the bracket wing, and the end is cut off flush. This places the twisted ends securely out of the way and eliminates the need for a separate tucking operation.

Preformed ligatures

Preformed ligatures with the ends formed to help engage the bracket wings may also be used. These are slipped under the bracket wings as shown in Fig. 15-16, and the tie is completed as before.

Ligature-locking pliers

The ligature-locking pliers (Fig. 15-17, *A*) may be used to twist the ends of the wires instead of twisting them by hand. While this will produce a tighter twist, it is seldom necessary. These pliers provide such a large amount of tensile force that they should not ordinarily be used with wires smaller than .010 inch (.25 mm) in diameter, and they must be used with care with any wire to avoid breakage.

In use, they are squeezed to pull the wire tight as in Fig. 15-17, *A*. Note that there is still some roundness as the ligature passes over the archwire on the side away from the pliers; this is as it should be, and efforts to pull it down too snugly will break or weaken the wire. After the wire has been formed in this way, *pressure is partially released* as the first half-twist is made in the wire. As the first twist is completed, pressure is relaxed even further, because the additional twists serve only to keep the first one from unwinding and so require only enough pressure to keep the pliers in place (Fig. 15-17, *B*). This avoidance of unnecessary stress on the wire is the key to breakage prevention.

A 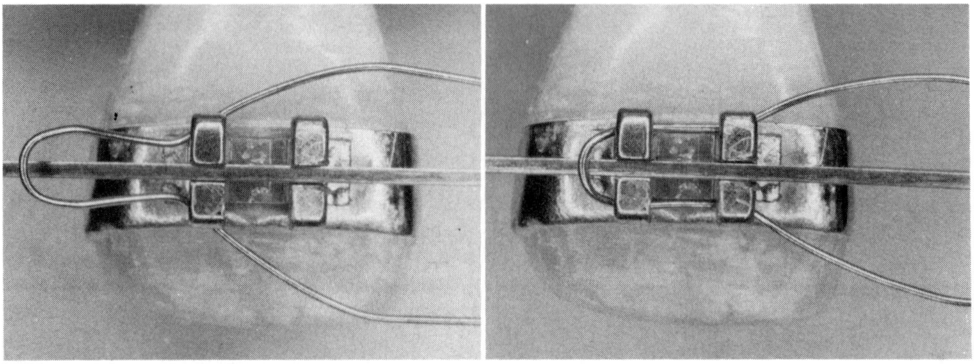 B

Fig. 15-16. A and **B,** Preformed ligature wires are placed directly under both wings; care must be taken to ensure that the loop conforms closely to archwire and bracket.

A 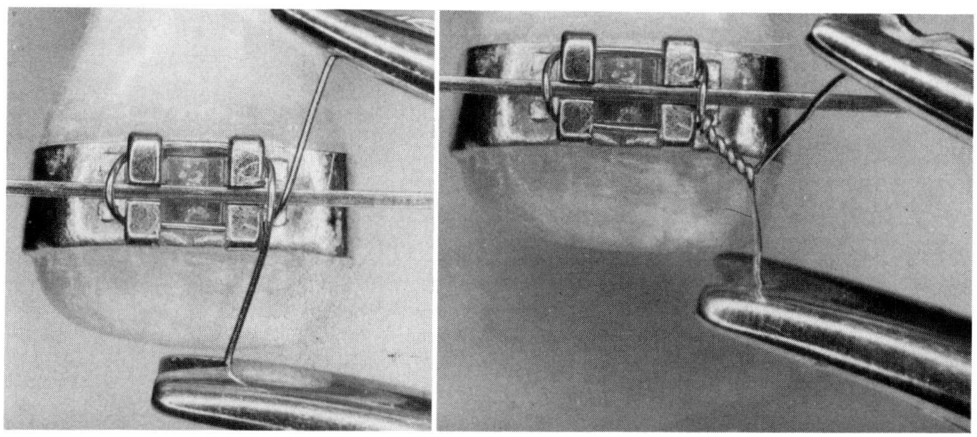 B

Fig. 15-17. A and **B,** Ligature-locking and tying pliers may be used to pull the wire tight and twist the ends.

Alternate methods of tying

With multiple brackets, several alternate methods may be used to lace the archwire in place.

A single bracket may be tied if it is desirable to leave the others free for rotation or for other purposes.

The archwire may be held more securely if the ligatures are crossed between the brackets, as shown in Fig. 15-18, *A* and *B*. *This is actually the optimum tie for most applications, because it provides added security as well as a convenient place for cutting the wire when the ligature must be removed.*

Additional twists may be made between the brackets, either above or below the arch, as shown in Fig. 15-18, *C*.

In some situations one wing of the bracket may be extremely difficult to engage.

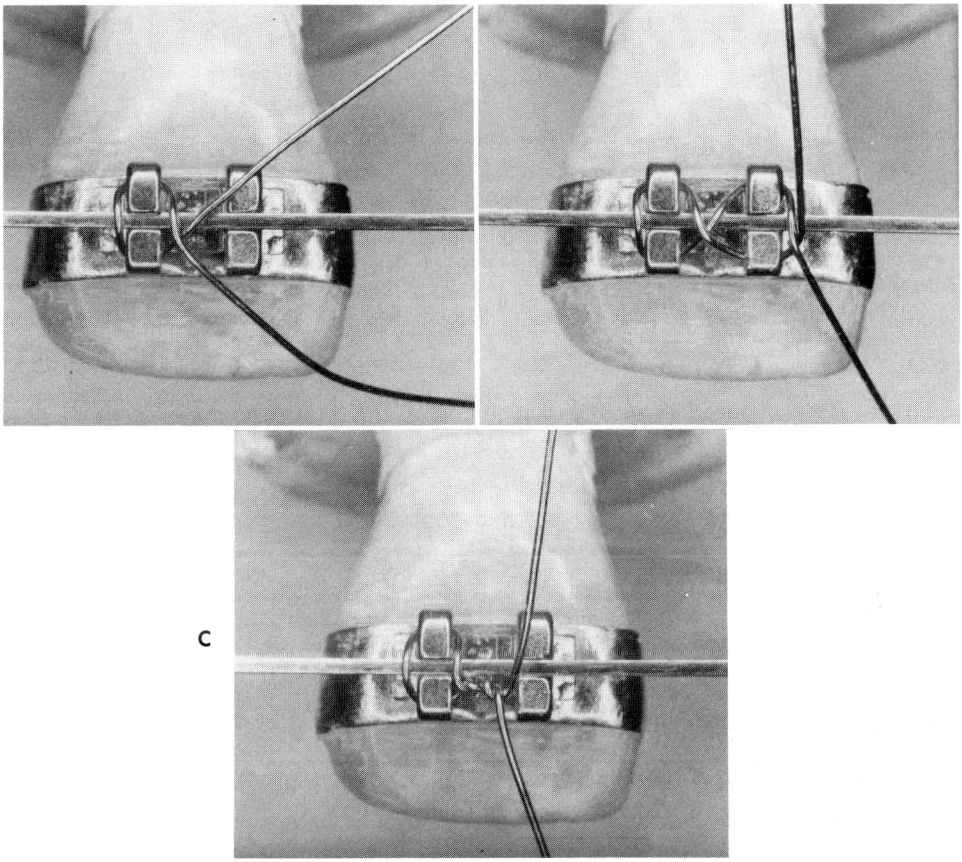

Fig. 15-18. **A** and **B,** For more arch control, wires may be crossed between brackets and tied in the usual way. This same tie may be used between adjacent teeth to hold them together, in which case it is often referred to as a figure-eight tie. **C,** For maximum security, the wires may be twisted into a "pigtail" between brackets. This is also useful between adjacent teeth.

This is frequently true of the gingival wing of a bracket that is rotated into the interproximal area. One can engage this wing more easily by first placing the wire over the occlusal wing and pulling it tight to form it to the exact contour of the bracket wing and then removing it and teasing it over the gingival wing. The remainder of the ligature is tied as usual.

Multiple-tooth ligation

Ligatures may also be used in a similar way to tie teeth together at the same time that the teeth are tied to the arch. This may be done either to close small spaces or to hold spaces closed. The most common method is to use exactly the same type of tie shown in Fig. 15-18 between the brackets of adjacent teeth. A separate ligature may be used at each interproximal space, or one wire may be extended across several teeth (usually called a figure-eight tie). A half-twist between the twin brackets on each tooth will secure such a wire on intermediate teeth, finishing on the last tooth the same as a single tie.

This multiple figure-eight tie is not only useful for holding teeth together, but also is easily and rapidly placed, so much so that there may be a temptation to overuse it. The following characteristics and precautions should be kept in mind in the use of this form of ligation:

Space closure with this ligation is minimal—limited to the immediate movement allowed by the periodontal ligament at the time of tying.

Additional space closure by other forces may be inhibited—the stiffness of the ligatures is sufficient to maintain the teeth in their position as tied.

Other movements may be inhibited by the rigid trusswork of the combined arch/ligature/contact point structure. A good rule is to avoid this type of ligation on any teeth that are not already in their final position.

It is very useful in consolidating anchorage. Elastic ligatures or springs to move another tooth may be attached to the last tooth of several tied together in this way to serve as anchorage.

It takes longer to remove than to place them, sometimes longer than individual ligatures.

Elastic ligatures

Molded or extruded elastic ligatures may be substituted for wire ligatures to good effect in most situations. These ligatures may be applied with a small-tip explorer, needle holder, or any of a number of specially designed applicators.

Where rotation control is a consideration, wide double brackets are an even greater necessity with elastic than with wire ligatures. Rotation control with the short moment arm of narrow brackets requires higher force levels than can be applied by the elastomeric material.

Elastic ligatures provide important advantages over wire ligatures for both doctor and patient. Ease of application is a help for both. The added comfort provided by the smooth elastic module, with no sharp ends that might cause irritation between visits, is a major plus for the patient.

Their elasticity also aids comfort and tooth movement by easing individual teeth into full engagement over an extended period between adjustments, rather than with the instantaneous heavy force application typical with wire ligatures. Used in this way, the elasticity of the ligature serves the energy storage function instead of or in addition to the archwire.

With wide double brackets this action can correct a slightly rotated tooth by bringing the partially engaged bracket into full archwire engagement. In these cases it is absolutely essential that both brackets of the pair be at least partially engaged at the time that the ligature is placed; an elastic ligature cannot be expected to bring a wire into the slot, and in most cases a tooth that is already tipped too far for engagement will tip even farther from the bracket slot before the next patient visit.

The smoothness of an elastic ligature, along with its limited strength, make it the ligature of choice in most cases that require sliding of a bracket on the archwire.

The superficially simple sliding action usually involves a collateral rotation effect that must be resisted by the ligature. This tends to tighten a wire ligature and so inhibit the motion; with an elastic ligature the movement is more free, but it is important to adequately control the rotation, as discussed in Chapter 18.

The major disadvantage of elastic ligatures is their relatively low strength. They are sufficiently strong for most applications, but for situations requiring heavier force levels or for patients who abuse appliances, the added strength of wire ligatures may be required. The strength and inflexibility of wire ligatures may also provide more secure ligation where appliance design calls for using a wire loop or other flexible arch component as the energy storage component.

MOLAR CONTROL

As the last tooth on the arch, a first or second molar is subjected to the resultants of many of the forces applied to other teeth in the arch. These may cover the complete range of possible tooth movements. Since the molar is a large tooth immediately adjacent to one or two relatively small bicuspids, it is difficult to move the molar significantly without either bypassing or adversely affecting those teeth. Management of these problems depends entirely on the attachments, so their selection is a critical decision that will govern many actions throughout treatment.

Problems in molar control are twofold: more unfavorable forces requiring control, combined with a limited mechanical advantage available through the cantilevered arch end for accomplishing that control.

The added forces are the collateral tipping and rotation moments that accompany space closure and intermaxillary traction (Fig. 15-19). These effects directly relate to the location of these teeth and are in addition to original orthodontic

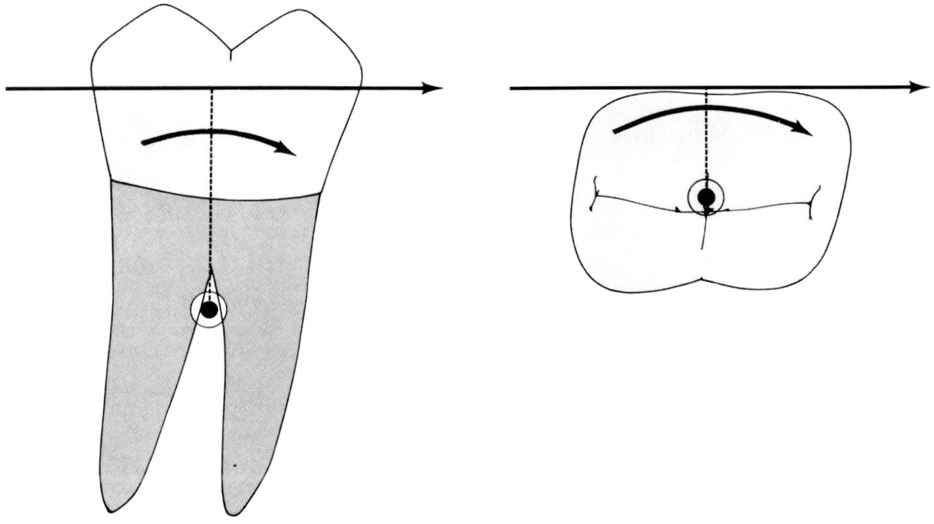

Fig. 15-19. Mesial traction on a molar produces collateral mesial tipping and axial rotation moments. Moment arms for these effects extend from the line of force to the center of resistance, as shown by the broken lines.

problems such as crossbites, which may also need control. Mechanical problems are those related to the cantilevered position of the molar on the arch, with no tooth available on the distal side to provide archwire support.

A wide variety of attachments and associated mechanisms are available for molar control. These will be discussed here in sufficient detail to understand the function of the attachments, with additional coverage where it is appropriate in the discussion of therapy.

Buccal tube or sheath

This is the basic molar attachment of the edgewise and most other arch mechanisms. The inside dimensions ordinarily match those used for the bracket slot, either .0185 × .025 inch (.46 × .63 mm) or .022 × .028 inch (.55 × .70 mm), although an oversize lumen can be used to advantage in some situations. Length is a critical factor that varies over a broad range.

If suitable auxiliaries are used, the dimensions of this tube may be of little importance, but if it is the only source of molar control, this mechanical advantage must be exploited.

Lumen size. The discussion of slot dimensions for brackets applies equally to molar tubes.

Precision of fit between the wire and the opening in the tube is important only in torque control applications, and even for this purpose a slight bend or "wave" in the arch can provide the necessary arch engagement for many undersized wires (Fig. 15-20). Brackets do not have a continuous inside surface of sufficient length to provide this option.

Looseness of fit in a molar tube can be a very important asset, in that it provides freedom for the arch to slide through the tube. The same light irregularity in the archwire that can engage the wire for torque control can also inhibit desirable sliding movements.

Tube length. Tube length is extremely important to adequate control over tipping and rotation. It provides the same advantage in rotation and tipping control as is provided by bracket width, so control in these functions is directly proportional to tube length.

The optimum position for the mesial end of the molar tube is near the center of the mesiobuccal cusp (Fig. 15-21). This provides adequate space for arch adjustment and a solid base for attachment in a relatively flat area of the band.

An extended distal end can provide easy clearance for insertion of elastics and ligatures without the need to extend the sharp end of the arch. Care should be exercised to avoid excessive extension when the next molar has not yet erupted. In the upper arch especially, this tooth may erupt in a buccal overlapping position, and it can become impacted on a long tube.

Machine-formed weldable tubes are not available in the optimum long lengths (8 to 10 mm) because of manufacturing limitations and the inability of long thin-wall tubes to hold dimensional accuracy and shape in service. Only heavy-wall extruded tubing is available in these lengths.

Weldable tubes in shorter lengths require auxiliary means of control, but even in these situations the longest available tube is usually the best choice. In selecting

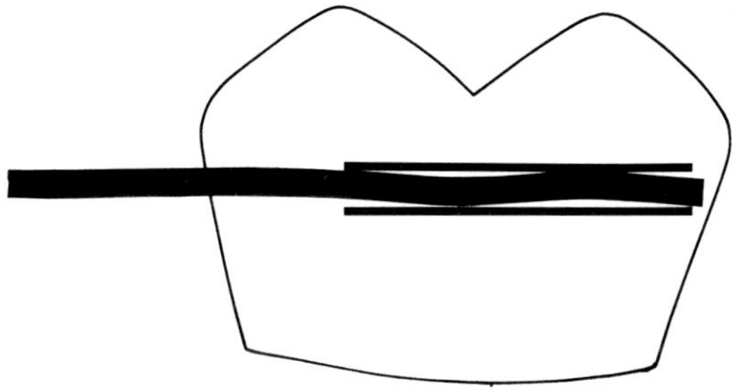

Fig. 15-20. A slight "wave" in a free-fitting rectangular arch can engage the opposite walls of the tube as securely as a snug-fitting wire.

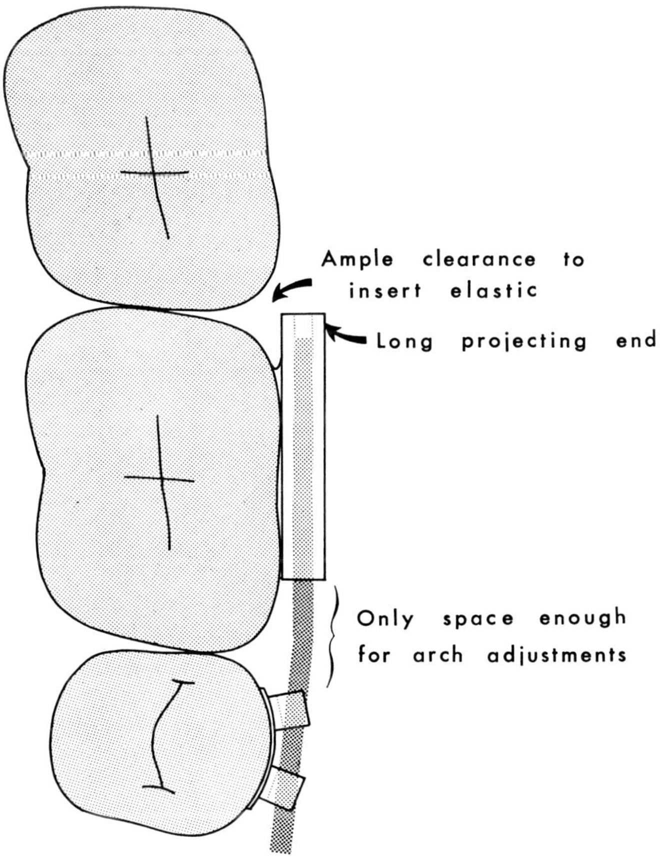

Fig. 15-21. Molar tube placement for maximum control.

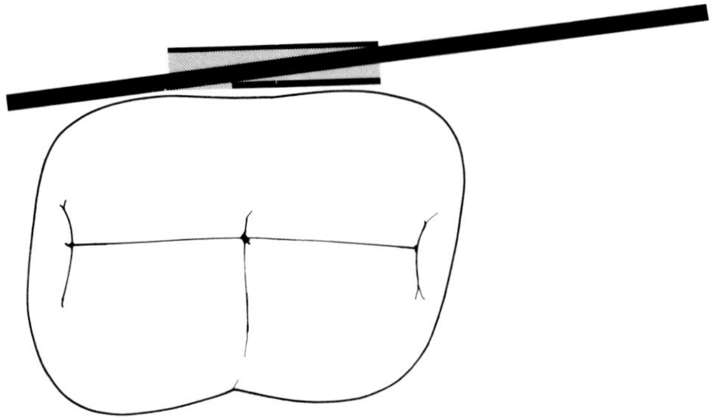

Fig. 15-22. An opening at the distolingual end of a molar tube reduces its effective length for mesial rotation control to the length of the remaining closed tube. This is inadequate with all but the heaviest wires.

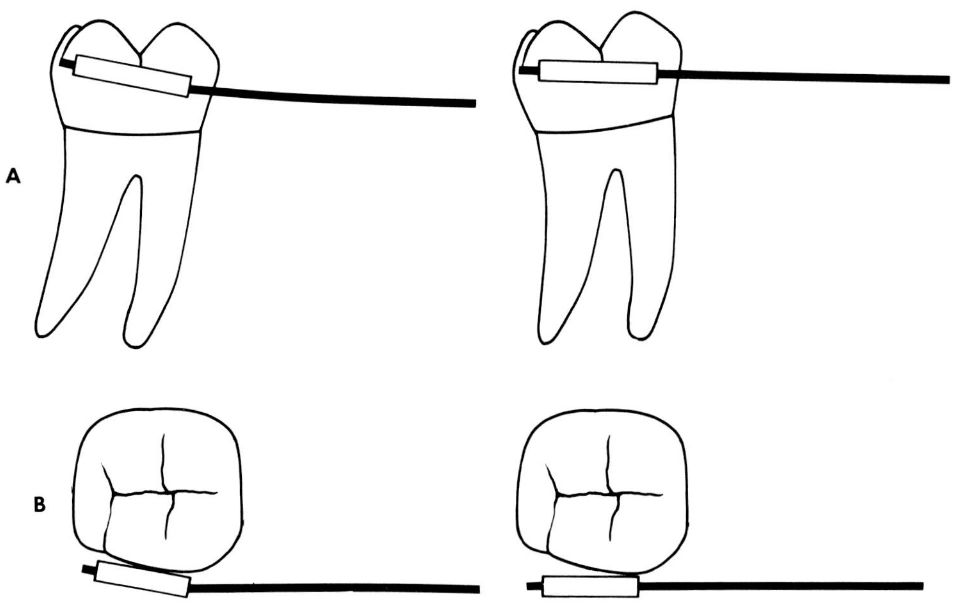

Fig. 15-23. A, Angulation of molar tubes with the distal end inclined occlusally introduces a distal tipping moment that will help control mesial collateral moments introduced by auxiliary traction. **B,** Control over mesial rotation requires either a bend in the archwire or distobuccal angulation of the tube.

these tubes it is the effective length that is important, and many tubes are formed in such a way that the effective length for distal rotation is reduced in order to provide a distal notch for ligation (Fig. 15-22). Other means for ligation are available without this penalty. Control over rotation is important for almost every case, and only the heaviest archwires can provide it with these attachments alone. Such wires can provide stabilization of rotations but are very awkward for use in active rotation correction, so a lingual arch or other adequate auxiliary is recommended.

Angulation. Angulation of tubes is a very valuable aid in molar control because these teeth are often subjected to collateral mesial tipping and rotation moments. Elevating the distal end of the molar tube will greatly augment control over tipping effects (Fig. 15-23, *A*). In the lower arch care is required to avoid occlusal interference from the upper molar, especially when long tubes are angulated.

Tubes may also be angulated buccolingually to aid in rotation control (Fig. 15-23, *B*). This angulation reduces the need for an arch bend for first molar rotation, but it introduces new considerations that cannot be ignored. Molar rotation and arch form are a part of the same anatomic pattern, and tube angulation provides only part of the necessary adaptation. Each arch must be carefully formed with anatomy, not attachments, as the governing criterion.

Buccally angulated tubes can compromise patient comfort, especially with long tubes or arches extending out of the distal ends. This is only one of the disadvantages of angulating headgear tubes; buccal angulation of headgear tubes is definitely not recommended, as explained below.

Special mention should be made here of buccolingual angulation of first molar brackets where the second molar is fitted with a tube to engage the archwire. Such angulation is definitely contraindicated because it severely distorts the dental arch form. Buccal surfaces of first and second molar should follow a smooth curve (Fig. 14-7). Angulation of a first molar bracket directs the archwire buccally and results in an excessively buccal relationship of the second molar to the first.

Multiple tubes. An additional buccal molar tube can be useful in many ways throughout treatment. This tube may be the same size as the archwire tube (my preference), or it may be a different size. The second tube provides two options for archwire level, minimizing many adjustments, and it also provides an attachment for a supplementary hook or a host of other auxiliaries that may be used for control of other teeth.

Extraoral attachment tubes may also be angulated, but only in the occlusogingival direction for mesiodistal tipping control. Buccolingual angulation requires an excessive flare angle on the archwire of the extraoral appliance, making insertion difficult. This often leads in turn to compensation by incomplete passivation of the appliance in the fully seated position, with resultant constriction in molar width that is contraindicated for most patients.

An extraoral attachment tube that parallels the buccal surface of the molar is not only easier to insert; it also provides clearance for bicuspid attachments (Fig. 15-24).

The extraoral attachment tube may be located either occlusally or gingivally in relation to the rectangular tubes. Anatomy and personal preference should govern. The occlusal position may make patient insertion of the appliance and oral hygiene somewhat easier, while the gingival position tends to impinge less on the buccal tissues and provides more clearance in chewing.

Preference for the gingival position is sometimes expressed on the basis of mechanical advantage in distal tipping control, but this is illusory. The orientation of the extraoral components is what governs tipping, regardless of the attachment position on the tooth.

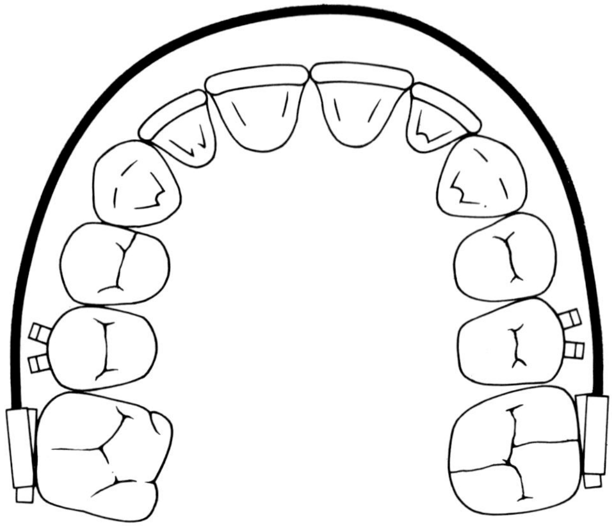

Fig. 15-24. Angulating extraoral tubes as shown will provide clearance between the removable extraoral arch and bicuspid brackets. This angulation also tends to parallel the right and left tubes, making insertion of the appliance easier for the patient.

Many different tube combinations are available as weldable assemblages. When an extraoral attachment tube is a part of such an assemblage, the added strength provided by soldered reinforcement can add greatly to durability.

Buccal hooks

It is often necessary to attach ligature wires, springs, or elastics to a molar to provide intermaxillary or intramaxillary traction. If the buccal tube includes a distal extension, it will serve this purpose very well, but other alternatives are available. When the second molar is banded, gingival interference usually makes it impossible to use a long buccal tube. In this situation and in others in which a shorter tube must be used, a soft wire hook can be welded and soldered as shown in Fig. 15-25.

The arch end may be extended beyond the distal end of the tube to serve as a hook. When two tubes are used, a small section of archwire can be placed in the unused tube to provide a semipermanent hook (Fig. 15-26).

The cutout tube shown in Fig. 15-22 provides sufficient space to tie a ligature wire or coil spring, but the small space and sharp edges make most of these tubes unsuitable for use with elastics.

Lingual hooks

The usual rotation problem with molars is excessive mesial rotation. Applying a mesial force to the lingual surface provides a distal rotating moment (as viewed from the buccal) that provides effective control. This traction is usually applied from a cuspid that has also been fitted with a hook (Fig. 15-27). Since the opposite rotation problem is most common with that tooth, such an arrangement can work out very well, even though care is required to avoid overrotation of one of the two teeth.

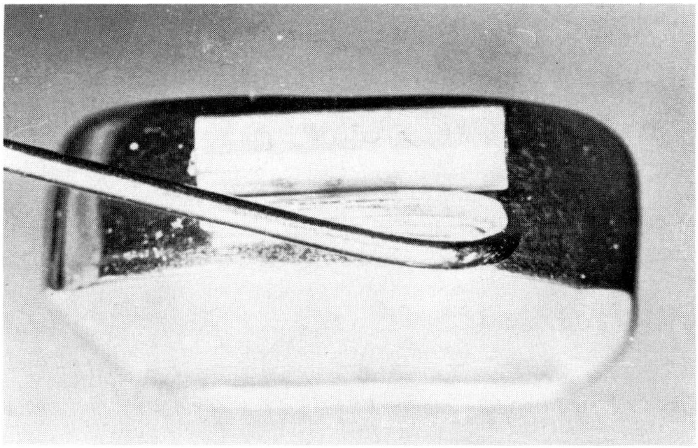

Fig. 15-25. Lower second molars are usually too close to the ramus to allow distal tube extensions for elastic attachment. A soft wire about .025-inch (.6-mm) can be placed gingivally as shown to serve as a hook. This is cut to the desired length and finally contoured after soldering.

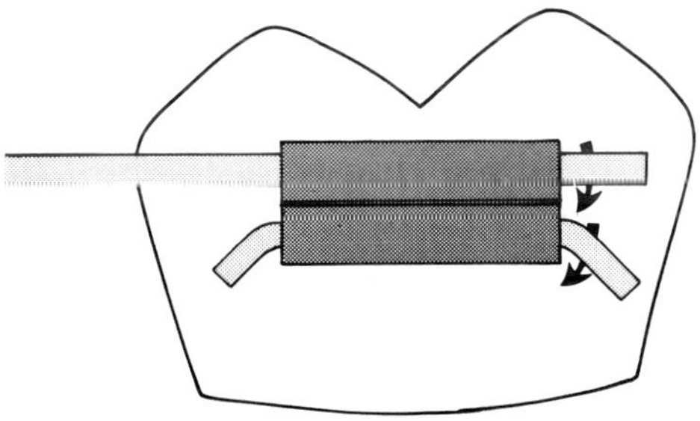

Fig. 15-26. Short molar tubes do not provide an extension for engagement of elastics or ligature wires. This function can be achieved by letting the main archwire extend behind the tube, or by inserting a small section of rectangular wire in an auxiliary tube and bending the ends to keep it in place.

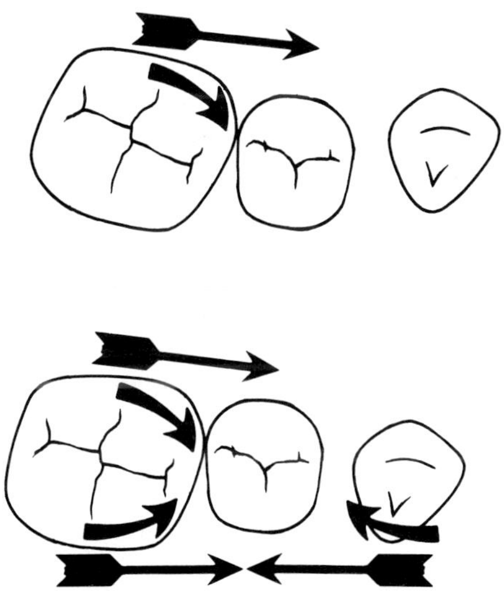

Fig. 15-27. The collateral mesial rotation of buccal traction on the molar can be balanced by lingual traction from the cuspid. This will place a mesial rotating moment on the cuspid, which is often a desired effect.

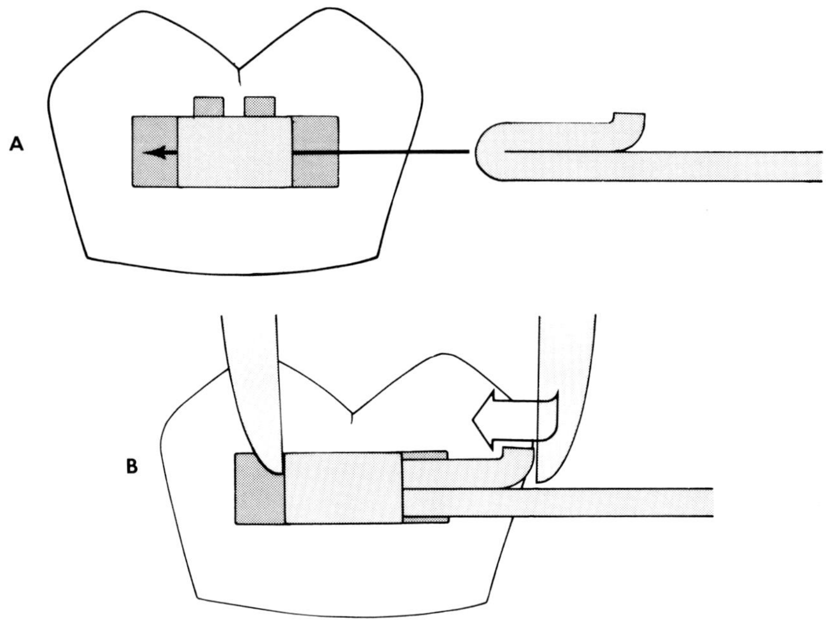

Fig. 15-28. A, The working wire of a horizontal lingual arch has no bends in the attachment area. The folded occlusal end provides retention only, with no flexing in the bend. **B,** The lingual arch is seated by engaging the stop lug and the distal end of the tube with an angled How or similar pliers.

The major limitations of this method of rotation control are the collateral space closing and tipping actions, which may be undesirable.

Lingual arch

One of the most effective means for molar control is the lingual arch. When the objective is simple stabilization, lingual arches are sometimes soldered directly to the bands. This provides the ultimate in stability, but their usefulness is limited due to lack of adjustability. The two molars are rarely in the precisely ideal positions required for effective use of nonadjustable lingual arches.

Removable lingual arches provide much more versatility, and of those available in stainless steel the horizontal sheath type as developed for the Universal technique provides a most desirable combination of mechanical properties (Fig. 15-28, *A*). The critical section in a lingual arch lies at the point where the arch enters the tube. Placing a right-angle bend at this point for a vertical tube greatly increases the possibility of fracture of the wire. The horizontal placement eliminates this critical point and also provides space for a longer tube. This in turn provides more positive control over mesiodistal tipping and the vertical position of the arch in the incisor area. Looseness in those applications is a common problem with shorter vertical steel tubes.

Insertion may appear to be a problem, but the .036-inch (0.9-mm) arches have ample flexibility and are easily placed with an angled How or similar pliers. Full engagement of the arch in the tube is most easily accomplished by engaging one plier beak at the distal end of the tube and the other at the short mesial stop and closing the pliers (Fig. 15-28, *B*).

Lingual arches of this type will overpower most buccal arch actions on the molar and provide full control over buccolingual tipping, axial rotations, and intermolar width (Fig. 18-5). Control over mesiodistal tipping is essentially limited to reciprocal actions between the molars. It is possible to equalize their inclinations by tipping them in opposite directions, but a lingual arch is ineffective in tipping both molars in the same direction.

16

Banding and bonding

Controlling the movement of a tooth in all directions requires a firm attachment to that tooth. The orthodontic band, cemented to the tooth, is one practical means of obtaining such an attachment for most purposes. The continuing development and refinement of materials and techniques for direction cementation (bonding) of orthodontic attachments to the teeth offers a viable alternative to banding in many situations.

A vital secondary function of the orthodontic attachment is protection of the tooth from carious attack. Any covering that provides a sheltered area for accumulation on the surface of a tooth can encourage plaque formation and increase the caries hazard, so bands and bonding attachments must be carefully designed, fitted, and cemented to control this problem.

Modern bands and bonding techniques have brought many improvements in the ease and comfort of the placement, as well as in esthetics and protection of the tooth. These are not without new disadvantages of their own, but with a properly adapted technique the gains are clear.

BAND OR BOND?

There is no difference in the clinical management of orthodontic therapy with banded or bonded attachments, provided that the attachment slots are of the same dimensions and bear the same relationship to their respective teeth. The choice between the two attachment methods involves four very different considerations: attachment options, separation, tooth protection, and overall ease and efficiency. As with most such choices, they are clouded by many often conflicting variables.

Attachment options

The nature of a band, with its broad surface, places no limitations on the type or number of attachments that may be used. Welding secures most attachments to bands, and soldering is also available as an alternative means.

Attachment options are more limited with bonding. Single attachments of small and medium size present no serious problems, but wide attachments are another matter. Bonding bases are not easily adapted to large areas, especially to the sharply curved surfaces near the mesial and distal surfaces, so there is a tendency to avoid wide attachments for bonding. This is doubly unfortunate because wide attachments provide better control and require lower force levels, which can be especially advantageous with bonded attachments.

Limitations on bonding lingual attachments are more serious. Since lingual attachments are ordinarily used in combination with buccal attachments, they usually require multiple bonding procedures. Bands facilitate such operations because any number of attachments may be positioned with precision in an extraoral environment, followed by a single cementation procedure. The two-stage operation required to bond both lingual and buccal attachments to most teeth may be more an inconvenience than an actual limitation on options, but it can be an important consideration.

The higher gingival levels found on the lingual side of many teeth can make the bonding of lingual attachments practically impossible for many patients. Bands can generally be expected to provide the most dependable retention and easier placement for lingual tubes, hooks, or buttons.

Interproximal space and arch length

Bands occupy interproximal space and so add to arch length during the time that they are in place. This is obviously recovered at the time that the bands are removed, and in most but not all cases it presents little difficulty.

The time of appliance removal brings many adaptations, including a considerable change in labial and lingual tissue pressures on the teeth. Labiobuccal attachments can increase labial pressures by their protrusion from the tooth surface, and they can reduce pressure by their rough, irritating contours. Which effects will dominate depends on the individual patient, but it will have an effect on posttreatment adaptations. The spaces occupied by bands are typically closed during the time that the dentition is also readapting after all of the other changes, and the process usually continues uneventfully.

Where arch length is extremely critical, the small space occupied by bands can be very important. Bonding can provide a great advantage in such cases by not compounding the space problem with the interproximal width that would otherwise be added by bands.

Tooth protection

Protection of the tooth is a collateral function of all means of securing orthodontic attachments to the teeth. There is no question that decalcification and caries patterns are altered by orthodontic attachments, but their relative contributions to protection or hazard are difficult to evaluate. Orthodontic treatment is often deferred until the age period when caries is most active, and the caries cannot be expected to halt during the treatment period.

A securely cemented band provides protection for the underlying tooth, with only the adjoining exposed areas subject to carious attack. These will not be protected by the band, and poor oral hygiene can take its toll just as it does in the absence of appliances. The only difference will be in the distribution pattern that is modified by the protection of the band. A damaged band with loss of cement seal can occasionally provide a sheltered area that will also be subject to decalcification or caries, but this is the exception.

On the positive side, interproximal areas are well protected by a cemented band, and caries in these areas is very rare in banded teeth.

Bonding adhesive can be extended into the gingival areas to protect those surfaces, but much larger areas are still left unprotected. These include the critical interproximal surfaces, where the caries process will tend to go on as usual. As with a damaged band, a microscopic loss of adhesive seal at the bonding margin may also expose additional areas.

Bonded attachments also expose the enamel to possible scarring in the removal of remaining adhesive after debonding heavily filled, highly adherent bonding agents. These materials require much heavier instrumentation than the more easily removed, less adherent bonding agents or oxyphosphate cement.

Ease of placement and removal

Ease of placement must be evaluated in both a general way and in relation to specific local factors.

Securing bands to the teeth with oxyphosphate cement requires very different procedures than securing attachments directly with a bonding adhesive. Relative ease of these procedures differs little overall, so the choice is more one of personal preference than a technical decision. Each has its own unique areas of large and small time requirements, ease and difficulty, elation and annoyance.

Bonding is better suited to mass application by the indirect technique, but this presents problems as well. Full efficiency with this technique requires routine use, which can easily lead to full appliance placement in cases where incremental placement would be more appropriate.

Individual attachments can be placed with comparable ease with either technique, with any advantage usually lying with banding.

Removal is easiest for bands and the lightly filled bonding materials that respond well to normal scaling technique. Heavily filled adhesives may require abrasive removal, which has attendant destructive potential.

DIRECT OR INDIRECT?

Both banding and bonding offer the option of direct and indirect techniques for selection and fitting. Indirect techniques transfer a part of the procedure to the laboratory, where it may be accomplished by auxiliary personnel. Chair time is reduced, even with the additional patient visit that is required to produce the working casts.

Advantages of the indirect technique largely depend on the availability of skilled technical personnel for the laboratory phase of the procedure. There is little benefit if the orthodontist merely moves the area of operation from chairside to laboratory, although the mass placement that is a part of indirect bonding techniques may also be considered advantageous in some cases. Training, supervision, and periodic replacement of key personnel are important ongoing considerations in such operations.

Cementation patterns following the laboratory phase differ considerably between banding and bonding techniques. Bands that have been fabricated and fitted in the laboratory may be cemented at the same time or in groups as required. Most indirect bonding techniques are based on simultaneous placement of all attachments.

Immediate placement of attachments on all teeth at the start of treatment is not the method of choice for many patients, so full reliance on this method can seriously compromise treatment options.

Use of auxiliary personnel for actual cementation to the teeth should not be a factor in the choice of techniques. Technical demands of the cementation procedures are comparable for either method; local practices in this regard depend more on legal interpretations than on actual treatment requirements, so they are beyond the scope of this review.

ANATOMY

Anatomical variations impose many limitations on fitting attachments to specific teeth. These may involve coronal anatomy that affects retention or gingival anatomy that establishes the area of the crown that is exposed and available for bonding.

Coronal anatomy

Coronal anatomy can create problems for effectively securing attachments by either banding or bonding.

The six upper anterior teeth present the most frequent difficulty in band retention. Certain tapers and contours of crown form offer little or no retention for bands, making a bonded attachment much more effective. In other cases good band retention is attainable only by compromising attachment levels, which again can make bonding the more attractive choice.

Upper lateral incisors can present difficult problems in attachment retention by either method, especially when these teeth are abnormally small. It is virtually impossible to contour attachments for bonding so that they will fit such a small-radius surface as closely as is necessary for secure bonding. A band may or may not provide reasonable retention on such teeth. An open mind is necessary, and it is sometimes desirable to evaluate both methods for certain teeth before making a final decision.

Cuspids can be attractive candidates for bonding when their crown form offers little or no band retention or dictates an excessively gingival attachment level. On the other hand, sharply pointed cuspids can present anatomical constraints similar to those described for lateral incisors that compromise optimum position as much with bonding as with banding.

Buccal teeth generally offer good retention for bands, so coronal anatomy is seldom a reason for bonding. On the other hand, short crowns and round buccal surfaces can make bonding to bicuspids difficult, especially when the wide brackets that give most effective control over tipping and rotations.

Gingival anatomy

Most orthodontic patients are young, with many teeth only recently erupted. Gingival margins can be very high on such teeth, especially the bicuspids, leaving clinical crowns often too short for secure bonding. Bands can be much more effective than bonding in these cases.

The last molar may also have extremely high gingival margins, or even a distal operculum, that can even make band placement a questionable procedure. In extreme cases these teeth may need to be controlled by removable appliances or extensions from an appliance cemented to other teeth.

THE CHOICE

The choice of attachment means is clearly one of personal preference, but it should be based on serious consideration of all of the factors discussed above as they apply to the case at hand. Every orthodontist should be prepared to use either, or a combination of the two, to best meet the needs of the individual patient. The key factors are tabulated below.*

	Band	Bond
Dental anatomy		
Tapered teeth	−	+
Cuspids	?	+
Upper lateral incisors	?	?
Buccal teeth	+	0
Short crowns	+	−
Attachment selection		
Wide attachments	+	−
Lingual attachments	+	−
Multiple attachments	+	?
Fitting and placement		
Separation	−	+
Level control	−	+
Replacement of loose attachment	+	−
Decalcification and caries		
Facial	?	?
Interproximal	+	−
Removal and cleanup		
Removal	+	+
Cleanup, heavily filled adhesive		−
Cleanup, lightly filled adhesive		+
Cleanup, bands (oxyphosphate cement)	+	

BONDING TECHNIQUE

Attachments should be contoured to adapt as closely as possible to tooth contours. All bonding adhesives attain maximum adhesive strength in thin layers, so adaptation is no less important in bonding than in banding.

Adhesive handling is material specific, so the manufacturer's instructions should be carefully followed. This adhesive technology is still advancing at such a rate that relative merits of the many variants may change at any time. It would be presumptive to attempt to evaluate the technical details of such a fluid technology at this stage of its development.

*+ or − indicate an overall favorable or unfavorable effect; 0 indicates little importance in selection; ? indicates a variable effect, depending on the case.

BANDING TECHNIQUE

Banding technique requires attention to many details that have evolved over years of practical experience. These cover all stages of the procedure, from selection of materials to final cleanup of excess cement.

Band materials

The ideal band material for fitting and adaptation to the teeth must have physical properties almost exactly opposite to those that can best meet the demands of service conditions in the mouth.

To be easily formed into a band, a material must be soft and ductile, like 24-carat gold. Such a material is easily deformed to adapt it to the contours of the tooth, and once adapted, it will keep its new shape. Edges of such a band can be burnished to a perfect fit at all the margins. The finished band can be truly beautiful, but it will be just as easily deformed in service as it was in formation.

In the mouth, under the many stresses of occlusion and accidental trauma, a band must be strong, stiff, and well able to hold its shape. Ideal properties for this purpose are more like those of a rigid casting.

Castings can also be made to a beautiful fit, but between the actual forming of the band and its service in the mouth there is one more short but important operation: seating of the band on the tooth. This operation requires a material with properties different from either of those just mentioned. Here we need a springy material that will stretch over the contours of the tooth and return to its original shape as the band is seated in its final position.

A band of soft material would distort in passing over the wide parts of the tooth and overhang at the gingival margins. If resistance is encountered in pushing a soft band into place, the edges may also crumple or tear.

Castings are ruled out for band construction, since the tooth cannot be prepared to eliminate undercuts as can be done for a crown. The orthodontist is expected to use the tooth as he finds it and to leave it in its original condition at the end of treatment, and he must adapt his techniques accordingly.

A springy material with optimum properties for band placement actually comes close to an optimum compromise between the extremely soft and hard materials, even though springiness can be a problem in initial formation. No metal has sufficient elastic range to pass over the widest parts of all teeth and return to a good, tight fit at the gingival margin.

During the period when gold alloys were the preeminent band material, alloys with superior hardness and strength were developed for this application. Since that time, stainless steel, with its own unique properties, has become the overwhelming choice for orthodontic band material. In spite of its superiority, stainless steel still requires careful handling, and some of its properties can be misleading if they are not fully understood in relation to band placement.

Thickness and hardness

Manipulation during the manufacture of stainless steel bands can produce varying degrees of work hardening, which affects both adaptability and working life.

Preformed seamless bands are usually manufactured by drawing a flat sheet into a cup shape, cutting off the top to leave a ring, forming that to band shape, and sometimes stretching to size.

All of these operations work-harden the material, requiring carefully controlled annealing during fabrication to produce a band with sufficient softness for adaptability and durability. Softness is required for durability because an overhardened band is also brittle and much more likely to split or crack in service.

A band that has not been adequately annealed after manufacture will *feel* stronger in the fingers than an annealed band, but this apparent strength is altogether illusory. Even a small amount of deformation is too much in a band on a tooth, and in this working range there is *no difference* between an annealed and a work-hardened band. The differences noted by "feel" are the gross deflections at the upper end of the elastic curve, which are far outside the range of actual service conditions. These gain nothing for the work-hardened band but reduced adaptability in fitting the band to the tooth.

The descriptions of wire properties in Chapter 17 apply equally to stainless steel band materials. The key point is that temper or hardness does not alter physical properties in any way that will compensate for a reduction in thickness or improve retention or durability.

Because of the rapid work hardening of stainless steel and the difficulty of annealing adequately in a clinical situation, there is a distinct advantage in the use of performed bands that are fully annealed. Final shaping can then be easily accomplished without excessively hardening the material.

Loosening of bands

When a gold band has been subjected to occlusion or other distorting forces, the malleable metal is rapidly pounded thin in the affected area. The metal from this thinning spot spreads in all directions, increasing the size of the band and breaking the cement bond. This is often only a local effect, because the adaptable surrounding material tends to absorb the spreading action, taking up the slack without affecting the parts of the band that are farther away. This can cause a local loosening of the band without causing the entire band to become loose. Detection of such loosening may be difficult, for the band can still be tight when tested. If the process continues, the entire band will eventually loosen. Then, of course, detection becomes relatively easy.

Because of the stiffness and toughness of stainless steel, bands made of it tend to loosen in a different manner under the impact of occlusion. In a stainless steel band, the tendency is for the stiff material to transmit the displacement over a larger area of the band, breaking the cement seal and loosening the entire band. This complete loosening may sometimes be easier to detect, but the same elastic properties may also cause a well-fitted band to hold tightly to the tooth, even with the broken seal, and thus escape detection for some time.

Loosened bands of either material can thus in their own way escape detection in a limited number of cases, but the number should be extremely limited if the clinician is alert to the problem and understands the characteristics of the material being used.

Joining the metal

Soldering or brazing is the only practical method for joining gold alloys. Stainless steel can also be soldered, but this is often not the method of choice. With gold materials, high-fusing, corrosion-resistant gold solders may be used with impunity. These may be used with stainless steel only if the entire piece is heated to soldering temperature and annealing is not undesirable. When this is done, a very sound joint is the result, but the metal is heated beyond the sensitizing temperature. When a large steel band is to be soldered, it is not always easy to heat the entire piece, so low-fusing silver solder is generally used. At silver-soldering temperature the operation must be carried out quickly and the piece quenched immediately to avoid sensitization and later intergranular corrosion. High-temperature electrical instruments of the "soldering gun" type are very useful for this controlled local heating, as are electrical resistance soldering units and various small-flame torches.

The bond between solder and stainless steel is a relatively weak one, so joint design is an important consideration. In general, there should be some mechanical locking effect, as when solder wraps around a wire. On flat surfaces, such as attachments on bands, reinforcing with several welds before soldering is very helpful. Welds have great tensile strength but are easily twisted off, so the solder provides rigidity to enhance the strength of the weld while the weld augments the adhesion of the solder.

The method of choice for joining most stainless steel band materials and attachments is resistance welding, a technique completely impossible with gold because of the latter's low electrical resistance. Properly carried out, welding produces a neat, strong joint that is highly resistant to corrosion. For additional strength and

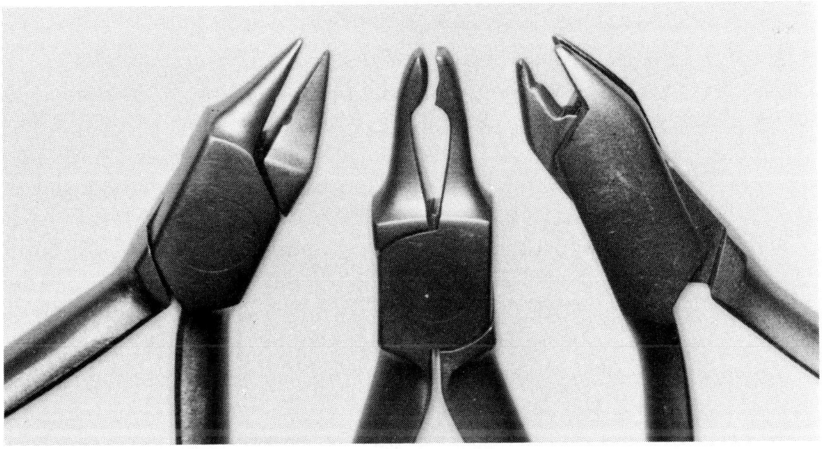

Fig. 16-1. Band-shaping pliers. Left to right, round tapered point "bird beak" pliers, ball-and-socket or similar contouring pliers, and triple-beak clasp-adjusting pliers with center beak relieved to facilitate bending of multiple brackets to fit tooth contours (Fig. 16-7, **B**). The latter two are also useful for adapting the contours of brackets to be bonded to the teeth.

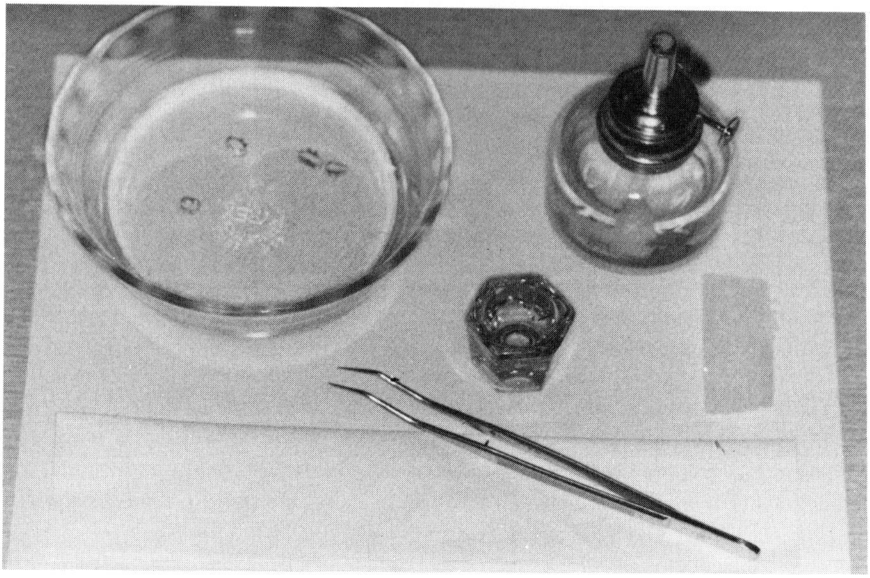

Fig. 16-2. Auxiliary equipment for band fitting: alcohol lamp or other flame, alcohol, dish of water, facial tissue, soft utility wax, and cotton pliers.

rigidity, such welded joints may be reinforced with silver solder. This is a very effective means for attaching extruded molar tubes to bands. For maximum corrosion resistance and long life, welded and soldered joints may be electropolished before they are placed into service.

BAND FITTING

Banding is most readily accomplished with preformed bands, with attachments welded to the bands in advance wherever possible. Such assemblies are available for all teeth, but molar variations often make individualization desirable.

Three kinds of pliers, shown close up in Fig. 16-1, are used for shaping bands. The triple-beak clasp-adjusting pliers are modified as shown by relieving the middle beak to facilitate the adjustment of bracket curvature without distorting the band margin. The outside beaks of this plier must be spaced the same as a double bracket. The remaining two pliers are used to contour margins of different-sized bands. Other pliers, band pushers, or automatic mallets may be used as desired.

The following are also at the chair when teeth are being banded (Fig. 16-2):

1. Alcohol lamp or other flame for igniting alcohol and warming bands
2. Dappen dish of 95% (190 proof) alcohol for drying and sterilization
3. Dish of water for rinsing bands
4. Soft white utility wax for filling grooves of attachments prior to cementation
5. Cotton pliers

Separation

Spaces between the teeth to be banded should be checked three to seven days before handing. This is done by passing a strip of heavy band material (.007 inch or

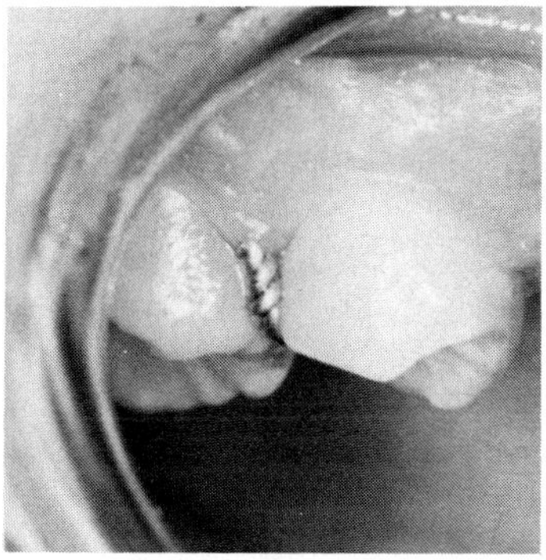

Fig. 16-3. Separating wire in place.

.16 mm) through each contact point. Where this strip will not pass through the contact point, the teeth must be separated to facilitate later placement of bands. It is impossible to fit bands well if contacts are excessively tight.

Special separating spring clips may be used for this purpose, or .020-inch (.5-mm) soft brass wire can be wrapped around the contact point and twisted tight. This wire is threaded below the contact point, wrapped around, and twisted moderately tight with pliers into a rather long "pigtail." The excess wire is cut off, and the twisted ends tucked toward the gingivae (Fig. 16-3). This long twisted end facilitates removal immediately prior to the fitting of bands.

Metal separators can be inserted into almost any contact area. The only exception is where adjoining teeth are tipped so that the roots are unusually close together in the cervical region. They apply pressure for only a short time, after which the teeth move in response and the pressure is rapidly dissipated.

Elastic separators are of value only where overseparation is desired, such as for complete arch indirect banding. A contact that is too tight for a metal band to pass through will also be too tight for an elastic separator, so these are unusable in the situations where separation is most needed. Elastic separators apply pressure over an extended period without the self-limiting action of metal separators as the teeth move. This increases pain and trauma, making the time of their application much more critical.

Separation is usually the first actual experience of a patient with active tooth movement, and it can be a tense and painful experience. It is best used sparingly, only as required, rather than as a routine for all teeth to be banded. Separation of all teeth or placement of all bands at one visit is rarely necessary. One of the many advantages of sequential placement of attachments as treatment progresses is a great reduction in the need for separation; developing dentitions rarely require separation of more than molar teeth with this approach.

Band selection

All separators are removed immediately before the bands are fitted and the teeth are cleaned. Recent fluoridation is also desirable.

Preformed bands are stocked in all sizes, with the proper attachments prewelded to all with the possible exception of the molars. The plaster casts of the teeth

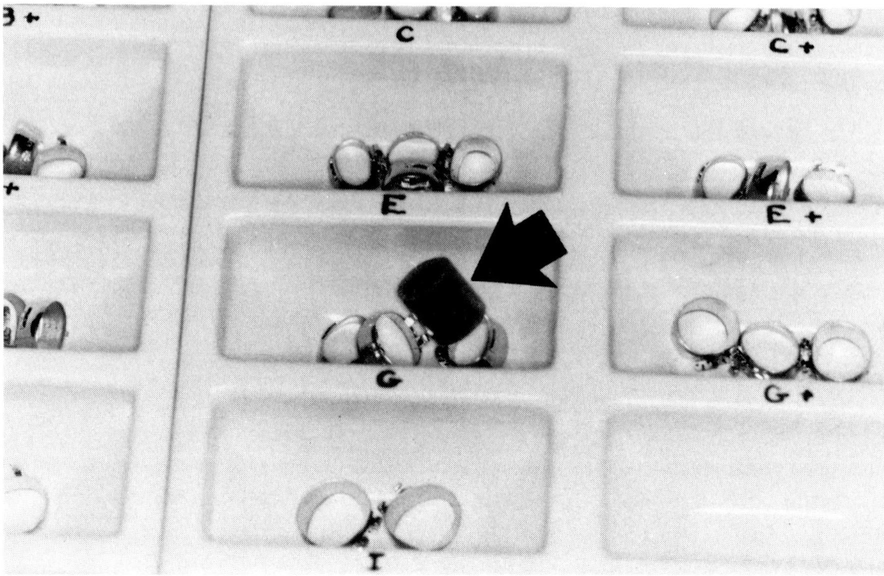

Fig. 16-4. A foreign object in the band tray helps to identify the size first tried in the mouth for later replacement of unused bands in the proper compartments.

may be used for preliminary selection if desired, but final selection must be based on fitting the band to the individual tooth. A small foreign object in the band tray (Fig. 16-4) can serve as a convenient reminder of the size of the first band that was tried, facilitating the return of unused bands to their proper compartments.

Bands of unsuitable size are placed in the dish of water, rinsed clean, and then placed on absorbent paper to remove excess water. They are next dipped in the 95% alcohol, which is immediately burned off. This sterilizes the band rapidly without overheating the metal.

The band is returned to the stock of unused bands as soon as the alcohol has completely burned off, care being taken not to contact the sides of plastic compartments with the hot band. This procedure eliminates the problems of sorting unused bands later.

Bands that are to be welded or soldered should not be sterilized in this way because a layer of oxides will be formed on the surface. Electropolishing will quickly remove this layer and provide a chemically clean surface for welding or soldering, but alternate methods of sterilization are usually more expedient.

Placement and fitting

Levels. The ideal goal in band placement is the location of all bracket slots at the same level. This makes it unnecessary to use compensating bends in the arches to control tooth levels. Such level arches are much easier to form. They avoid the many secondary effects of vertical arch adjustments, and they slide more freely through the brackets in space closure. These advantages are well worth the effort required to keep levels constant wherever possible and to control band levels as accurately as possible. However, levels should not be pursued blindly at all costs.

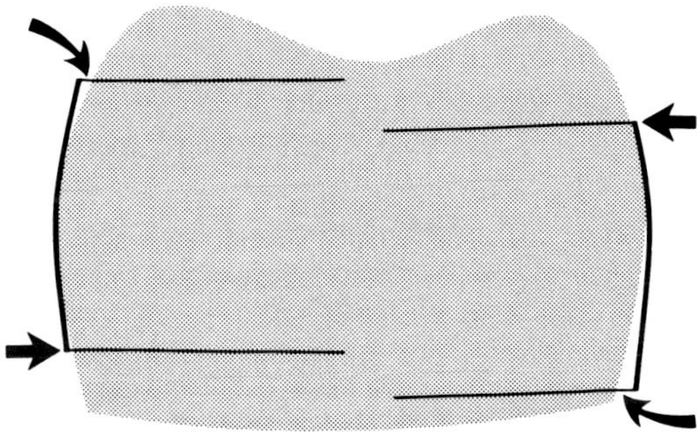

Fig. 16-5. Band elasticity cannot fully accommodate to tooth contours, so open margins are inevitable; the important option is deciding where they will be placed. A deeply seated band (right) can have an esthetic occlusal margin while the hidden gingival edge traumatizes the periodontal attachment with its deep position and open margin. A band positioned more occlusally (left) is much more compatible with periodontal health, while the open margin is more conspicuous and readily inspected for integrity.

Band levels can be measured and compared with a height gauge. Different clinicians use different reference points for height measurements, usually the cusp tips or marginal ridges or some combination of these. Such factors as wear and tooth anatomy must be considered, and no rigid reference will be suitable for all patients or even all teeth in some arches. The important consideration is the ultimate vertical relationship that is desired between adjacent teeth.

In some difficult situations, especially in the banding of cuspids or of teeth where occlusion interferes, it may be necessary to place a band at a different level in order to obtain adequate retention. When this must be done it is important that care be taken to adjust *all* arches from the very first, to keep such a tooth at proper level and buccolingual position.

Care is essential to avoid seating a band so far onto a tooth that the periodontal attachment is jeopardized. The occlusal margin is exposed for all to see, while the gingival margin is out of sight, creating a strong temptation to overseat bands to provide the most visually satisfying occlusal margin. There is a real risk of periodontal injury with this approach.

The geometry of the teeth combines with the physical characteristics of the metals used for band construction to make all seating of a band beyond the greatest convexity of the tooth cause a progressive degradation of the unseen gingival fit (Fig. 16-5). Dividing the unavoidable compromises in fit between gingival and occlusal margins provides the most physiologic environment during the active phase of treatment.

Rotations. Normally, bands should be placed on all teeth with the brackets centered on the labial or buccal surface. Where this is impossible because of severe rotations, the bracket should be placed in a position as nearly correct as possible and repositioned later when conditions permit.

On rotated bicuspids it is often helpful to position the bracket *slightly* toward the lingual contact point to aid in overcorrection of the rotation. Such overcorrection must be very subtle, not over .5 mm in bracket position.

Molar brackets should either be centered on the buccal groove or positioned with the mesial end near the center of the mesiobuccal cusp.

Contouring. When a band is first placed on a tooth, it will probably fit very poorly (Fig. 16-6, *A*). It is only partially seated at this stage, to give guidance for major adjustments in margins and bracket curvature.

The bracket often needs adjustment to adapt it to the buccal contours of the tooth. When this is necessary, the band is removed from the tooth and the bracket is adjusted with the triple-beak pliers (Fig. 16-7, *B*) before any other fitting.

When the band is returned to the tooth, it is seated with the plugger, which alternately engages the bracket-mounting flanges and the lingual seating lug (Fig. 16-6, *C* and *D*). Mesial and distal margins may also be used for seating when necessary (Fig. 16-6, *E*).

The sides and end of the plugger are used to adjust all occlusal margins to the contours of the tooth (Fig. 16-6, *F* and *G*).

The band may be adequately fitted at this point, or it may need repeated fitting and adjustment. When it is adapted so that it fits well and exhibits good retention when it is removed from the tooth (Fig. 16-6, *H*), it is removed once more for final contouring and cementation.

Most margins, especially gingival margins, are contoured further at this point to provide the best possible adaptation to the tooth. Contouring on the tooth gives general form, but the springiness of stainless steel makes it necessary to do the final forming off the tooth. Two kinds of very effective pliers for this purpose are shown in action in Fig. 16-6, *I* and *J*. In actual practice, the band is held securely in the fingers for this procedure. It must be held in such a way that the action of the pliers results in constriction of the margins and not in stretching of the center of the band.

After final contouring, the band is placed in water to prevent saliva from drying on the surface. It may be left in the water while other bands are formed or it may be rinsed vigorously at once and placed on absorbent paper or tissue to dry.

Incisors. The procedure for handling incisors is much the same as for the bicuspids just shown, except that brackets usually require less adjustment to the contours of the tooth.

The gingival proximal areas of incisors will sometimes overhang and thus require additional contouring. This must be done without bulging the band excessively at the contact point, for such a bulge adds width and leaves excessive space when the band is removed. Contouring labially and lingually and tilting the bracket so as to narrow the incisal thickness and widen it gingivally in the labiolingual dimension can help pull this proximal margin into position without creating an excessive bulge in the contact area.

Cuspids. The procedure for fitting cuspid bands is similar, but the anatomy of these teeth often makes it more difficult. Band retention is a problem on many cuspids with any banding technique. Bands must be adjusted and formed much more with the pliers as they are fitted over large cingula and other aberrant contours.

It is sometimes necessary to place a cuspid band farther gingivally than the adjacent bands to gain adequate retention. Using wide bands or incisal aprons and locating the bracket toward the occlusal margin of the band will relieve this prob-

A B

C D

E F

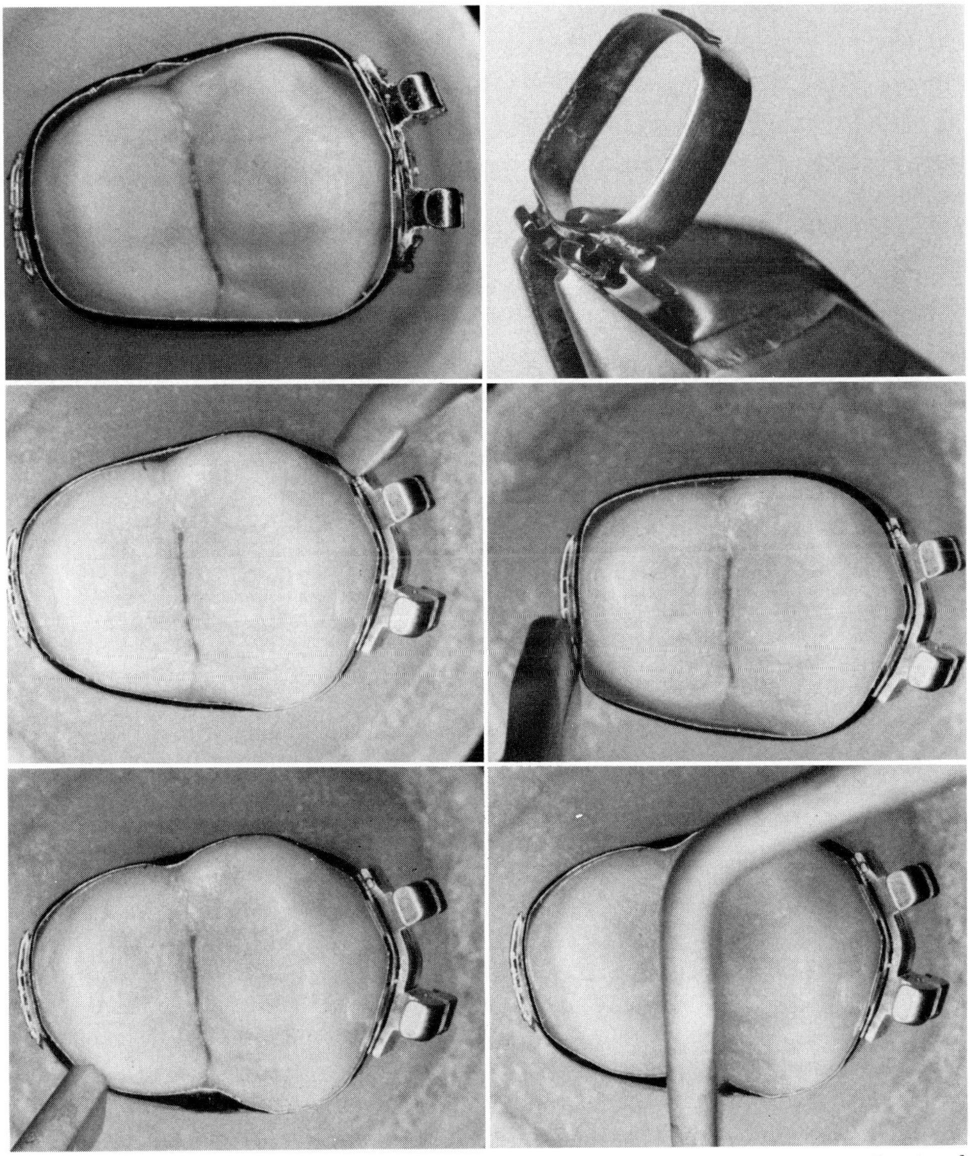

Continued.

Fig. 16-6. A, Bracket as supplied may not conform to the buccal contours of the tooth. **B,** The modified triple-beak pliers will very effectively adjust the bracket curvature. **C,** Seating recontoured bracket with pressure on the bracket flange—*never* on the bracket itself. **D,** Lingual seating, using welded seating lug (not band margin). **E,** Care must be exercised in seating bands by direct pressure on the band margin. **F,** Edge of plugger can also be used to contour band margins. **G,** Side of plugger will smooth band margins. **H,** Fitted band, ready for removal and gingival contouring. **I,** Pliers with a round, tapered beak are very useful for adjusting the margins of small bands. The tip that is used inside the band should be smoothly rounded, not sharp, for this application. **J,** Ball-and-socket contouring pliers are most effective for bands that are large enough to accommodate them.

G H I J

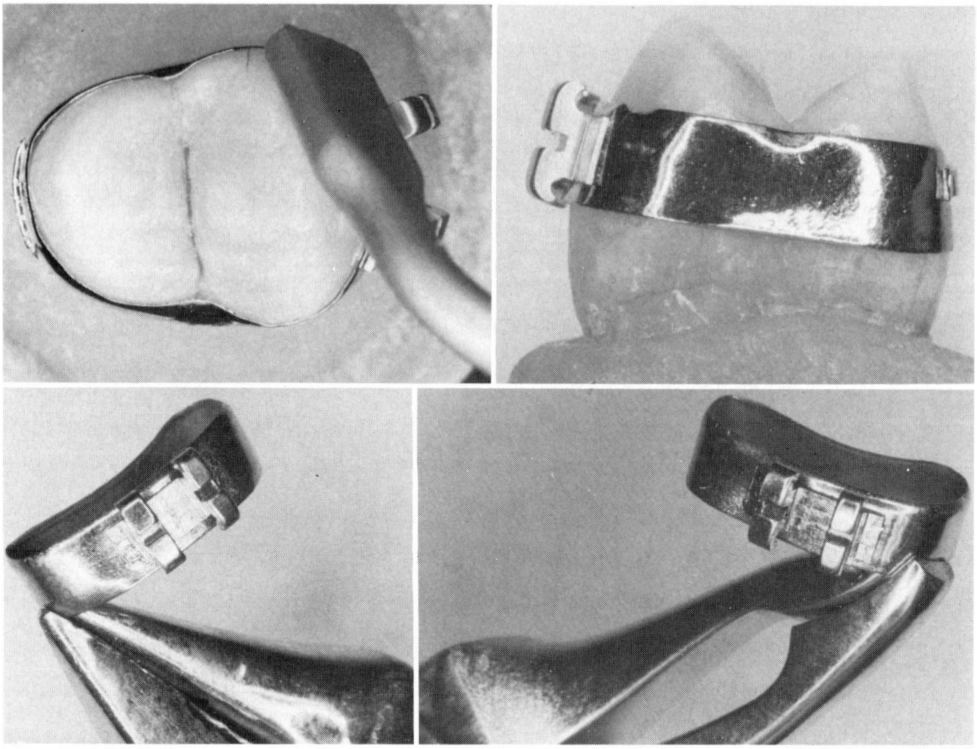

Fig. 16-6. cont'd. For legend see p. 209.

lem but it will not solve it in all cases. Good band position is important, but retention is even more important; therefore the position of the band in each case must be decided on the basis of the specific alternatives.

Molars. The fitting of molar bands follows the same pattern as with other teeth, varying only to adapt to the nature of the attachments. With prewelded attachments the band is fitted for optimum attachment orientation to the tooth and contoured accordingly.

In many cases custom welding of attachments after initial band fitting will provide the best orientation. Even the specially positioned right and left, upper and lower, first and second molar attachments cannot cope with the wide variability of molar anatomy and treatment requirements.

Individualized welding can be especially useful where both buccal and lingual tubes are being used, because the optimum relationship between buccal and lingual tubes is asymmetrical and varies with individual tooth anatomy. A combination technique, with one of the two tubes prewelded, may prove most effective in many cases.

The rigidity of welded attachments will alter the shape and tighten the fit of preselected bands to which they are welded, so initial selection must anticipate this change of fit.

Molar attachments are very useful in removing the bands after trial fitting.

A

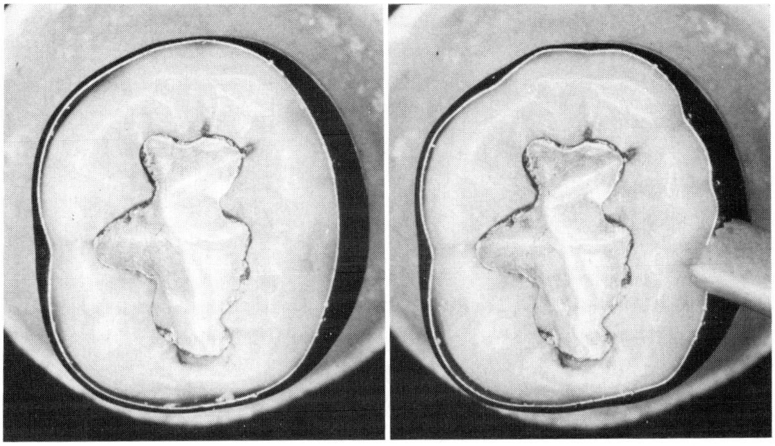

B

Fig. 16-7. A, Molar band when first placed on a tooth, before fitting. **B,** Preliminary contouring of the margins with a plugger.

A

B

C

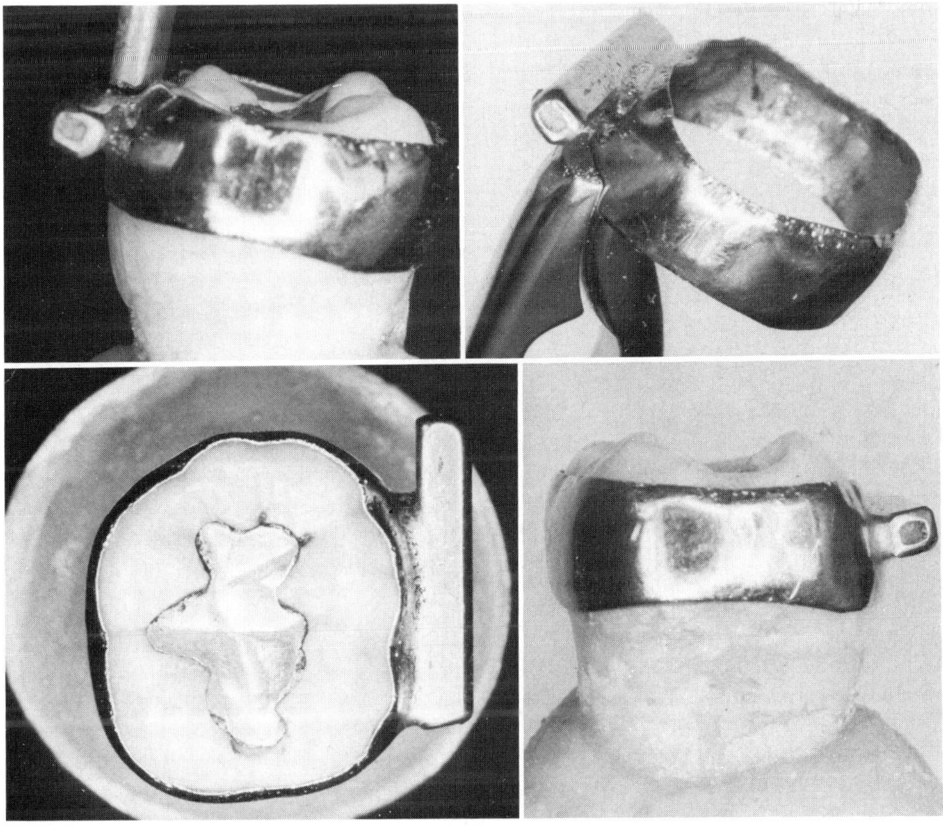

Fig. 16-8. A, Lower molar bands are seated first lingually, then buccally. **B,** Final contouring of gingival margins. **C,** All margins completely adapted for cementation.

When bands are being fitted before welding any attachments, it is important that they not be fully seated in order to avoid a difficult removal that requires engaging and possibly distorting the gingival band margin.

The partially seated band (Fig. 16-7, *A*) is roughly contoured to the form of the tooth with the plugger (Fig. 16-7, *B*). Final band position is judged at this time to serve as a guide to positioning the attachment.

The band may be contoured further with pliers after its removal from the tooth. Brackets and weldable tubes can be attached by welding alone, but solid tubes without flanges require additional reinforcement with solder.

All welded attachments, buccal and lingual, should be placed before any attachments are soldered. The heat of soldering will cause surface oxidation that adversely affects any welds made later unless the surface is carefully cleaned and electropolished. All welding flanges should be secured with as many welds as space will permit—usually four to six for each flange.

Lower molar bands are always seated first on the lingual and then on the buccal side (Fig. 16-8, *A*). Upper molar bands are seated in the opposite way, buccal side first and lingual side last. Margins are contoured as required (Fig. 16-18, *B*) until the band is fully adapted to the tooth (Fig. 16-18, *C*). At this stage the band may be fully seated, or in some cases it may be almost seated but fully contoured so that it will fit tightly when finally positioned.

• • •

Gingival margins should be contoured once again before the bands are cemented. Bands should not be placed on a tooth, removed, and then cemented without being recontoured. Placement and removal always stretch the margins, and this must be corrected before cementation.

Contouring and fitting of performed stainless steel bands should be done with dispatch; the band should be formed to its correct contours with a minimum of reworking of the metal. These bands are supplied in an annealed, workable condition. After the work hardening of excessive manipulation, they will no longer respond easily to additional contouring, and the increased springiness will reduce adaptability and retention.

CEMENTATION

Cementation is a critical procedure that should be carried out with all possible care. The safety of the tooth is at stake, along with uninterrupted treatment. Every loose band that must be recemented in the course of treatment is an additional burden to patient and orthodontist alike.

Preparing bands

As bands are fitted, they are placed in the dish of water to prevent saliva from drying on them (Figs. 16-2 and 16-9, *D*). This dish can be large enough to permit easy separation and identification of bands for upper and lower, right and left, or they may be placed on a separate rack after rinsing. After vigorous rinsing, the bands are placed on absorbent paper to remove excess water (Fig. 16-9, *A*). Individual bands are then dipped in 95% alcohol (Fig. 16-9, *B*) and set afire (Fig. 16-9, *C*). This will not heat the band beyond the stress-relieving range.

While the band is still hot, brackets and tubes are touched to a piece of soft white utility wax (Fig. 16-9, *D*) to fill holes and grooves with melted wax. This will prevent cement from filling these areas during cementation. Softer materials will also serve the same purpose, but there is a greater risk of contamination of the inside of the band or the tooth, where they can affect adhesion of the cement.

Bands are next placed on transparent surgical adhesive tape or masking tape, occlusal side down, and oriented for proper positioning on the tooth. The tape is folded as shown in Fig. 16-9, *E*, to expose only a small square of sticky surface.

This adhesive tape serves several purposes. It helps keep cement off the fingers and facilitates passing of the cement-filled band from assistant to orthodontist. It orients the band as it is placed in the mouth. It permits simultaneous placement of two or more small adjacent bands. The seal at the occlusal margin helps force cement gingivally as the band is seated. The protection afforded by the tape makes it possible to apply stronger finger pressure and seat the band farther on the tooth while the occlusal tape seal is still forcing cement out around the gingival margin.

Mixing cement

An instrument tray for cementation is shown in Fig. 16-10, *A*. It holds only the essentials: mixing slabs, spatulas, clear plastic adhesive tape, adhesive tinfoil, cement powder and liquid, and a small plastic measuring scoop.

When prepared for cementation, these are arranged as shown in Fig. 16-10, *B*. Bands are placed so that each group to be cemented with a separate mix of cement is in a separate vertical row. Adhesive foil is ready for use as the bands are cemented, with one end turned up so that it can be picked up easily when needed. Two small scoops of powder are placed together on the cool slab for each mix.

A

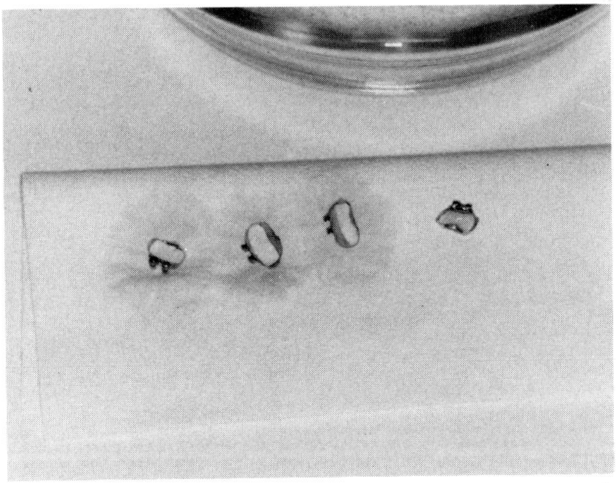

Continued.

Fig. 16-9. A, Placing bands on absorbent paper after rinsing will quickly remove excess water. **B** to **D,** Clean band is dipped in alcohol, set afire, and hot bracket touched to soft utility wax to fill grooves with wax before cementation. **E,** Bands on adhesive tape, ready for cementation.

B C D E

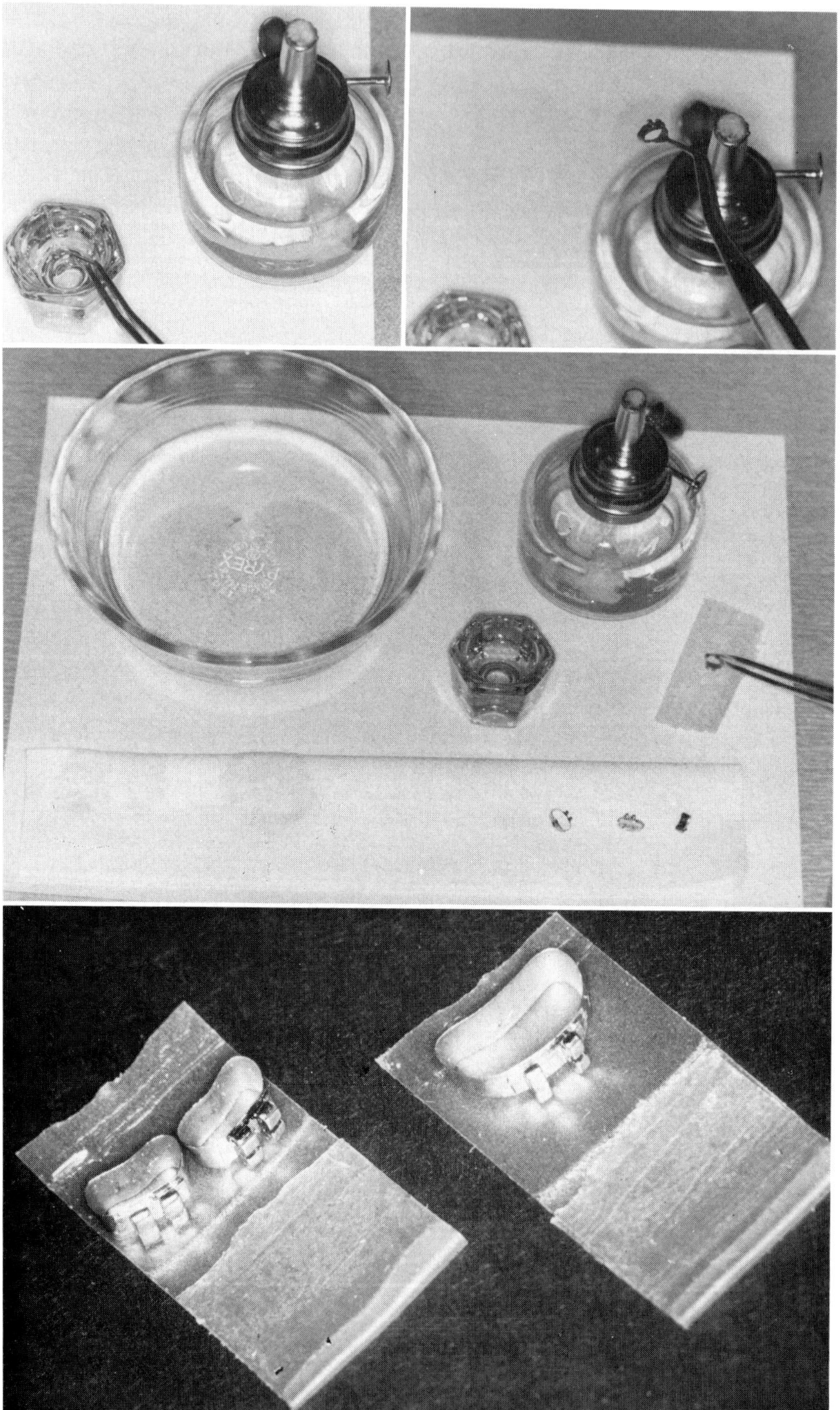

Fig. 16-9, cont'd. For legend see p. 213.

A

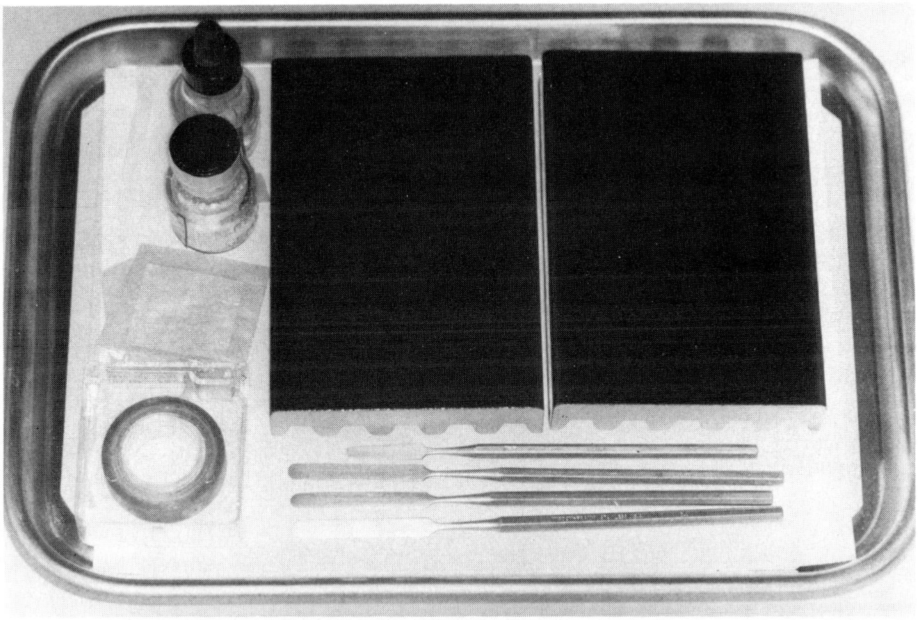

B

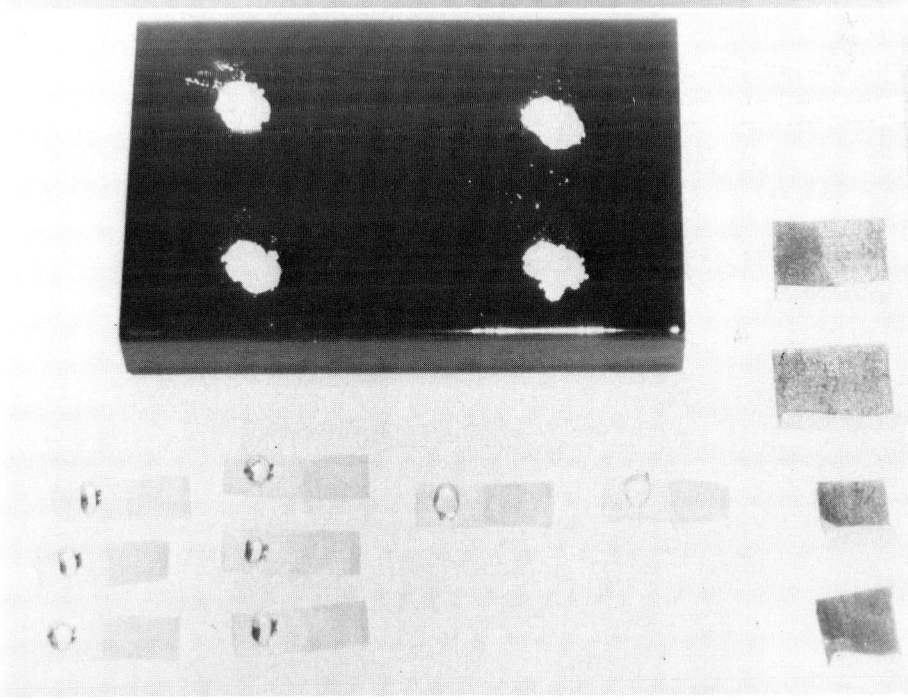

Continued.

Fig. 16-10. A, Cementation tray holding mixing slabs, spatulas, cement, adhesive foil, and transparent adhesive tape. **B,** Bands ready for cementation, aligned in order of insertion, with cement and adhesive foil prepared for use. Each vertical row of bands is to be cemented with a separate mix of cement. **C,** Correct amount of liquid is added to measured cement powder. **D,** Mixture is rapidly spread over slab as powder and liquid are mixed, to prevent buildup of heat in the material. **E,** Cement is spatulated rapidly to a uniform consistency, which should draw out in a thread as spatula is lifted. It is important that the mix be well spread over the slab surface. Spatula is "rolled" from side to side, so all mixing is done with one side of the blade. **F,** Cement is gathered on the spatula so that it is evenly distributed along the blade. **G,** Bands are filled immediately with the same motion that would be used if the objective were to clean the spatula with the band.

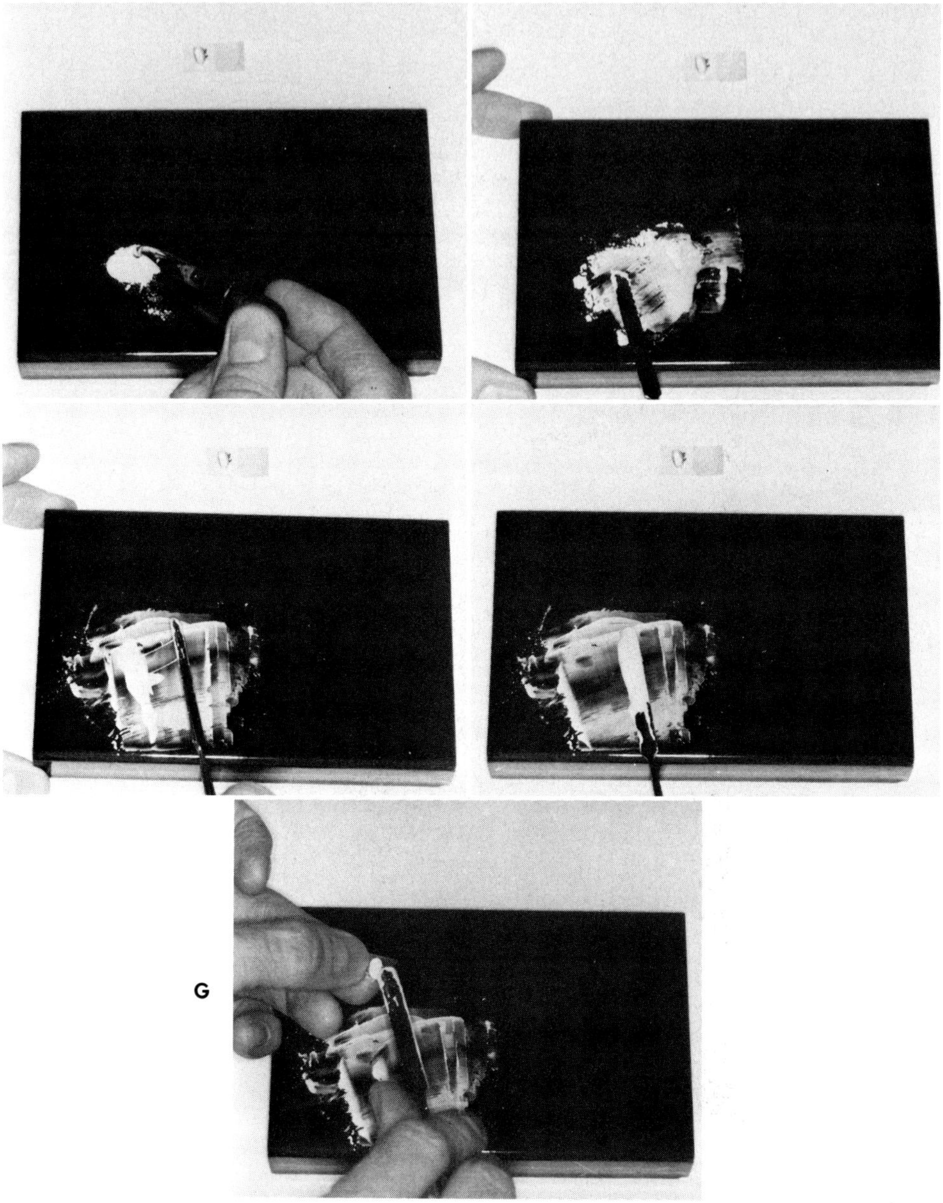

C D E F G

Fig. 16.10, cont'd. For legend, see p. 215.

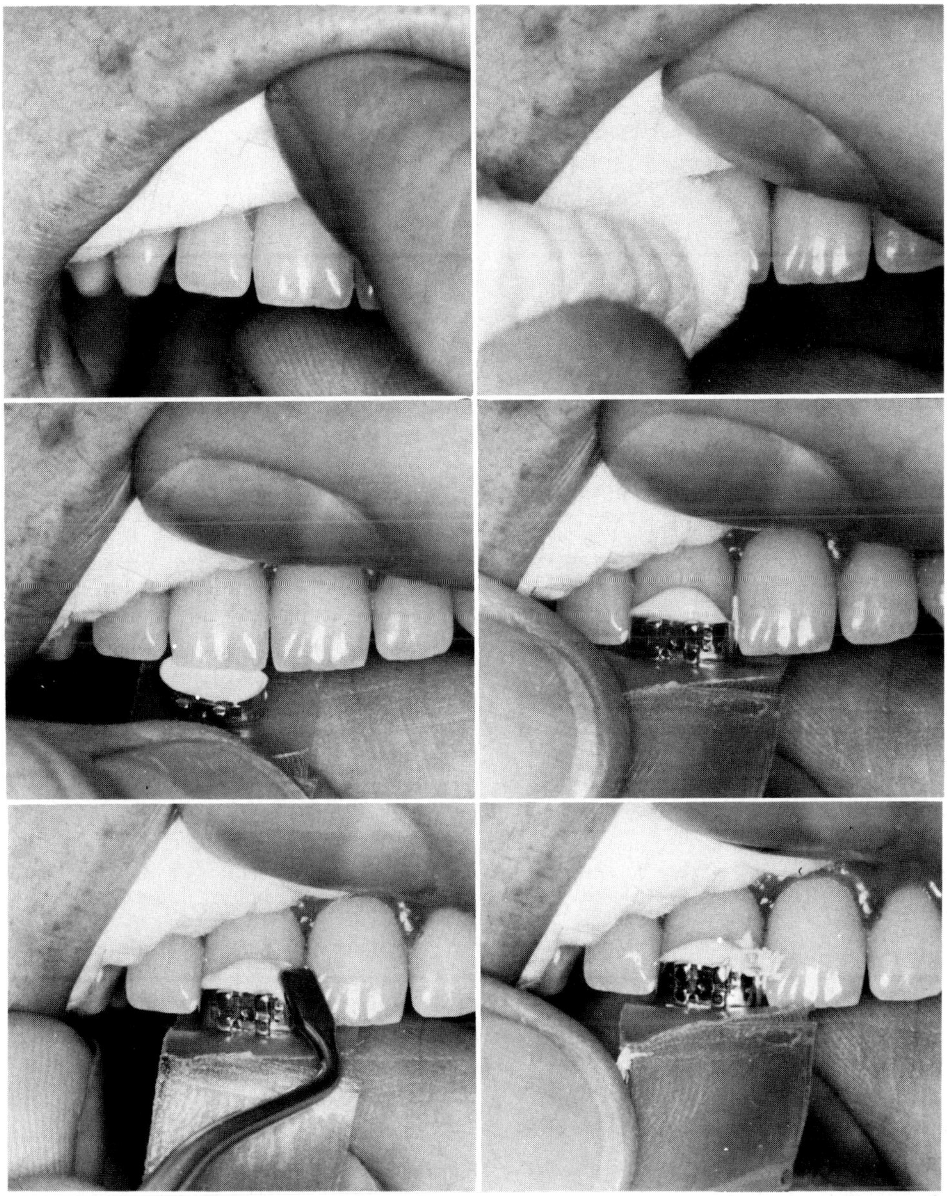

Continued.

Fig. 16-11. A, Tooth isolated with cotton rolls. **B,** Tooth is wiped dry with end of unstarched cotton roll, followed by an air blast if required. **C,** Cement-filled band, ready to place on tooth. **D,** Band placement is suspended if cement bead is depleted at any point. **E,** Cement is moved with plugger to deficient area. **F,** Band is placed as far as possible with finger pressure; then tape is removed. **G,** Seating is completed, using either end of plugger as required. **H,** Entire band is covered with adhesive foil until cement is set.

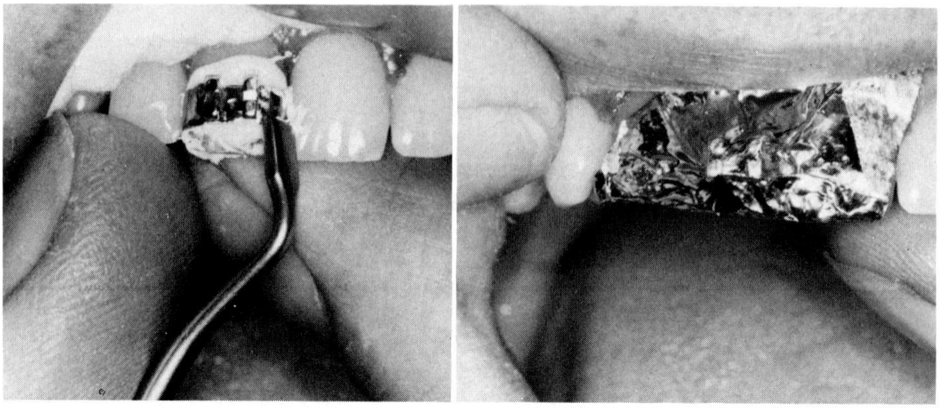

G H

Fig. 16-11, cont'd. For legend see p. 217.

With everything in readiness, the assistant begins to mix the cement while the orthodontist prepares the teeth.

Four to six drops of cement liquid are added to the measured powder (Fig. 16-10, *C*) and quickly spatulated so that the mix is spread in a thin layer on the slab (Fig. 16-10, *D*). This is important in achieving a smooth mix and ample working time. The cement is rapidly spatulated to a suitable consistency (Fig. 16-10, *E*) and gathered on the spatula (Fig. 16-10, *F*), and the bands are filled (Fig. 16-10, *G*).

Proportions of powder and liquid may have to be adjusted for different cements and for variations in liquid-dispensing droppers. The same dropper should be used consistently with this technique, and it should always be held with the dispensing tip exactly vertical to ensure uniform drop size.

Anterior and small bicuspid bands should be completely filled with cement. Larger bands may have only the inside periphery covered, but the entire gingival margin must always be fully covered with an ample bead of cement.

Band placement

By the time the band has been filled with cement, the orthodontist has isolated the tooth with cotton rolls (Fig. 16-11, *A*), wiped it dry with the end of an unstarched cotton roll (Fig. 16-11, *B*), and completed the drying with air.

The cement-filled band (Fig. 16-11, *C*) is placed on the tooth only as far as is possible without losing the bead of cement that advances ahead (Fig. 16-11, *D*). In the illustration there is little cement ahead of the band near the mesial contact point; this is not unusual. Additional cement is moved to this area with the plugger (Fig. 16-11, *E*) before the band is advanced farther (Fig. 16-11, *F*). The tape is removed for final seating with the plugger (Fig. 16-11, *G*). The band should be firmly seated, bucally and lingually, mesially and distally.

When the band is completely positioned, it is covered with adhesive tinfoil to protect the cement from moisture until it is completely set (Fig. 16-11, *H*).

When the cement has set (it must be hard and brittle), all excess is removed and banding is complete.

17

Wire selection

The orthodontist faces a continually expanding variety of wires for almost every application. This variety in both size and material is a benefit, but it creates baffling problems of selection. Choosing by "feel" can be grossly misleading, and standard physical test data are mostly irrelevant in spite of their more scientific basis.

The present trend in materials testing is away from sole reliance on standard tests, such as the tensile test, in favor of simulated-use tests that measure the actual performance required in service. This approach has much to offer in the evaluation of orthodontic wires.

In use, orthodontic wires are subjected to bending and to torsion, but not to pure tension. A realistic evaluation of the performance of these wires is very difficult without information about their response in bending or in torsion.

The following information about the performance of orthodontic wires has been derived from tests with a device specially designed and constructed to measure forces and deflections in the orthodontic ranges. The heart of the device is a laboratory balance, accurate to .01 gm, with a maximum capacity of over 1000 gm. This balance has been built into a mechanism for supporting a test wire in such a way that it can be loaded by the balance.

In the tests that will be reported here, the test wires are suspended between supports spaced .5 inch (12.7 mm) apart and subjected to a load applied at the center. The ends of the wire are free to tip in a simple beam arrangement. A span measured in inches instead of metric units was selected because wire sizes are normally stated in inches, and diameter and span must be considered together in some calculations. The test span is approximately the distance across a central incisor, measured between the brackets of the two adjacent teeth, so it simulates the deflections and forces on a single tooth.

In relating these test forces to practice, one should remember that the test wires are suspended as a simple beam with ends free. If the ends were rigidly supported, as is more nearly the case under actual conditions, force would be multiplied up to four times for the same deflections. Maximum deflection would also be reduced to as little as one-fourth of the reported values. Most spans in the mouth will be as short as the test span, or shorter; therefore, the forces found in these tests usually can be considered to be the lowest forces that might generally be encountered with these wires in a full-banded appliance.

Both force and deflection are measured as the load is applied to the test wire.

These are plotted in a curve that closely resembles the tensile test curve in appearance.

DESCRIPTION OF BENDING TEST CURVES

The difference between a stress-bending curve and a stress-strain curve made from a tensile test is in the region of the elastic limit and plastic deformation. In the tensile test, the entire test piece is subjected to the same strain or elongation so that the entire piece reaches the elastic limit at the same time. In bending, the outer fibers of the wire are strained (stretched or compressed) more than the inner fibers so that these areas reach the elastic limit first (Figs. 9-1 and 9-2).

The result of this unequal strain is that the straight-line portion of the bending curve ends when the *outer* fibers begin to deform plastically, even though the part near the center is still behaving elastically and following a straight-line response. The bending curve is a composite of the response of all these fibers; therefore the transition into the upper curved portion is much more subtle than it would be in the tensile test where the entire piece reaches this limit at the same time.

Drawn wires may be more work-hardened near the surface, which is subject to the most strain in bending. This effect can be very important in bending tests, but may be partly obscured in a tensile test that places an equal strain on all parts of the wire under test.

The form of the upper part of this curve is an indication of work hardening. The curve bends sharply for such metals as gold or moderately low-temper chrome-cobalt, which have undergone very little work hardening. After the elastic limit for these materials has been passed, the metal fails under a relatively small additional force. Stainless steel has been heavily work-hardened in drawing, and the result is a higher and more gentle curve as the wire resists much greater maximum loads (Fig. 17-1).

It can be seen from the curves that steel has a high reserve strength beyond the elastic range as a result of this work-hardening effect. This is a great advantage in wires of small diameters, but it can be a distinct disadvantage in wires of larger sizes.

Releasing the load from a wire in the plastic range results in a curve such as the descending line shown in Fig. 17-2. This more or less straight line shows slight curves at the upper and lower ends. On reloading, the curve ascends between and almost parallel to the original loading and unloading lines. The hysteresis loop formed by the unloading and reloading curves represents energy lost to internal friction in the wire and dissipated as heat. As the reloading curve reaches the original curve, it continues in an extension of that curve, following the same line that it would have followed without the interruption.

It is important to note that the force delivery curve is the lower unloading curve, *not* the upper loading curve. Because the stress-bending curve represents actual response of a wire under simulated clinical stresses, it gives information that can be directly adapted to clinical practice.

To facilitate interpretation and application of these curves, two marks have been made on most of the graph lines. The first is a short vertical line at the point where deflection reaches .022 inch (.56 mm). This is a deflection equal to the width of the wide .022-inch edgewise bracket slot. The second mark is a dot placed on the line where plastic deformation has added a 10% deflection from the straight-line elastic response. This deflection represents the reduction in applied force resulting from plastic deformation. This is a purely arbitrary point, which is used to suggest an upper limit to acceptable plastic deformation. No special virtue is claimed for the 10% value; in fact, an ideal index probably should provide a different offset for each material and perhaps for each size of wire.

The failure point in these curves, where they become horizontal, does not indicate fracture. Orthodontic wires will not normally fracture under an overload in bending. What occurs is that the bending wire is finally bent so far that it is pulled down between the supports, so that it is incapable of supporting the load. This

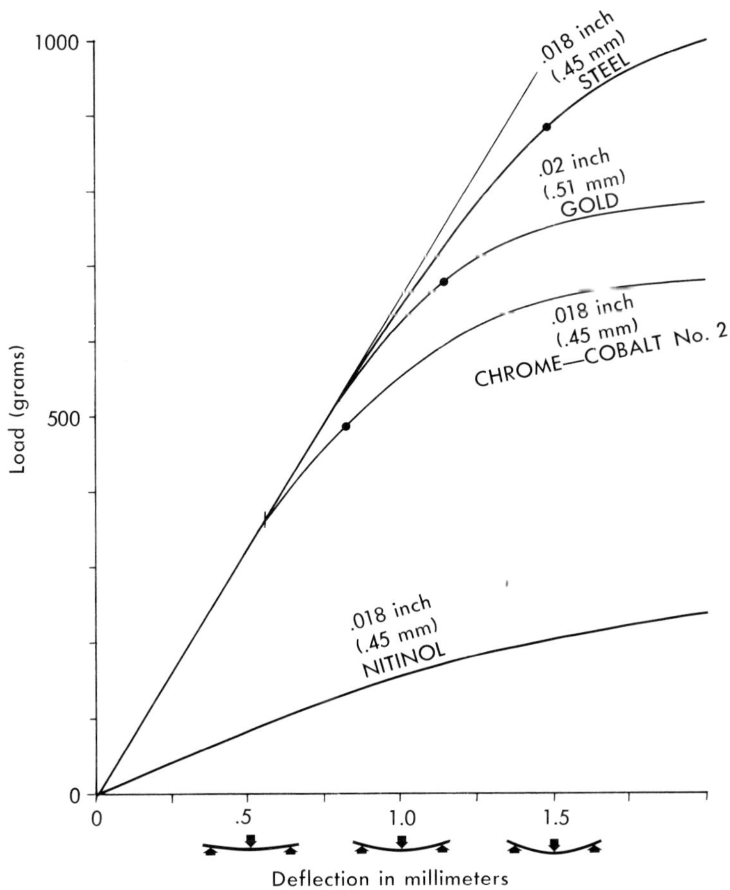

Fig. 17-1. Stress-bending curves for stainless steel, gold, and chrome-cobalt wires of the same stiffness and for nitinol wire of the same diameter as the steel and chrome–cobalt wires. Harder tempered (or heat-treated) chrome–cobalt wire would show a curve comparable to stainless steel. The small diagrams below the deflection values of 0.5, 1.0, and 1.5 mm show the span and deflection of the test wires in actual size. The short vertical mark at the .55-mm deflection point indicates the width of the wide (0.22-inch) bracket slot. The dot on the upper part of the curve marks a deflection 10% in excess of a straight-line response, indicating 10% permanent set.

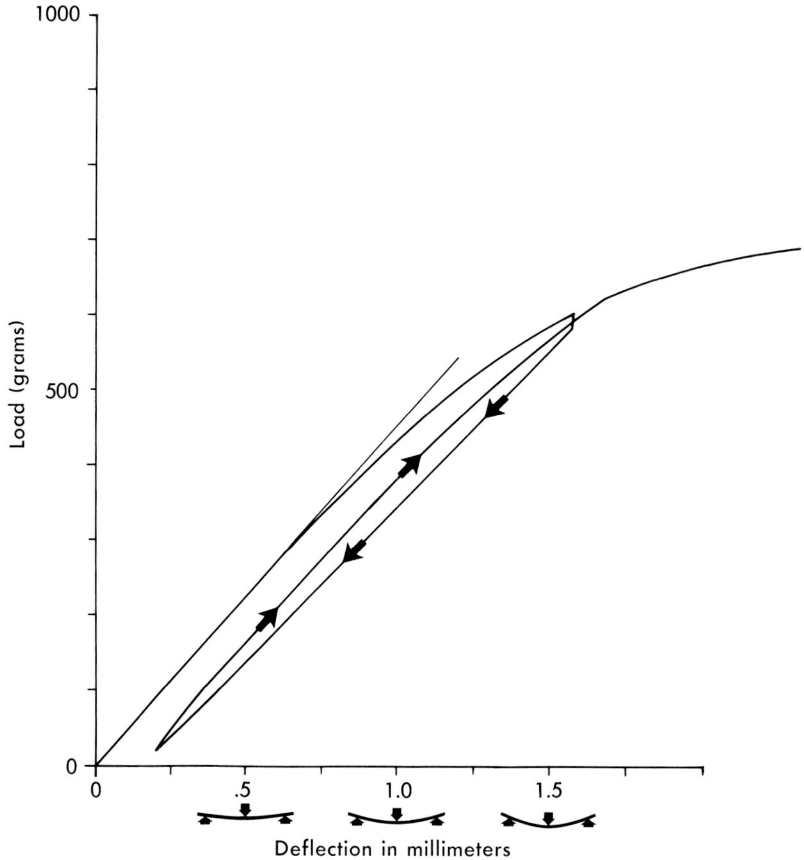

Fig. 17-2. Effect of unloading and reloading a bending wire after it has been stressed beyond the elastic limit.

change in the geometry of force application with large deflections is an important factor in both the clinical and test situations.

COMPARISON OF BENDING CURVES FOR DIFFERENT MATERIALS

Full comparison of different materials involves several considerations, which will be discussed individually. Before these individual characteristics are examined, it will be helpful to consider the more gross aspects of the curves for the different metals.

Fig. 17-3, a composite of several graphs, shows the ranges found for each class of metals in a single wire size (.018 inch or .45 mm). Each of these ranges is based on multiple samples of commonly used high-quality orthodontic wires.

Gold

The curves for gold are in the lowest range. One extremely hard clasp alloy accounts for the upper extreme of the range for gold. Only a few gold samples were

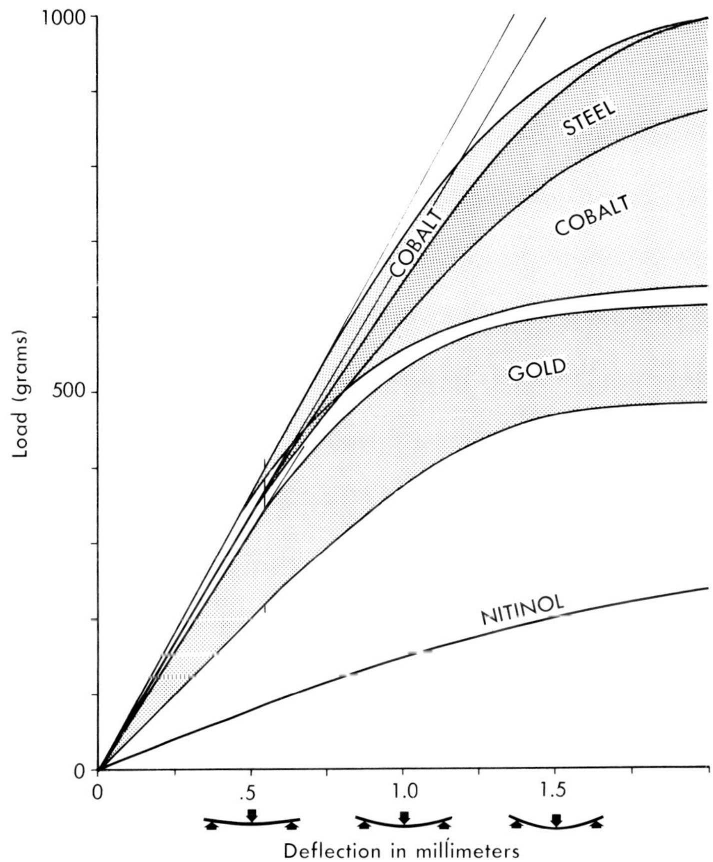

Fig. 17-3. Ranges of stress-bending curves for the four major classes of orthodontic wire material, comparing wires of the same size (.018 inch or .45 mm).

tested, all of high-spring orthodontic wires; therefore this range would undoubtedly be expanded in a downward direction if softer wires were added.

The most important points to consider in the graphs for gold wires are the low stiffness (steepness of the straight line) and the sharp drop-off after plastic deformation begins. One can completely compensate for the low stiffness by using wire with a larger diameter; if graphs for these stiffer wires were shown, the entire range for gold would be higher. The sharp curve in the plastic range has both advantages and disadvantages that will be discussed later.

Stainless steel

Steel shows the narrowest range of the three materials. The range shown in Fig. 17-3 is based on samples from several manufacturers and with different degrees of heat treatment. In comparison with the gold curve, the curve for steel arcs very gently after the elastic limit is exceeded. The curve begins to deviate from a straight line below 400 gm, only slightly above gold, but it does not approach the horizontal line that indicates failure until these forces are about doubled. This behavior is typical of materials that work harden appreciably, and it is one reason it is often almost essential that steel be used beyond its elastic limit.

Chrome-cobalt (Elgiloy)

The chrome-cobalt alloys are supplied in several tempers so that the complete range brackets steel on both sides. These alloys are slightly more stiff than steel, although much less than .001 inch (.025 mm) difference in diameter would compensate for this difference. The softest of the chrome-cobalt wires shows a working range almost as low as gold. This wire will fall well within the gold range if smaller wires with comparable stiffness are compared (Fig. 17-1). The hardest of the chrome-cobalt wires is comparable to steel. The hardest wire shown in Fig. 17-3 is the heat-treated form of the second hardest temper; heat treating the hardest wire could give a slightly higher curve, but such a wire would be too brittle for most uses.

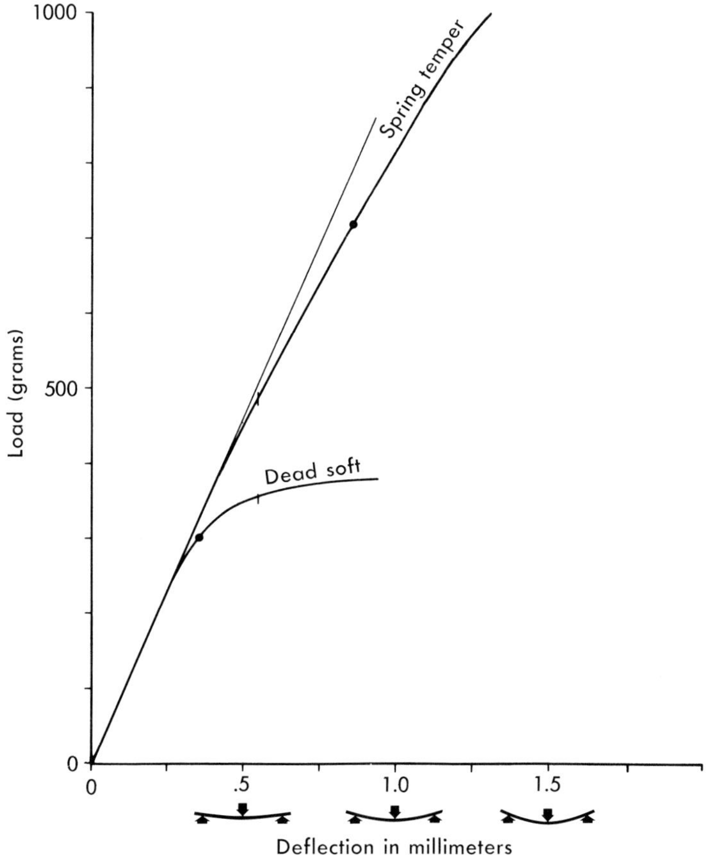

Fig. 17-4. Effect of hardness or temper on the bending properties of stainless steel, showing the extremes of dead-soft and hard-temper wires of the same diameter (.5 mm). Stiffness is identical, but strength and working range are much lower for the dead-soft material.

INFLUENCE OF WIRE HARDNESS ON STIFFNESS, STRENGTH, AND RANGE

Stiffness

Stiffness is dependent on the modulus of elasticity, which is not appreciably influenced by any hardening treatment. All wires of the same alloy will be equally stiff. Fig. 17-4 shows the bending curves for two stainless steel wires, each .020 inch (.5 mm) in diameter. The lowest curve is that of a dead-soft wire that can be bent with the fingers almost as easily as lead. The upper curve represents a hardened and stress-relieved wire with maximum spring properties.

In the lower force ranges, the curves for these two wires are identical; they respond exactly the same under stress. It is this straight-line section of the curve that indicates stiffness; thus these two wires actually are equally stiff. Both wires require 228 gm to produce a deflection of .010 inch (.25 mm).

It is important to remember that stiffness is the same for wires of the same material, regardless of their hardness, and that these wires behave identically below the point where plastic deformation begins for the softer wire. An exception is seen in certain gold alloys that do show some change in stiffness after heat treatment.

Importance of stiffness. Stiffness should be the first criterion in the selection of wires for a specific purpose, for it determines the relationship between force and deflection in the ideal working range. Stiffness tells *how far* the tooth will be moved by a specific initial force and, conversely, *how much force* will be applied at a certain deflection. The fact that soft wires apply the same force as hard wires of the same material in the lower working range is a very important consideration that is often overlooked in archwire selection.

If only stiffness is considered, any of the commonly used materials can be used interchangeably by merely selecting a suitable diameter of wire for each material. Wires of equal stiffness will behave identically below the point at which they take a permanent set, regardless of the material.

Working range and strength

The difference between the two wires that are compared in Fig. 17-4 lies in the upper force ranges where the curves diverge. This upper end of the curve is the part that is dependent on the strength and range of the wire.

Looking more closely at the graph, we see that the limit of proportional response for the soft wire was reached at a deflection of about .011 inch (.28 mm), half the width of a wide bracket slot. At this point it was exerting a force of about 250 gm. At a deflection of .022 inch (.56 mm), this soft wire was exerting a force of 350 gm, whereas the hard wire had continued proportionately to reach a force of about 500 gm. Even when it was bent near the point of failure, the soft wire applied more than two-thirds as much force as the hard wire at that same deflection. Bending these two wires with the fingers would give no hint of such great similarity, because we tend to feel for the upper limit. Beyond the proportional limit the similarity disappears and the dominant effects of strength and working range mask the identical stiffness.

Working range and strength combine to determine the upper parts of the curve. The problem in comparing these properties for different materials lies in the selection of a suitable reference point in that upper section of the curve. This entire end of the curve shows the effects of the higher forces and deflections; therefore what is needed is some meaningful reference point that can be accurately located on the curves of different materials.

Maximum limits. The maximum height of the curve will show the highest load that the wire can possibly sustain or apply to a tooth. This is ultimate strength, the limit that is approached when a wire is tied into place with a heavy permanent set.

The deflection at this extreme load will be the ultimate working range of the wire, but deflection changes so rapidly as failure is approached that a precise point for measuring this value cannot be determined.

For many reasons, the ultimate limits just described should not be approached routinely in applying force to a tooth, but they do give a good indication of the behavior that can be expected in two important clinical situations: arch formation and unwanted bending.

In arch formation and adjustment, a wire with a bending curve that drops off sharply will stay where it is put when it is bent, with relatively little springback. This is characteristic of most gold alloys and the soft temper chrome-cobalt. A wire with a gentle curve in the bending graph must be bent far beyond the desired form by the force indicated at the top of that curve to obtain an appreciable permanent set. This wire will then spring back a great part of that distance when the force is released. It may also tend to recover part of the permanent set later and change shape in the mouth unless it is stress-relieved. This behavior is typical of stainless steel.

The ease with which a wire in the mouth can be deformed by chewing and other patient-applied forces is related to ease of adjustment. Here the desirable ease of formation becomes undesirable ease of deformation. This is the reason that gold wires with diameters below .018 or .020 inch (.45 or .50 mm) were seldom used. These problems are all relative; no wire is patient-proof.

Working limits. The ultimate stress is unsuitable as a measure of strength and range in the clinical application of force to teeth, for permanent set is undesirable in this situation. A lower limit, based on minimum permanent set, is needed for orthodontic use, so the 10% plastic-deformation point previously described is used here as a guide. At that point 10% of the original adjustment will be lost to permanent set.

The curves shown in Fig. 17-4 show the marked differences in working range between the hard and soft steel wires. The soft wire failed at 485 gm, while the hard wire could have supported a heavier load than the 1000-gm limit of the test scale. This is more than 2 pounds. The dots at 10% deflection show a working range of .014 inch (.35 mm) for the soft wire and .034 inch (.86 mm) for the hard wire. Strength at these deflections was 305 gm for the soft wire and 720 gm for the hard wire.

EFFECTS OF WIRE SIZE

Stiffness

Fig. 17-5 shows bending curves for stainless steel wires of different sizes, along with the curves for two gold wires. Relative stiffness is most easily judged from

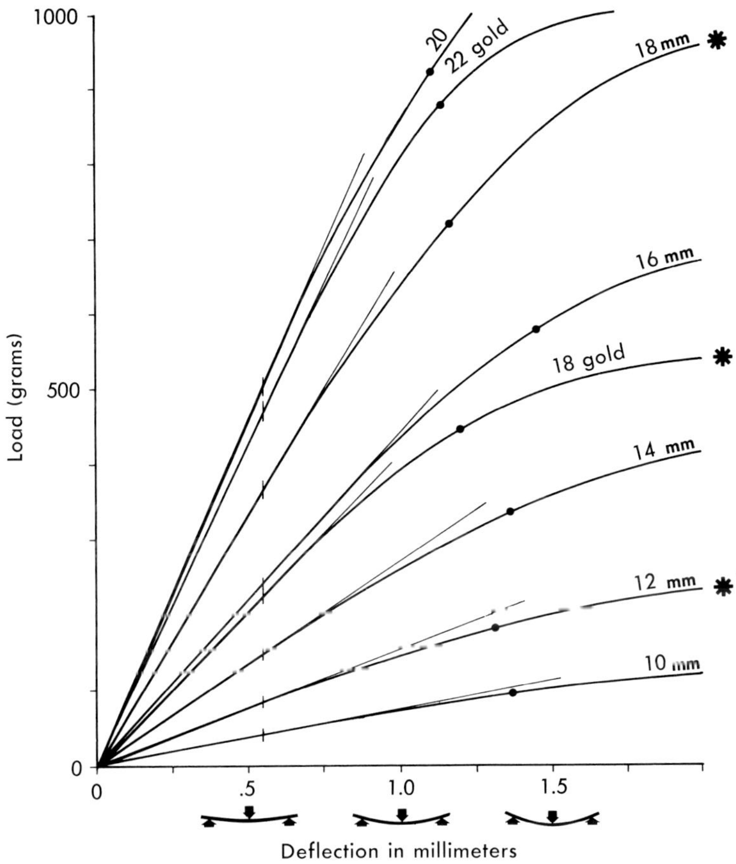

Fig. 17-5. Stress-bending curves for wires of different sizes of the same material (stainless steel), with gold and nitinol samples added for comparison. The curve for .018-inch (.45-mm) nitinol wire is essentially identical to that for .012-inch (.30-mm) steel. Asterisks mark the curves for .018-inch (.45-mm) wires of steel, gold, and Nitinol.

these graphs by comparison of the forces required for a .022-inch (.55-mm) deflection. This deflection is below the proportional limit of all the wires, and it is well within the range of clinical application. These forces are directly proportional to stiffness.

The gold wires shown in this graph are high-spring orthodontic wires that fall between and close to other gold wires that were tested. As a rule of thumb, gold wires .002 inch (.05 mm) larger in diameter can be expected to compare very closely with steel in stiffness. Such wires are somewhat below steel in strength and useful working range.

Strength and range

It is not difficult to stress wires of very small diameter to their limit with a heavy permanent set; therefore it is important to compare maximum stress levels.

These wires can apply surprisingly heavy forces, as shown by the graph. A .010-inch (.25-mm) wire can apply a 120-gm force over the wide span used in the test. With a shorter span and more rigid conditions at the ends of the span, more typical of the situation with an orthodontic arch, this wire could easily apply more than 1 pound of force to a tooth. The ultimate force for an .008-inch (.20-mm) wire on this test (not shown on the graph) was 65 gm, compared to 120 gm for the .010-inch (.25-mm) wire.

For heavier wires, the 10% deflection is a more useful criterion for judging strength and range. The locations of the 10% deflection dots on these graphs point up the variability in this criterion for measuring range and strength. With steel wires, the transition from a straight to a curved line is so gradual that even a very slight deviation will shift the 10% point a considerable distance up or down the curve. The straight portion of the graph for steel will often begin to curve almost imperceptibly at a very low level, especially when wires have not been stress-relieved. It is this difficulty in accurately establishing the straight-line reference that makes the proportional limit in bending so unreliable.

These graphs bear out the previously noted fact that working range varies comparatively little with wire size (only inversely proportional to the diameter). Strength (the height of the 10% dots) is affected much more (proportional to the cube of diameter), and stiffness is changed the most (proportional to the fourth power of diameter).

MULTIPLE ARCHES

Multiple arches, made up of several small wires, are sometimes used in the initial stages of treatment. These offer a combination of the low stiffness and long working range of small-diameter wires with the increased strength of numbers.

Multiple straight strands keep the same working range as a single strand while stiffness and strength are additive as strands are added.

Twisting the strands provides a cabled wire of larger diameter that will engage the bracket slot more fully. This will increase force levels and carry movements somewhat farther than loose-fitting single strands or bundles.

Actual force levels for a given deflection are about the same for twisted wires as for straight strands. Tightly twisted cabled wires introduce some added effects that may be significant in some applications.

Tight twisting introduces more wire length into a given length of cabled wire, effectively increasing span. This will reduce stiffness and increase range. The tight twisting increases the distortion of individual wires in bending and so increases stiffness. These two effects tend to cancel each other in their effects on stiffness, so twisted wires still offer essentially the same stiffness as multiple straight strands. Fig. 17-6 shows bending curves for a nominal .018-inch (.45-mm) wire and one strand of straight .010-inch (.25-mm) wire. In the lower stress range the two behave identically, but the proportional limit of the stranded wire is considerably higher, as can be seen by the long straight-line response.

The wire in the illustration was made up of three .008-inch (.20-mm) wires, twisted tightly to a .066-inch (1.68-mm) pitch (one full turn every .066 inch or 1.68 mm). With each wire twisted one revolution in .066 inch (1.68 mm) this means a

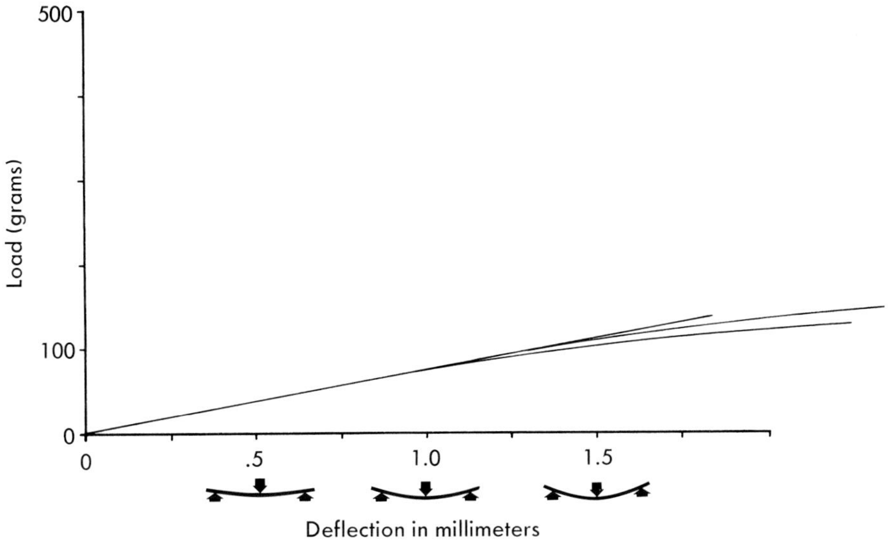

Fig. 17-6. Stress-bending curves for stranded and solid stainless steel wires. The top curve represents a tightly twisted 3-strand .0175-inch (.44-mm) wire. The lower curve represents a solid .010-inch (.25-mm) wire. Stiffness is identical, but strength and range are slightly higher for the stranded wire.

spacing of .022 inch (.55 mm), or less than three wire diameters, between wires as measured lengthwise along the cable. Actual outside diameter of the cabled wire was .017 inch (.43 mm). The smallest circle that will contain three wires .008 inch (.20 mm) in diameter is .017 inch (.43 mm), so it can be seen that there is virtually no free space for movement between these wires.

The moment of inertia for a .008-inch (.20-mm) circle is 181, or 543 for three wires. This compares closely to 491 for a .010-inch (.25-mm) wire, but not as closely as shown by the graph in Fig. 17-6. Two major contributions to the slight reduction in stiffness are the increased length of the wire and the change to a coiled configuration. Wires in a cable of this form actually flex in a manner approaching that of a coil spring, with tension and compression partially replaced by torsion loads.

HEAT TREATMENT

Effects of heat treatment on gold, steel, and chrome-cobalt wires are shown in Figs. 17-7 to 17-9. Heat treatment of all these wires increases strength and range but has little if any effect on stiffness.

Gold

Gold wires are extremely variable in their response to heat treatment. Some even show increased hardness after annealing, but such effects are small. The graph presented in Fig. 17-7, showing an increase in both stiffness and strength, is reasonably typical. Gold is the only orthodontic alloy that shows a significant increase

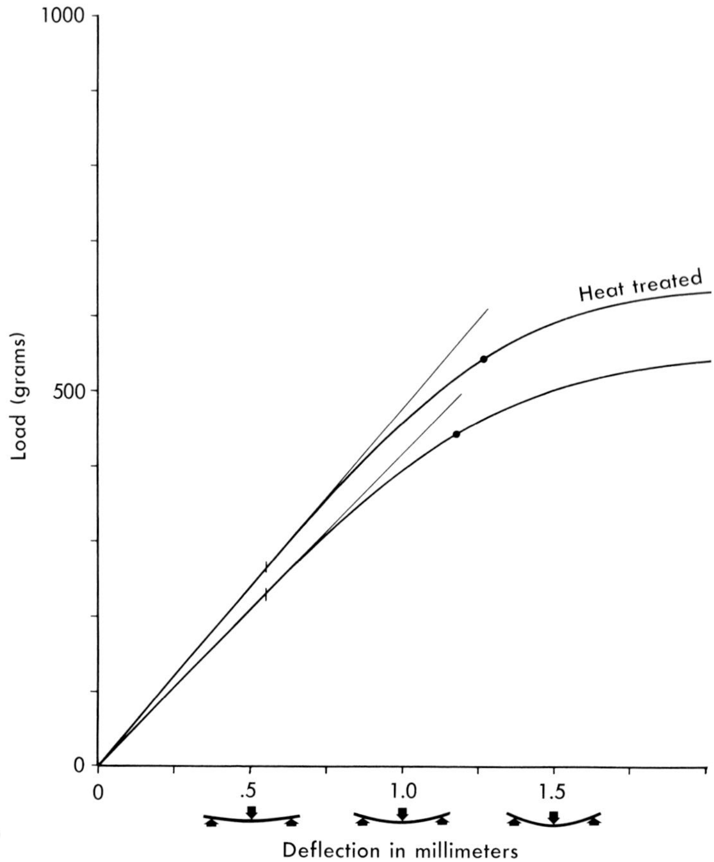

Fig. 17-7. Effect of heat hardening on one gold alloy. Note increase in stiffness, which is not found with stainless steel or chrome-cobalt.

in stiffness with heat treatment, and this is true only for some alloys of this group. Other gold alloys behave more like steel and chrome-cobalt, increasing in strength and range only. The effect of heat treatment, such as that shown Fig. 17-7, is merely to increase all properties to those of a slightly larger wire. This is really no advantage at all, for it would be much easier to use a wire .001 inch (.025 mm) larger than to go through the heat-treatment procedure.

There is seldom an advantage in heat treating any gold wires in view of the fact that orthodontists usually use only the larger sizes, in which the maximum strength is above the levels normally required. In these sizes gains in stiffness are usually disadvantageous, and gains in strength are seldon usable. In the unusual situations in which extreme strength is required, it is better to change to steel wire that has much greater strength than to try to gain a little extra strength by heat treating gold.

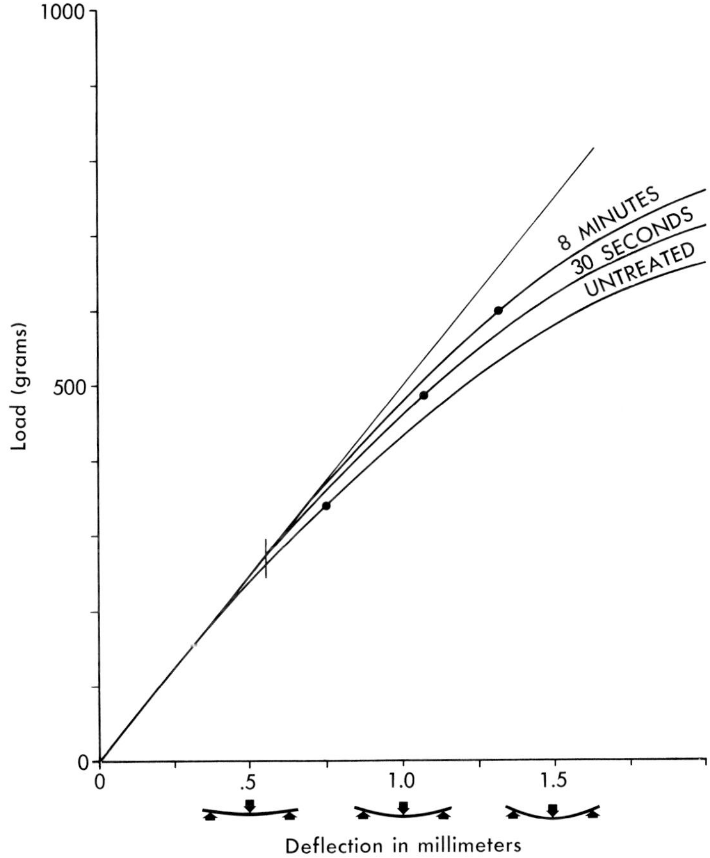

Fig. 17-8. Effect of heat treatment at 850° F (450° C) on stainless steel wire. Note that stiffness is unchanged, but strength and range are increased.

Steel

The major changes in the heat treatment of steel by stress-relieving are an elevation of the proportional limit (lengthening the straight part of the curve) and increases in strength and range (Fig. 17-8).

In large wires there is even less need for such gains in steel than there is in gold. In smaller sizes, where wires are stressed near their limit, these gains are valuable. As can be seen from the curves shown in Fig. 17-8, most of this gain is achieved rapidly; therefore short treatment times can be quite effective.

An additional advantage of heat treating steel, especially in wires of the larger sizes, is not shown in these tests. The stress-relieving effect makes a newly formed wire more stable in form, and this can be very important in the heavier wires. All large-diameter steel wires used in arches or retainers should be stress relieved to prevent later changes in shape that could affect their performance.

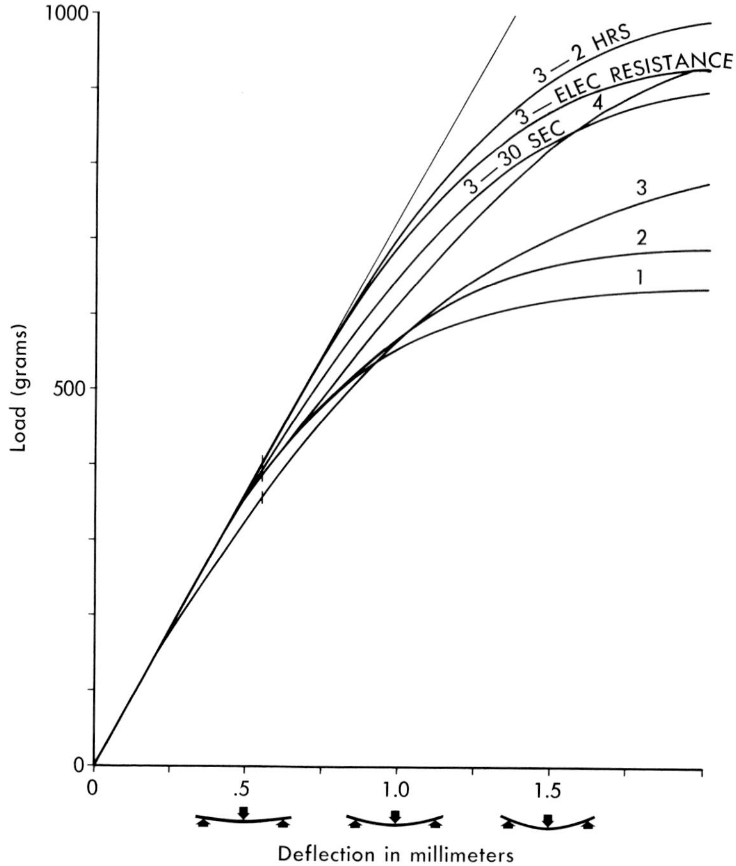

Fig. 17-9. Stress-bending curves showing the effects of initial temper *(B, Y, G, R)* and heat treatment on chrome-cobalt wire. The curves for the *G* temper wire show heat treatment in an oven at 900° F (480° C) for 30 seconds and 2 hours and rapid resistance heating with an electric current.

Chrome-cobalt

The curves for seven chrome-cobalt wires, all .018 inch (.45 mm) in diameter, are shown in Fig. 17-9. Those numbered 1 through 4 are the four basic tempers as received (blue, yellow, green, and red). Three additional curves show the effects of different heat treatments on the No. 3 temper wire.

Oven heat treatments used the recommended 900° F. temperature for the times shown. Electrical heat treatment was carried out with flash paste. Temperatures can be more variable with this method, but results in all cases provided a significant increase in strength and range. As shown in Fig. 17-3, however, these are closely comparable to stainless steel. The strongest of these wires was slightly stiffer than steel; the curve fell off more rapidly, however, so that it was below the level of steel near the ultimate load.

An interesting deviation appears in the curve for untreated No. 3 temper wire. Similar deviations were noted for other tempers in some other sizes. The curve for this untreated wire shows plastic deformation beginning much earlier than for the other tempers, but the difference disappears with heat treatment. This suggests a possible difference in heat treatment for these different tempers in manufacture to control ultimate strength. Ultimate strength for the four different tempers, indicated here by the highest part of the curves, is more evenly spaced than either usuable strength or working range. As with steel, these differences could vary with size and other production variables.

SUMMING UP

Stiffness

Stiffness is the first requirement that must be met in wire selection, since it determines the force acting on the tooth in the elastic range. Size is the most potent variable for controlling stiffness, and choice of material is of only secondary importance.

Differences in stiffness between steel and chrome-cobalt wires are negligible. No change in size is necessary in changing from one of these materials to the other.

Gold is about two-thirds as stiff as steel or chrome-cobalt. In round wires this must be compensated for by increasing the diameter for gold wires by about .002 inch (.05 mm) over steel or chrome-cobalt wires.

Stiffness of steel wires measuring .018 by .025 inch (.45 by .63 mm) and gold wires measuring .021 by .025 inch (.53 by .63 mm) is nearly the same in torsion and occlusogingival bending. In buccolingual bending, the steel is slightly stiffer than the larger gold wire.

Heat treatment and work hardening have little or no effect on stiffness.

Strength and range

Strength and range are also comparable for steel and chrome-cobalt wires if chrome-cobalt is used in the heat-treated medium-high temper or untreated high temper. In the untreated No. 1 or No. 2 tempers, chrome-cobalt is significantly lower in both strength and working range than steel or gold of comparable stiffness (Fig. 17-1). This provides a plus for workability in the larger sizes.

In larger sizes (over .018 inch or .45 mm) gold has superior workability, and its lower strength is still adequate for most applications. Torque control is especially facilitated by the use of rectangular gold wires. Gold is the material of choice in these sizes.

Heat treatment

Heat treatment for stress relief is important in steel wires to stabilize arch form, and in wires of smaller sizes it also gives a useful increase in strength and range. Chrome-cobalt wires must be heat treated to bring strength and range of all but the highest temper to the levels of the other materials. Heat treatment is of little value in most gold wires, for the gains in strength and range are not ordinarily usable in the large sizes where the use of gold is indicated.

18

Intramaxillary clinical force management

Intramaxillary forces are those which operate through either the upper or lower dentition. They may be applied by an archwire and fixed attachments or by removable appliances.

Corrective forces may be directed at a tooth from many different sources and directions. Response depends on the net resultant force as it reaches the tooth, regardless of the appliance or technique that may have brought it to bear.

Intramaxillary movements are best regarded as individual tooth movements, even though many individual teeth may be simultaneously involved. The four following factors must be considered for any tooth movement:

1. The required movement, whether it is translation, tipping, axial rotation, or some combination of those movements.
2. Points of application that are available and their usefulness for the desired movement—this is where the geometry of various appliance attachments plays a key role in appliance design.
3. Collateral movements of a tooth that will result from the application of force for the primary action—these critical secondary effects are discussed in Chapter 11 and illustrated in more detail in the *Atlas of Orthodontic Principles.*[34]
4. The energy storage and distribution mechanism (adjustable orthodontic appliance components) that is to be used—this evaluation must include the control of collateral movements and reciprocal effects on other teeth along with the desired effects.

SOURCES FOR ACTIVATING AND CONTROLLING FORCES

The actual source for most orthodontic forces is the fingers of the orthodontist or patient. Manual pressure is used to deform the elastic components of the appliance in such a way that those forces are stored in the appliance and delivered to selected teeth in a predetermined manner over a period of time. The orthodontist regularly adjusts and activates all storage components, and the patient provides supplementary forces through extraoral or intraoral elastic traction where frequent renewal of application is required.

Force storage and distribution elements may be either the archwire itself or any of a large variety of auxiliaries. These will be discussed individually, beginning with the simpler auxiliaries and progressing to the complete archwire.

STORAGE AND DISTRIBUTION ELEMENTS

Ligature wires

The usual application of a ligature wire is for the inelastic transfer of force from archwire to tooth and for holding the engagement of the archwire in the bracket. Ligature wires may also be used to tie teeth together or to draw them toward a stiff arch in small increments. Such movements are limited to the range of elasticity of the periodontal membrane, so they are of little use except for very small final positioning movements. Because of the short range of action, collateral movements are of no consequence in these situations.

Elastic ligatures

Molded elastic ligatures in sizes suitable for ligating individual teeth are a very effective means of applying force to individual teeth. This molded elastomer provides reasonably long-term action in the mouth, but with the loss of force that is typical of organic elastomers. Force levels will drop to about 40% in the first few hours, so it is important to allow for this as these ligatures are activated.

Single-tooth ligation. Single-tooth ligation with appropriate elastomeric ligatures will keep a bracket engaged on the archwire and can also be used to rotate some teeth into full engagement (Fig. 18-1). The limitations on rotation by this method are few but important:

1. The bracket must be wide, well over 3 mm for most teeth. The force available from these ligations is not sufficient to rotate a tooth with the short moment arm of narrower brackets.
2. The arch *must* be at least partially engaged in both brackets. If only one bracket of a pair is engaged on the arch, there is little possibility that the other will maintain alignment long enough to engage the arch as the tooth rotates. In most cases engagement will be even more difficult to attain at later adjustments.
3. The intended rotation must not require significant horizontal movement of

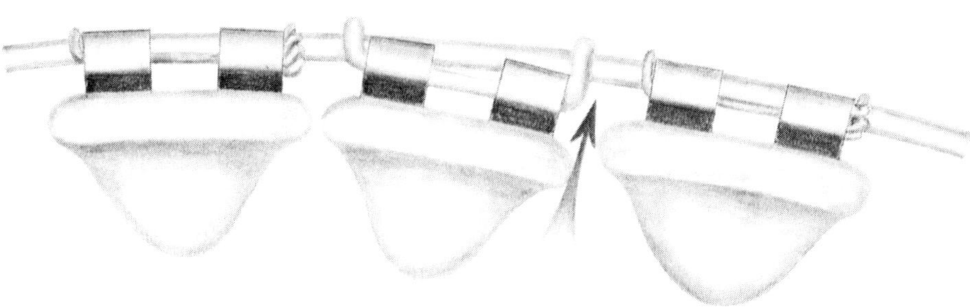

Fig. 18-1. An elastic ligature can rotate a tooth into position on the arch, provided that the bracket is wide enough to provide an adequate moment arm, space is adequate, and the arch is partially engaged in the bracket slots.

the bracket for accomplishment. As a tooth rotates on its axis, the bracket must often move mesially or distally, and the force available from a single elastic ligature cannot overcome this added resistance. A longer unit attached to provide the necessary simultaneous horizontal vector in combination with the rotating moment can be very effective in these cases.

Multiple-tooth ligation. Chains of two or more units can be applied to two or more teeth to apply a horizontal vector together with ligation. Any horizontal force applied to a buccal attachment will introduce a collateral axial rotating moment as well as a tipping moment. The tipping moment is easily controlled by the engagement of the bracket on the arch, but the axial rotation must be controlled by the ligature. When rotation is the object, it can be augmented by this means; otherwise, positive preventive measures are in order.

The moment arm for collateral rotation in this type of situation is approximately the same as the buccolingual radius of the root. For most teeth, this is about the same as the working distance between wide-spaced double brackets. This means that the proximal bracket must be held against the archwire with a force comparable to the closing force to prevent collateral rotation of the tooth (Fig. 18-2). This restraining force must be proportionately increased for brackets narrower than the radius of the tooth, so rotation control with the bracket alone becomes progressively more difficult if not impossible with the narrower bracket dimensions.

The application of a closing elastic ligature so that it engages only the proximal bracket, as in Fig. 18-3, *A*, provides a counter-rotating force equal to the closing force. This will control the collateral rotation for most teeth. Engaging both brack-

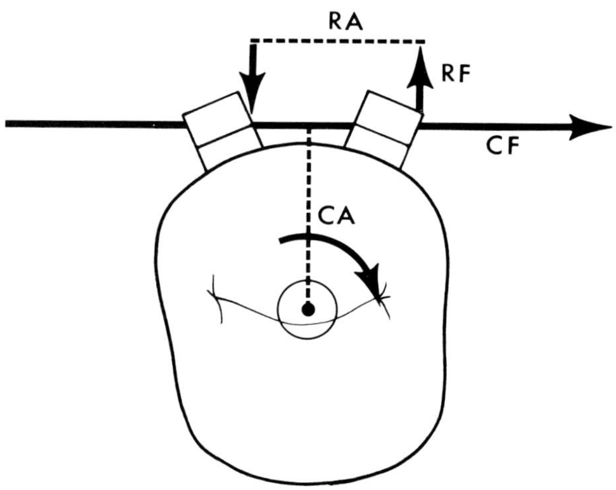

Fig. 18-2. Applying a horizontal force through a bracket introduces important collateral rotating effects. Such a horizontal force is also a collateral activating force, *CF*, working to rotate the tooth over the moment arm, *CA* where such rotation is not desired, control is applied at the bracket by the resisting force of a ligature, *RF*, working over the resisting arm, *RA*. When *CA* and *RA* are equal, a resisting force equal to the activating force will control the rotation. If *RA* is shorter than *CA*, *RF* must be increased proportionately to retain control.

A

B

C

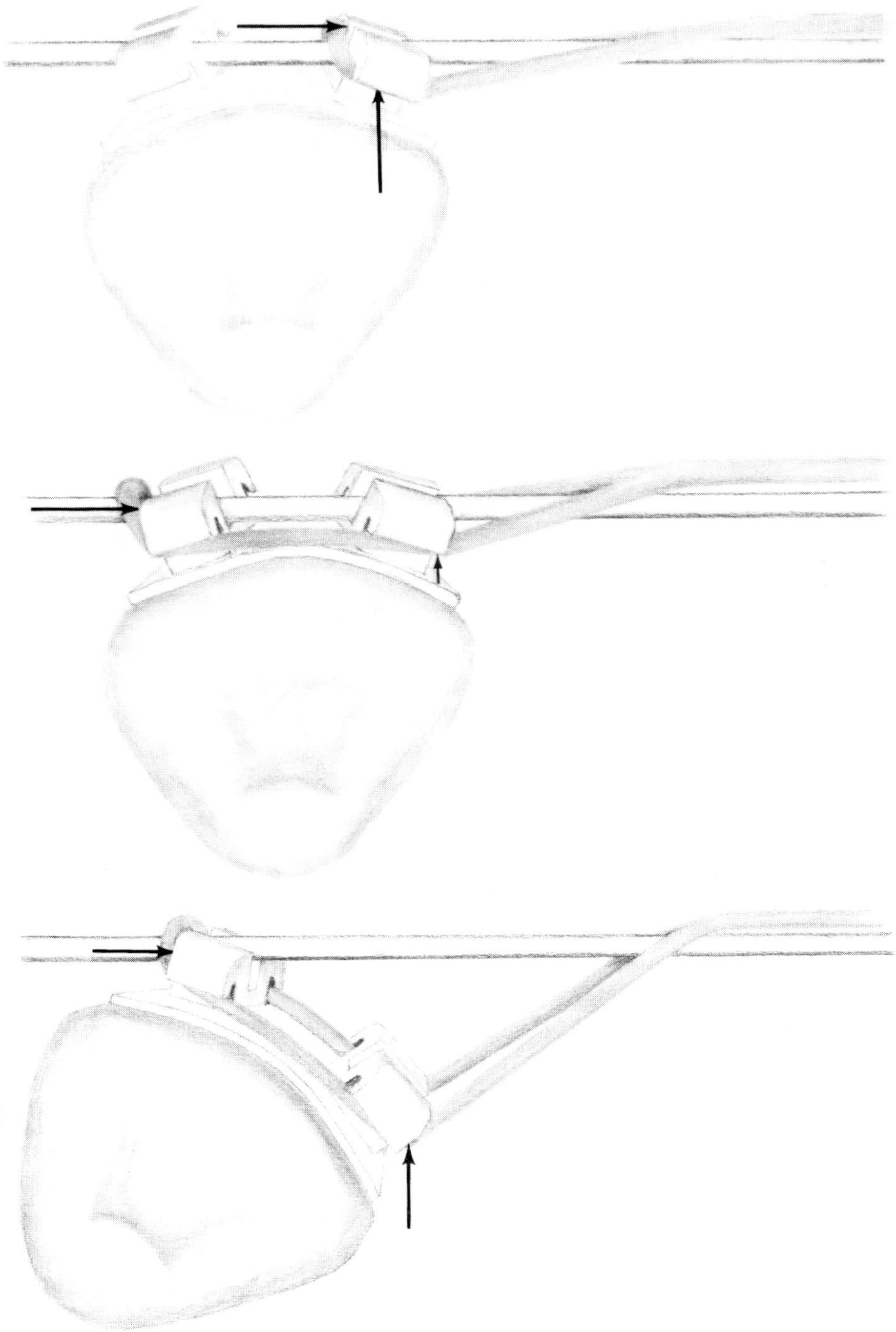

Fig. 18-3. Horizontal movement with an elastic ligature. Engaging the proximal bracket, **A,** provides a resisting force for rotation control equal to the activating force (Fig. 18-2). Engaging both brackets, **B,** provides almost no rotation control. As a tooth is rotated by this action, equilibrium is reached when the resisting and collateral rotation moments are in balance, **C,** usually at an extreme angle. It should be noted that before this point is reached, the proximal bracket is disengaged from the arch, and tipping control will also be lost.

ets, as in Fig. 18-3, *B*, places the point of application for the required counter-rotating action in mid-span, almost perpendicular to the ligature as it passes under the proximal bracket wing. The counter-rotating force is negligible in this configuration when both brackets are in contact with the arch. Such a tooth will rotate until the horizontal vector and the counter-rotating force reach equilibrium, which will occur at an extreme rotation (Fig. 18-3, *C*).

Intentional rotations can be very effectively accomplished with the configuration in Fig. 18-3, *B*, especially if the distant bracket is not fully engaged on the arch. The only added precaution is to be certain that the bracket that must be rotated into contact with the arch is engaged sufficiently to ensure that it can move freely into position.

A wire ligature can be used to control collateral rotations, but friction may inhibit the necessary sliding of the bracket along the arch. When wire ligation is used for this purpose, the archwire should be lightly pried out against the ligature with a scaler or other instrument after ligation to provide more freedom for movement. Even this may not prevent friction problems, because as the tooth begins to move and rotate, the rotation pressure against the ligature wire will build up to the level of the horizontal force and increase friction proportionately (Fig. 15-5).

Space closure with elastic ligatures is best accomplished one tooth at a time. Multiple units (chains) extending across several teeth will usually prove inadequate for closing intervening spaces. All teeth except those at the ends are in almost neutral positions on the chain. If they are not, the force is literally spread too thin, and local actions may even be reversed.

Whenever a chain unit is to be attached to more than two teeth, the ends should always be attached first. The positions in which the intermediate links are then found will indicate possible intermediate effects and serve as a guide to which brackets should be engaged. Failure to observe this precaution can lead to inadvertent space opening or other unwanted effects on intermediate teeth.

As with all sources of elastic force, these ligatures apply an equal reciprocal load at each end. Where it is desirable to move only the tooth at one side of a space, several teeth on the other side can be ligated together to provide a more stable anchor unit. The elastic ligature is then applied across the space, with the tooth that is to be moved attached only by the freely sliding elastic ligature.

An asymmetrical relationship can be corrected by sliding one tooth across a space with an elastic ligature, ligating it securely to those on the other side with a wire ligature, and then moving adjacent teeth one at a time in the same way.

Coil springs

Coil springs can store force for tooth movement through either extension or compression.

The extension (normally closed) coil functions the same as an elastic ligature or rubber elastic. The major advantage is that there is no deterioration of force level with time. There is only the normal loss through elastic force delivery as it shortens with tooth movement. On the negative side are the same frictional problems mentioned earlier with wire ligatures, along with the possibility that the patient may stretch and inactivate the spring.

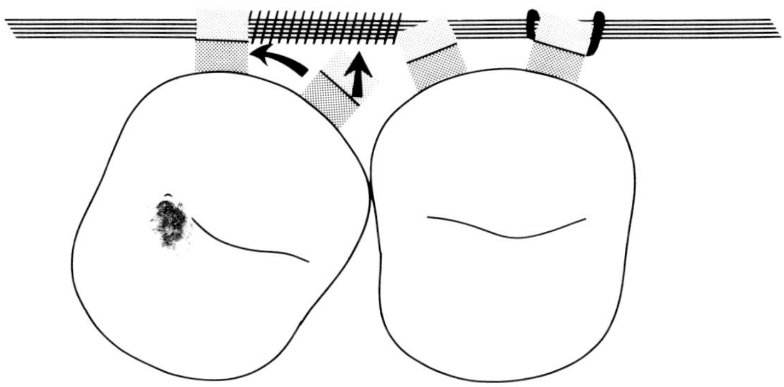

Fig. 18-4. A compression coil spring engaging the bracket of a rotated tooth is a very effective means for applying a corrective rotating moment. As the bracket under the spring approaches archwire engagement, the spring can be shortened to continue its action on that bracket. The tooth subjected to the reciprocal action (right) must be securely ligated to prevent unwanted rotation.

Compression (normally open) coils operate to open spaces instead of to close them. They have no counterpart among the auxiliary devices, although arch loops can be formed to perform the same function. These coils are threaded onto the arch and cut to a suitable length, so that they will exert an opening force when compressed between two attachments. Progressive adjustments can be made by grasping the coil with a Weingart or other curved pliers and then applying the flat side of a ligature-cutting pliers against it with the jaws lightly closed between the coils. Rocking the ligature cutter against the other pliers will permanently extend a short segment and so lengthen the spring.

Collateral rotation effects are the same with coil springs as with other horizontal forces, so measures should be taken to inhibit or encourage them as required. These springs are especially useful where the collateral rotating effect will correct a rotated tooth at the same time that a space is opened.

In severe rotations it can be applied across the tooth, from the adjacent tooth to the far bracket, until the proximal bracket rotates against the spring. Then the spring is compressed to engage the proximal bracket, shortening slightly if required, and the rotation carried to completion (Fig. 18-4). The adjacent tooth must be tied securely through this procedure to prevent unwanted rotation by the reciprocal force.

Rubber elastics

For intramaxillary action rubber elastics are usually attached between the molar and a hook in the cuspid region. This is a pure arch-shortening or space-closing action (Fig. 19-2) that is the same as that achieved with other elastic modules.

Arch hooks may be bent into the wire, soldered in place, or free to slide on the arch. A sliding hook will of course act directly on the tooth lying distal to its position, so its action will be the same as an elastic ligature or extension coil. Fixed

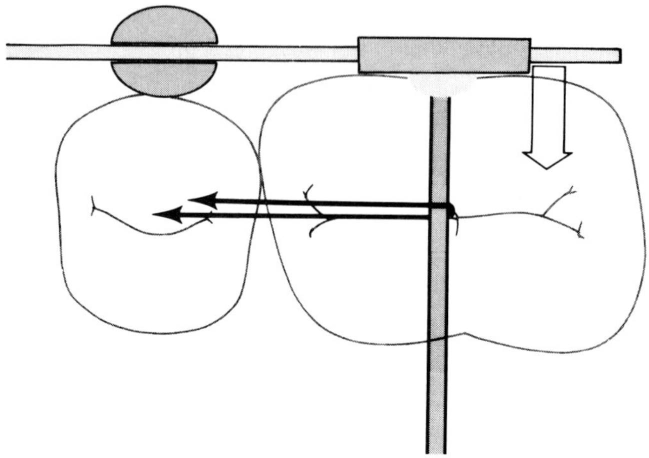

Fig. 18-5. Bending effects on different archwires can be seen directly with a simple mockup duplicating the force picture in the mouth. A stiff wire is soldered to a molar tube as shown. The archwire is slipped into this tube and grasped with pliers at the position of the first attachment mesial to the molar. Applying traction to the arm at a position comparable to the center of the molar will have the same bending effect on the arch as a mesial or distal force applied at the tube in the mouth. Not shown is a means for preventing the arch from sliding farther into the tube; this can be a coil spring, a bend in the wire, or even a finger.

hooks distribute their action across the entire anterior segment of the arch. Exact force distribution can be controlled by hook placement. For example, hooks in contact with the cuspid brackets will exert a distal action on the cuspids and move the incisors lingually only as the cuspids move; hooks spaced mesial to the cuspid brackets will concentrate action on the incisors and tend to close anterior spaces. Distribution becomes even more complex with loop hooks bent into the arch, as they change form under the elastic loading. This requires compensatory adjustments whenever elastic traction is used.

Collateral effects with sliding hooks are the same as with other forces applied to the same tooth at the same point, and they must be controlled in the same way. There are no important local collateral effects with a fixed hook on the arch, only those associated with the lingual tipping component on the incisors and the mesial vector at the molars.

Mesially directed elastic traction on a molar can cause extremely important collateral effects. Mesial tipping and rotation can both become serious problems, especially with light archwires. As mentioned earlier, the engagement of the archwire in a long tube is usually adequate for control, and it may be adequate with short tubes and heavy archwires. But light archwires, or medium weight wires (.016 inch or .40 mm) with short tubes, do not have sufficient strength to counter the heavy rotating and tipping moments developed by mesial traction on the long moment arm of a molar until after excessive movement has stored the required energy in the wire. The moment arm of a molar is at least half the root diameter, or twice the effective length of some molar tubes.

A graphic means for visualizing this rotating effect on the arch is to weld or solder a wire perpendicular to a molar tube and slide the tube on a section of wire that is held firmly in a pair of pliers at a point comparable to that occupied by the bicuspid bracket (Fig. 18-5). Attaching an elastic to this lever arm at a point $^1/_2$ root diameter away from the tube and applying the desired tension will demonstrate the bending effect on the archwire. Tipping effects can be demonstrated in the same way.

The only way in which an archwire can be adjusted to counter these effects is to bend the end lingually to resist the axial rotating moment and apically to resist the tipping, so that when the load is applied the wire will assume a straight configuration. These bends can be large in some cases; effects produced as in Fig. 18-5 can be used as a guide in this adjustment.

It is essential that these bends be made whenever mesial traction is imposed on a molar *and that they be removed when it is discontinued.* If this is not done, the unbalanced arch adjustment can severely tip and rotate those teeth.

Lingual hooks and elastic traction

Lingual hooks, spurs, or buttons may be used to attach traction between pairs of teeth to provide countermoments for the control of collateral rotations or the correction of preexisting rotations. Most commonly, they are used on cuspids and molars in extraction cases, but they may be used anywhere. Unusually rotated teeth may be fitted with these attachments as required to aid in their correction. One variation of the edgewise technique uses narrow incisor brackets to provide more flexibility in the archwire between the teeth. These brackets are inadequate for rotation control, so the teeth are fitted with lingual attachments that can be tied to the arch for this function.

Traction is usually provided by rubber elastics or elastic ligatures. Wire ligatures are sometimes used to hold a rotation, but they are not effective for major movement except when tied to very light arches that provide the energy storage.

The most typical application of lingual traction is in the closure of extraction spaces. Distal traction applied to a buccal attachment to move the cuspid distally imposes collateral rotating moments on both the cuspid and the molar. Elastic reaction applied between these teeth through a lingual attachment will counter both rotations at the same time that it augments the closing action.

One disadvantage that must be considered in the application of this mechanism is that the rotating moments are not available without the concurrent reciprocal closing action. The actions come in an inseparable package, and where this is helpful it is a most useful combination. However, not all cases require rotating and closing effects combined in just the right measure.

An additional and very important disadvantage lies in the collateral tipping moments. The lingual traction not only fails to counter them; it actually introduces added tipping moments of its own. Arches must be carefully adjusted to counter this added tipping effect.

Lingual arch

The lingual arch is a ubiquitous device in orthodontics. It came into its own very early, becoming one of the primary components of the Labiolingual appliance, and this identification was so strong that it was long avoided by those who were oriented toward the newer labial arch appliances (including the Edgewise) that followed.

One of the early applications of the lingual arch in combination with a full-banded appliance was in the Universal appliance. The .036-inch (.90-mm) steel arch in a horizontal sheath attached to the first molars, as used with that appliance, provides an exceptionally well-balanced combination of flexibility and strength for molar control.

A lingual arch, with its endless variations and auxiliaries, can be used for many purposes. Many of these are self-sufficient procedures unrelated to full-banded therapy, but the discussion here will be limited to its applications as an auxiliary in combination with the full-banded edgewise type of appliance.

The unadorned lingual arch, operating only through molar attachments, provides full control over intermolar width (Fig. 18-6, *A*), along with rotation around two of the three major dental axes. Axial rotation (Fig. 18-6, *B*) and buccolingual tipping (Fig. 18-6, *C*) of the molars are under complete control with this arch.

Tipping around the third axis—mesial or distal tipping—can be controlled only by a reciprocal tipping action between the two molars. Tipping one molar distally will tip the other mesially so this action is limited to equalizing the angulation of the two teeth.

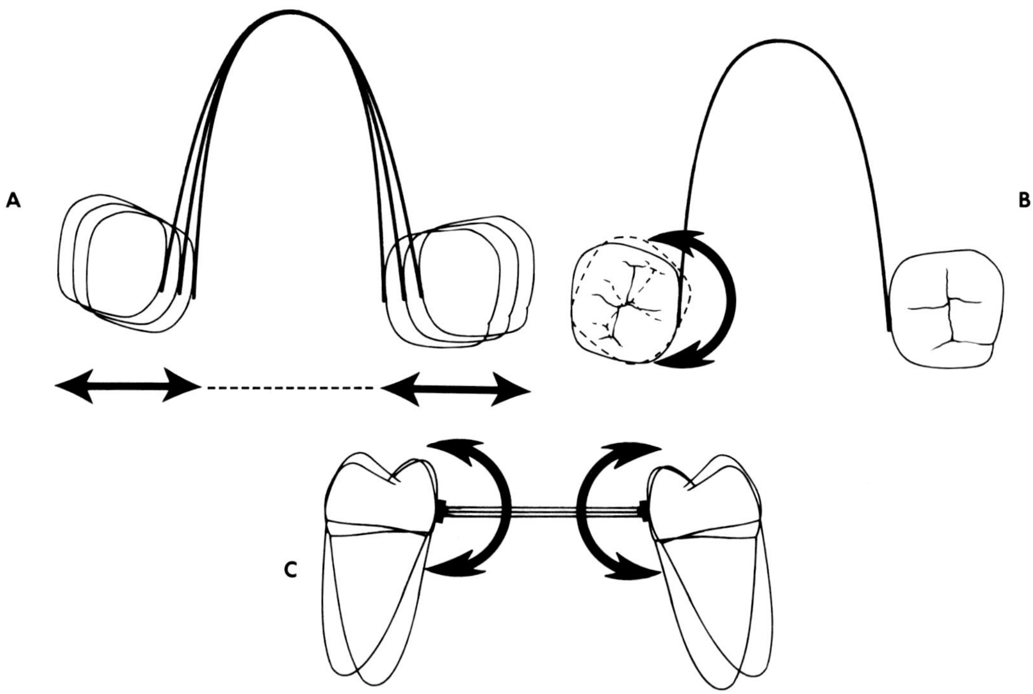

Fig. 18-6. A lingual arch provides full control over lateral linear movement and over rotation in two of the three planes of space. **A,** Buccolingual linear movement, which is reciprocal. **B,** Axial rotation. **C,** Buccolingual tipping rotation.

Further tipping requires anchorage on other teeth. It may seem tempting to use the incisors for anchorage in this way, allowing the lingual arch to rest on the cingulum to aid in tipping the molars distally, but the undesirable effects on the incisors usually far outweigh any benefit to the molars. In most cases, this action can be better accomplished by means of the labial arch, with reciprocal effects distributed over more teeth, but a carefully balanced coordinated action of the labial and lingual arches can prove very useful.

Buccal movement of bicuspids can be accomplished by contouring a lingual arch to engage their lingual surfaces and moving them buccally along with the molars or by adding fingersprings to move them independently, but these are limited applications in edgewise treatment.

A typical application of the lingual arch in edgewise therapy is in the attainment of correct molar rotations, buccolingual tipping, and intermolar width in the initial stages of treatment. In the course of treatment the arch then continues to serve as required to maintain those relationships against the collateral effects imposed by the buccal arch and auxiliary forces.

These actions also lie within the capabilities of the edgewise appliance alone. The virtue of the supplementary lingual arch lies in accomplishment of the results without dependence on heavy labial arches and, more important, without imposing reciprocal actions on any teeth other than the molars. Comparable actions with full buccal attachments will impose large reciprocal forces in the bicuspid segment. A lingual arch makes it possible to correct molar positions, including crossbites, at the same time that light or sectional archwires are moving other teeth.

Distal molar rotation will illustrate the difference between control with labial (edgewise) and with lingual arches. Fig. 18-7 shows a mesially rotated first molar typical of many of these teeth at the beginning of treatment. Rotating this tooth into its correct position requires a counterclockwise movement, as shown by the heavy arrow. The reactionary resultant force produced by this activation will be directed clockwise along an arc of a circle centered on the molar, as shown by the series of arcs. If the rotating force is derived from a single attachment, its intensity will be inversely proportional to the distance from the molar (a longer moment arm requires a smaller force).

A lingual arch attached only to the opposite molar will accomplish the rotation by placing a distal force on that tooth. This is a desirable action in most cases. A heavy edgewise arch will distribute the resultant load over many teeth, but only if it is adjusted gradually in many small increments. A light arch, a short arch segment, or a heavily adjusted heavy arch will concentrate the necessarily heavy load (shorter moment arm) at the second bicuspid.

Arch adjustments can mitigate some of the adverse effects of these reactive forces, but the first tooth engaged mesial to the molar will always receive the heaviest initial load. It will move lingually in response and then complete a round trip as the molar turns and the arch regains its passive form. This may be repeated several times with successive adjustments before a molar rotation is fully corrected in this way. These effects are eliminated with the lingual arch.

A few precautions should be noted in the use of the lingual arch. Detailed adaptation to the other teeth is not required for such auxiliary applications, so pre-

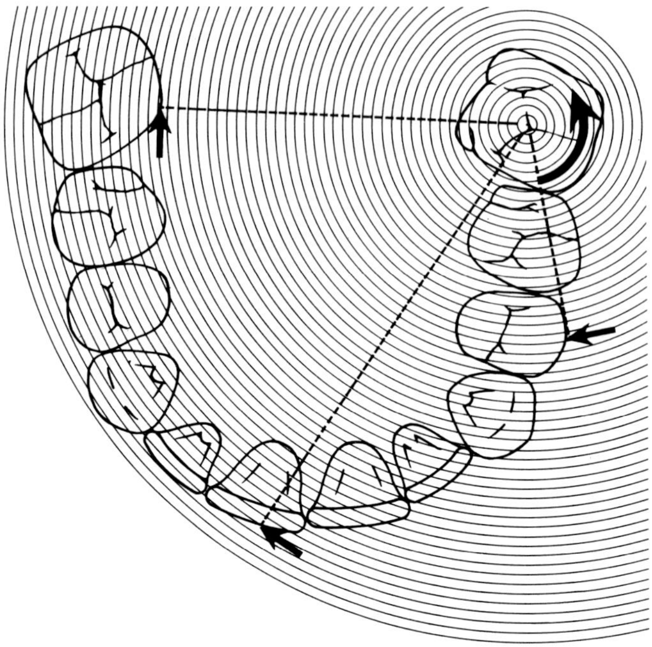

Fig. 18-7. Molar rotation places reactionary forces on the resisting (anchor) teeth along the arcs of circles centered on the tooth. This force is lingual on the bicuspids lying mesial to the tooth, distolingual on incisors, and distal on the opposite molar. It should be noted that the distal effect on the opposite molar is not a "free ride" in terms of anchorage; it is balanced by an equal mesial component (not shown here) on the rotating molar, so the mesiodistal effects will cancel each other when this action is applied bilaterally.

formed arches are easily fitted. However, they must be adjusted carefully for action (or inaction) in all planes. Ideally the arch should lightly or nearly contact the anterior teeth near the gingival margin, provided that those teeth are not to be moved lingually.

Clearance must be provided for lingual incisor movement when this is required, but this opens up the possibility for the tongue to play with the arch and either disengage it or drag the molars forward. This is probably the most serious complication in the use of the lingual arch, and it may require its removal during some stages of lingual incisor movement.

Size for preformed arches is determined by forming one end of a length of brass separating wire about .025 inch (.6 mm) into a form resembling the end of a lingual arch, so that it may be inserted into one of the tubes with the stop against the tube. The wire is then placed in arch position and grasped with pliers at the position of the other tube. A bend with the pliers will mark this point so that the wire can be straightened and the distance between tubes measured.

Using the dental casts as a guide, the anterior segment is reshaped as required. Bicuspid and molar width are then established approximately. The triple-beak clasp adjusting pliers is excellent for these adjustments, because it uses many successive small bends to maintain a smooth arch form.

Final adjustments are made by engaging one end of the arch at a time in its molar tube, noting the changes required to bring the anterior segment into position and the free opposite end into alignment with its molar tube.

Before inserting in the tube for the first time, the arch is held in approximate position to determine the orientation of the end to the tube. Some arches may be inserted immediately; others need adjustments in all three planes.

Mesiodistal tipping and axial rotation bends are made with all three jaws of the triple-beak plier positioned mesial to the folded stop that engages the molar tube. This keeps the bends well away from that critical section area. Buccolingual tipping is adjusted by securely holding the folded section in sturdy pliers and bending the entire free arch up or down as required. A firm grip is essential for this adjustment; if the plier jaws separate even slightly, the arch will twist at the tightly folded end, making breakage at some time almost certain.

If the free end lies in exact position at the molar tube, the adjustments at the engaged end will provide for an essentially passive arch. Repeating the procedure on the opposite side will complete the adjustment with one possible exception: exact position in the anterior area should be reevaluated after both arch ends have been seated in their tubes, and additional fine adjustments made if required.

If active adjustments are required, these are evaluated by inserting one end at a time in its tube. Deviation in position of the free end of the arch in relation to its tube will clearly show the activation that will be accomplished when it is seated there. A displacement of about one-half tube length will provide effective axial rotation correction. Slightly greater displacements may be used for correcting arch width and buccolingual tipping.

Tipping and axial rotation auxiliaries

An endless variety of tipping and rotating auxiliaries are available for use not only with the edgewise appliance but also with practically all others that use fixed dental attachments. The operating principles of all of these auxiliaries are the same, regardless of variations in attachment.

All use a two-point engagement on the tooth providing a moment arm for application of the rotating couple. The engagement points may be the opposite ends of an edgewise or vertical slot or tube, or the diagonally opposite wings of a pair of edgewise brackets (Fig. 18-8). Spacing of the two contact points has the effects discussed in Chapter 15 in the section concerning bracket width, but all of the commonly used methods provide adequate spacing for the delivery moment arm.

The distance from the nearest dental engagement point to the point of outside force application establishes the length of the activating moment arm and so determines the required activating force. The longer the arm, the lighter will be the force required to produce an adequate tipping moment. This distance typically spans about two teeth, but there are no rigid requirements. The most important considerations are the distribution of the reciprocal force and patient convenience and comfort.

Fig. 18-9 shows the force picture for a typical cuspid uprighting spring. The reciprocal force from the activation is in an apical direction. This is usually applied to an archwire that distributes it over several nearby teeth. The way in which it is

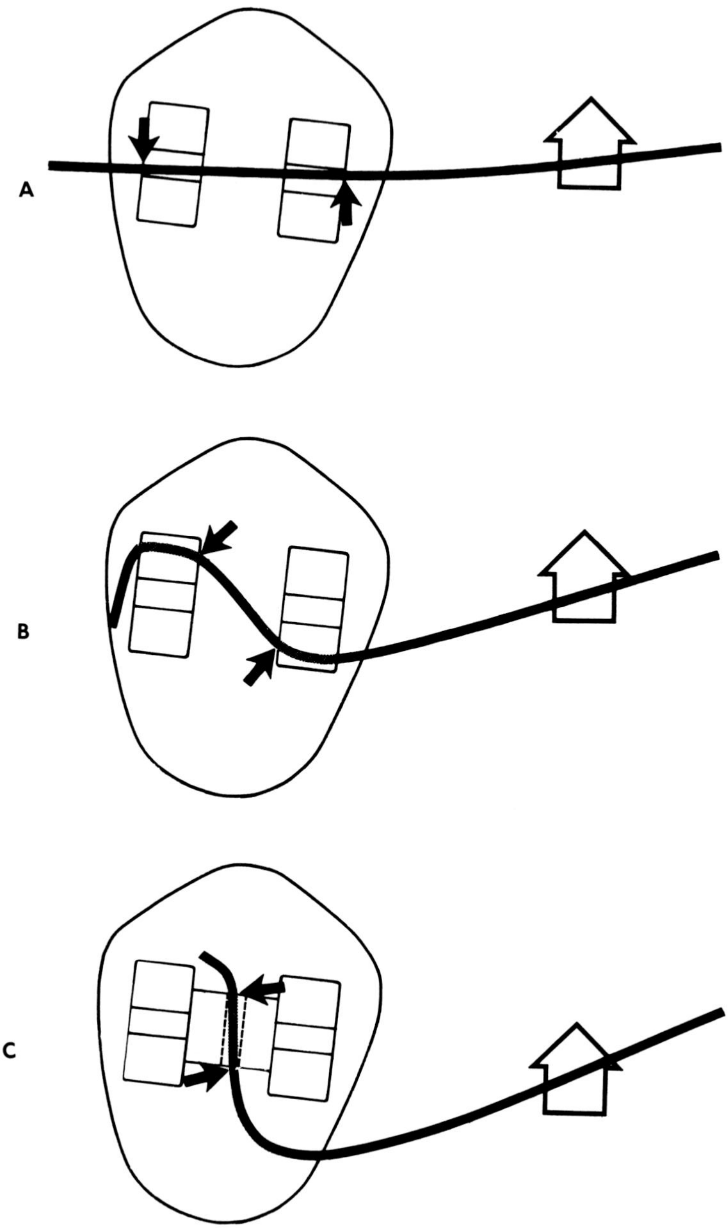

Fig. 18-8. All tipping (and rotating) auxiliaries use a two-point contact to apply the required moment to the tooth. Three of the most common are shown. **A,** Conventional bracket slot engagement. **B,** Engagement under opposite bracket wings. **C,** A vertical slot milled in the base of an edgewise bracket. This type of slot or tube is used as a principal attachment in the Begg and universal appliances. All may be used as a part of or in conjunction with a conventional archwire.

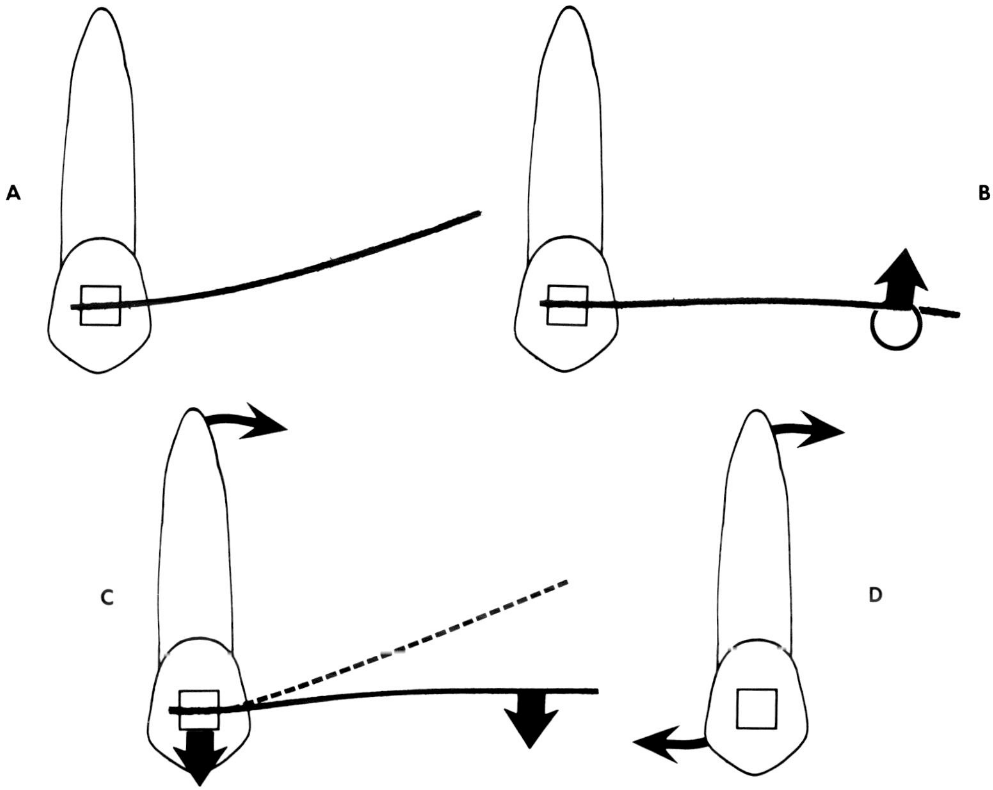

Fig. 18-9. Principal actions of a simple cuspid-uprighting spring. **A,** Passive. **B,** Activated by engagement on the arch at some remote point. This applies an apical force at the point of engagement. **C,** The vertical (downward) force applied in activation also applies a similar vector to the tooth, completing the balance of vertical forces. The resultant effect on the tooth must be controlled by another appliance component. **D,** The tipping moment introduces a collateral mesial crown vector along with the desired distal root action.

distributed depends on the point of application and on the stiffness of the archwire. A very flexible wire can distort enough under the load to concentrate this force on one or two teeth.

Collateral effects on the cuspid are two, each with its own secondary effects. One is the occlusal vector that is directly introduced by the activation (Fig. 18-9, *C*). The other is the mesial vector introduced by the tipping action (Fig. 18-9, *D*).

The occlusal vector is normally controlled by engagement of the cuspid on the same archwire that is engaged by the activating end of the auxiliary. So what is the net effect? One way of describing it is to say that the occlusal vector at the cuspid (Fig. 18-9, *B*) and the apical vector at the point of engagement of the auxiliary on the arch (Fig. 18-9, *C*) form a couple that rotates the entire archwire down anteriorly and up posteriorly.

These tipping effects on the arch are minor in many cases, but when two large cuspid roots operate as anchorage to tip an arch in concert with other forces that

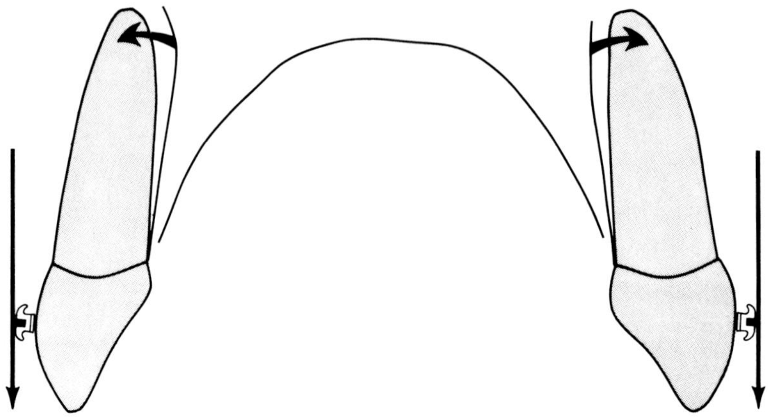

Fig. 18-10. An occlusal vector at the cuspids, as from intermaxillary elastic traction, applies a lingual tipping moment to these teeth. Since the archwire usually prevents lingual crown movement, this effect is typically expressed as buccal root movement if it is not otherwise controlled.

may be operating at the same time, they can be extremely important. Countermeasures where required must provide an apical vector in the anterior region from some other source.

The occlusal vector on the labial surface of the cuspid produces its own collateral lingual tipping action (buccal root movement), but only as the tooth actually moves occlusally (Fig. 18-10). Control of the occlusal movement will also prevent this very undesirable tipping effect.

The remaining collateral effect (the mesial crown vector on the cuspid) always requires positive countermeasures. Arch engagement with suitable arch restraints elsewhere, intermaxillary or intramaxillary traction, and ligating the cuspid to the molar are common methods. In any case it is a matter of shifting and distributing the mesial component of force to some area where it will not be too detrimental to the treatment objectives.

Intermaxillary traction requires special caution in this application, because its vertical component augments the occlusal vector and its very undesirable effects that were discussed above.

Rotating auxiliaries. Rotating auxiliaries behave in exactly the same way as the tipping auxiliaries, except that all forces are horizontal instead of vertical. Resultants can influence buccolingual positions of nearby teeth and alter arch form, depending on the way in which they are applied and distributed. This depends again on the nature and the adjustment of the archwire and auxiliaries that are used to distribute the reciprocal forces.

Helical loops. Helical loops and other variations in the shape of the activating arm of a tipping or rotating auxiliary of this type *have no effect* on the force picture discussed thus far. These tipping and rotating actions depend only on the straight-line length of the moment arm and on the activating force that acts through that arm to produce the moment on the tooth.

The function of loops in the activating arm is to reduce stiffness and extend working range. They affect force level and duration, but not distribution. An activating arm modified in this way must be deflected farther to attain the same force level, and the reduced steepness of the elastic curve means that the force will decay at a slower rate as the tooth moves. These can be important aids to effective application, even though they do not affect the ultimate force distribution.

Force modifying loops

Loops may be incorporated into any orthodontic wire that functions in the elastic storage of force, from the simplest auxiliaries described previously to a full edgewise arch. The basic principles of loop design and function will be described here, with specific applications discussed in following sections in connection with use of the different appliance components.

Orthodontic wires are formed into loops for only two reasons: (1) to alter the elastic properties of the wire and (2) to serve as hooks or stops, in lieu of welding or soldering additions to the wire. In using loops for the second reason, one should not lose sight of the fact that those same loops will also alter the elastic properties of the wire, and the inevitable side effects can play an important part in the design and application of loops for any purpose.

The only limitation on loop design is the imagination and dexterity of the operator, and they may be used in many forms and applications. Some of the more complex may be practical only when they are manufactured with standardized jigs and fixtures.

Most loops will perform as advertised, and their complexity can serve a real purpose; but like almost all orthodontic devices, they do not represent the only means to any desired end.

Loop mechanics is based on some of the simplest of the engineering principles presented in Part I, and even the most complex are little more than combinations of a few basic types.

Loops of the types commonly used, including most multiple combinations, function by elastic bending of the wire (not torsion), and the loop form can contribute four effects: (1) reduce stiffness, (2) increase working range, (3) control the direction in which the first two effects operate, and (4) reduce strength. The third of these effects may often add new control problems of its own, and the fourth is usually an undesirable side effect rather than an objective of loop function.

Loop anatomy. The effects listed previously are accomplished by altering the bending moment arms and the length of wire that is subjected to bending action. The parts of a loop can be divided and identified on the basis of these functions, as shown in Fig. 18-11 for two loops.

Function of loop components. In opening and closing loops of the type shown, the two arms are usually the same length, but this is not always the case. Most loops are designed so that they are activated perpendicular to the arms, in which case the activating arm also represents the moment arm of the loop. In cases in which the loop is activated at some other angle to this arm, the moment arm is measured from the line of the activating force, the same as shown in Fig. 2-4. This is important, because the effectiveness of most loops diminishes progressively as the angle of activation deviates from 90 degrees.

The base of a loop ordinarily functions under a uniform bending moment. It

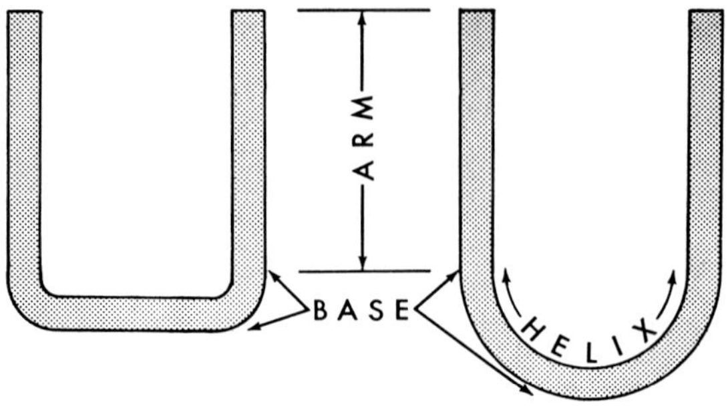

Fig. 18-11. Basic parts of orthodontic arch loops. The base lies in the area of greatest stress, so it is here that multiple helices and other wire-lengthening devices are most effective in reducing force and increasing range. The elasticity of the arms makes a relatively small contribution, so the most significant effects of arm length are those which depend on the distance that the arm moves and the moment that it applies to the base.

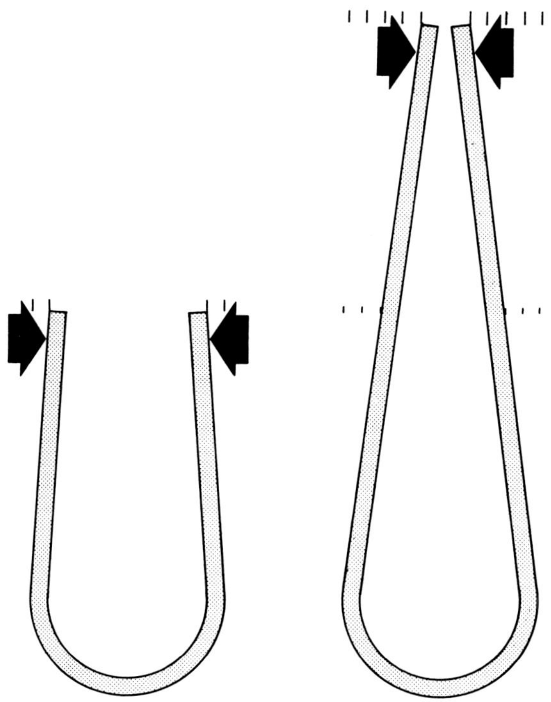

Fig. 18-12. Stiffness of a loop is inversely proportional to the square of arm length. The direct effect of doubling the length of the arms is to double the distance traveled by the arm ends under the same loading of the base. The additional deflection results from the fact that the doubled length will also apply a doubled moment to the base, giving a fourfold total increase in deflection.

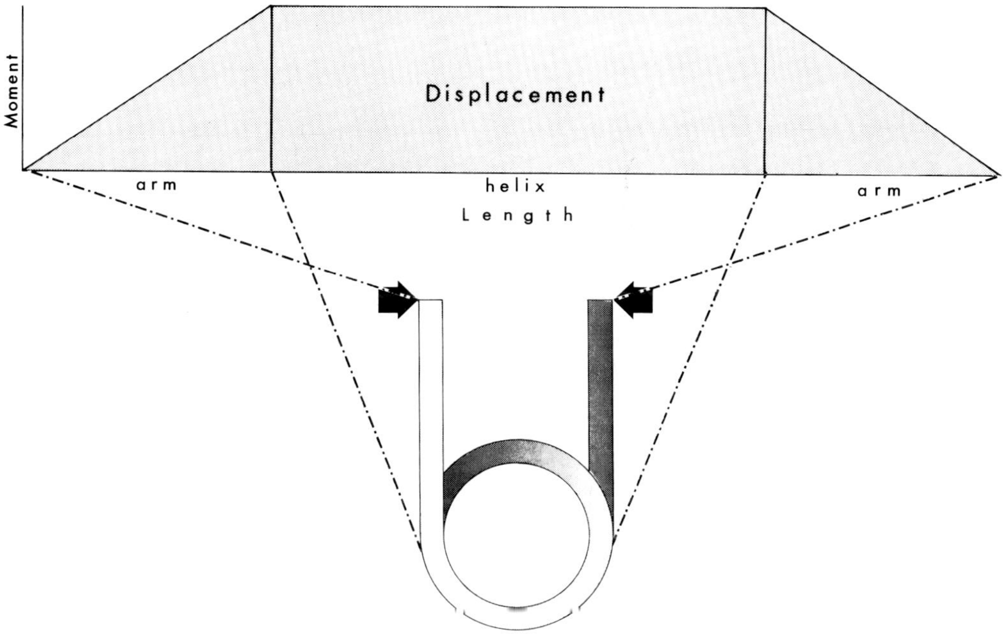

Fig. 18-13. Factors involved in loop elasticity. The horizontal scale of the graph represents the length of each arm and of the wire in the helix. The vertical scale represents the bending moment, which is a function of the applied force and the length of the moment arm. Bending moment rises from zero at the arm ends to a maximum in the helix. The area subtended by the graph is proportional to total displacement. Increasing arm length will have the effect of "lowering" the base line by extension of the sloping ends, thus increasing moments and displacement "across the board." Adding turns to the helix will extend the central rectangle laterally without affecting the contribution of the arms.

may be straight, curved, or coiled into several helices. A helical coil, even one of many turns, is loaded with a uniform moment that is determined by the length of the moment arm and by the applied force. The arm for a helix is measured to a point opposite the center of the coil.

A simple helix formed in an archwire, such as that shown distal to the cuspid in Fig. 18-28, is nothing more than the same loop with the arms folded out to a straight line. Arm length in this case is determined by the points of force application on either side of the helix.

Length of arms. The arms of a loop function essentially as cantilever beams. Their major effects depend on the bending moment that they apply to the base, even though their own bending also contributes to the action.

Increasing the length of the arm increases the moment on the loop *and* the distance that the end of the arm will move, so the stiffness of a loop is inversely proportional to the *square* of the length of the arms. Doubling the length of the arms will reduce stiffness to one-fourth (Figs. 18-12 and 18-13).

Range is directly proportional to the length of the arm, *not* the square, so that increasing arm length will increase working range much less than it will reduce stiffness. Working range of the base or helix is not affected by changes in the length of the arm, so the only important contribution of arm length to range is in the distance traveled by the end of the arm as the base is stressed to its limit.

Loops with low stiffness may have a theoretical working range, based on the elasticity of the wire, that exceeds the limits of movement imposed by the configuration of the loop. If the ends of a loop touch and prevent further movement before the limits of the wire are reached, the loop will never reach or exceed the proportional limit.

Strength (or maximum force) is inversely proportional to arm length for the same reason that range is directly proportional to length.

If the two arms are of different lengths, the force operating at the end of each arm will be different, in inverse proportion to arm length. The moment on the base must obviously be the same, regardless of the relative lengths of the arms. In Fig. 18-12 the moment in the loop at the right has been doubled by moving the points of force application upward. If only one point of application were moved to the higher point, the force at that long end could be only half that at the original level to maintain a balance between the two sides. To maintain the doubled moment shown in the helix in the loop at the right, a force applied to either arm at the original lower level would have to be twice as great as that at the longer ends.

The arms of a loop also contribute a share to the overall deflection. The significance of this contribution depends on the relationship between arm length and base length, as shown in Fig. 18-13. A long loop with a simple half-turn helical base like that in Fig. 18-11 will derive a large part of its deflection from the arms. A loop with a multiturn helical base and short arms will derive almost all of its effect from the helix.

Function of a helix. The length of wire incorporated into a helix has an inverse effect on stiffness and a direct effect on working range, but it has no effect on strength.

Length can be controlled by changes in either the diameter of the coil or in the number of turns; the effect is the same. Note that increasing the diameter or number of turns in a helix that is loaded by bending in this way has only a linear effect on stiffness (the center section of the graph in Fig. 18-13 is merely extended lengthwise). Loading a helical coil lengthwise, as in an extension or compression coil, subjects the wire to a torsion load. In these cases coil diameter has a third-power effect on stiffness because the torsion moment arm is dependent on the diameter (Fig. 3-1).

Selecting helix diameter. When coils are made extremely small in proportion to the diameter of the wire, internal strains become somewhat greater and risk of failure goes up. Such tight loops have a lower range and less strength than would be expected on the basis of wire length alone. Loop diameter should be at least six times wire diameter for optimum service.

When coils are made extremely large, it is often necessary to reduce arm length to fit the loop into an available space. Where space limits the total height of arms and helix combined, the net effect of changing the size of the helix is relatively slight. Stiffness is changed very little; strength and range are lowered somewhat by a smaller helix, but not enough to make this an important consideration in design.

The simplest way to decide upon the diameter of a helix is to make it fit the available space most conveniently without making the diameter of the helix less than six times the diameter of the wire.

Number of turns. The number of turns of wire in the helix affects elastic properties in the same way as the diameter of the helix. Using extra turns of wire is merely another means of increasing wire length.

Adding one full turn of wire to a simple U-shaped loop will about double its working range and reduce stiffness by half. The working range of the helix itself will be tripled (one and one-half turns have been substituted for one-half turn), but the effect of bending in the arms is unchanged by this alteration, so the overall effect is less.

Opening versus closing actions. A loop that works in the direction of winding can function more efficiently than a loop that is unwound as it is activated. Part of the reason for this is explained in Chapter 9. A second significant factor is that the bending moment on the helix is increased in unwinding by the addition of the radius of the helix to the moment arm.

The moment arm is measured to the point opposite the center of the helix when activation is in the direction of winding, but it is measured to the outside diameter of the helix (bottom of the loop) with an unwinding activation. This difference results in lower stiffness in unwinding, which may sometimes give a false impression of relative weakness in this application. Stiffness is not an indicator of strength or range. Design compensations can easily adjust for this difference, and there are some situations in which it may even be used to advantage.

Where there is no sacrifice of other advantages, it is good practice to form loops so that they are activated in the direction of winding. When occlusion or other space considerations present problems that can be avoided by winding in a direction opposite the direction of activation, this should be done without hesitation but with suitable compensations.

Tipping action of opening and closing loops. As a helical loop opens or closes, the arms will tip. This in turn will have a tipping effect on teeth (Fig. 18-14).

This tipping action can be reduced only slightly by adding helices where the arms join the horizontal arch. Extending a second loop in an occlusal direction so that the two loops form an S will produce an equal tipping action in the opposite direction, but occlusal interference limits the usefulness of this modification. Some of the more complex special-purpose loops are designed to accomplish a similar (but smaller) effect in a more compact configuration.

Loops with short arms will cause more tipping than those with long arms (Fig. 18-14), so arms should be made as long as possible where tipping is a consideration.

Loops with tipping action should be adjusted so that the inclination of the adjacent teeth will be correct at the *end* of the movement. In space closure this will tip the roots together before the crowns. Tipping freedom of the wire in the brackets will help dissipate part of this action, and the remaining tipping effect should be kept small. Such an adjustment may require an additional stress-reducing loop, such as a simple helix, on the other side of the tooth in question.

Torsion in loops. Where a loop is activated perpendicular to the plane of the loop, as in a buccolingual movement, the lower part of the loop will be in torsion

(Fig. 18-15). The arms will still be subjected to bending, the same as in opening and closing actions.

When a typical loop with a helical base is subjected to this type of stress, there is a gradual transition from pure bending in the arms to pure torsion at the base of the helix. With one or more full turns, the top and bottom of each will be in torsion while the sides will function in bending.

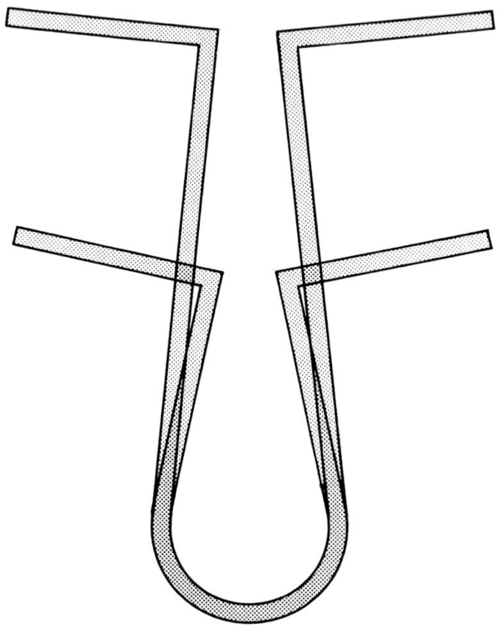

Fig. 18-14. Teeth adjacent to an opening or closing loop will be tipped as the loop opens or closes. This tipping is greater with shorter arms.

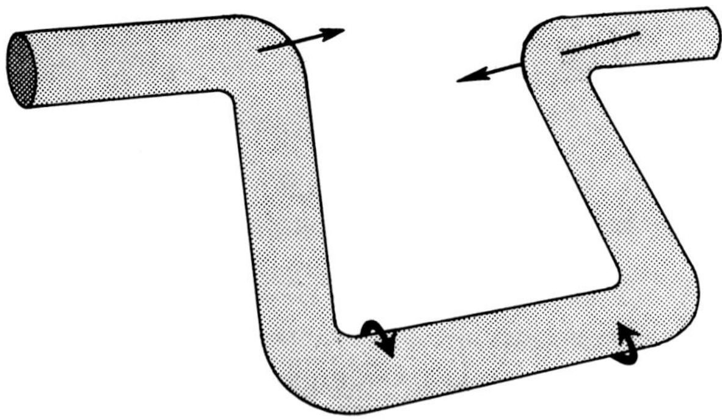

Fig. 18-15. Activating a loop perpendicular to the plane of the loop, as in buccolingual movement, will cause a torsion strain in the base of the loop. In a round loop there is a gradual transition from pure bending in the sides to pure torsion at the bottom (and the top as well, in a helix with one or more full turns).

The maximum moment in such a loop is at the base of the helix, where the stress is pure torsion. Working range in torsion is directly dependent on the length of the wire, and this is inadequate in a typical U-shaped loop. It is essential to provide adequate length in the high-moment region of these loops to prevent overstress and failure of the wire.

Necessary length can be provided either by a long horizontal section, as shown in Fig. 18-15, or by large or multiple helical coils. In a helical coil subjected to torsion in this way, the strain changes gradually from pure torsion at the top and bottom of the helix to pure bending at the sides. The load and the deflection are thus distributed over the entire helix in one way or another. It makes little difference how the stress is distributed, as long as it is distributed over enough wire to keep the maximum torsion strain at a safely low level. A helix must be loosely wound for this application, so that all coils are free to flex; if the coils are tight together, bending is restricted and the stress is still concentrated in the critical torsion sections.

Summary of properties of loops

Stiffness. There are several possible means available for controlling the stiffness of loops. The most potent is wire diameter, which has an effect proportional to the fourth power. This holds true in loops that function in bending as well as in straight wires.

The length of the working arm of the loop is the next most effective means for varying stiffness, with reductions proportional to the square of the length of the arm.

The least effective variable is the length of wire in the base. Its effect is proportional to the length of wire, whether that wire is in a straight section or in a helix. Reducing the arms of a loop by one-third will more than double stiffness. Compensating for this would require that the length of the helix be more than doubled.

Using a loop so that the coils are opened instead of closed in activation adds the radius of the loop to the moment arm, reducing stiffness accordingly. This effect is easily compensated, but stress relief is especially important.

Range. In addition to the effect of wire size, working range depends on the length of wire in the base and on the length of the arm. There is no squared effect

		Stiffness	Strength	Range
Arm length	A	$\frac{1}{A^2}$	$\frac{1}{A}$	A
Base length Diameter of helix Number of coils	B	$\frac{1}{B}$	No effect	B
Wire diameter	D	D^4	D^3	$\frac{1}{D}$

Fig. 18-16. Factors affecting the mechanical properties of a wire loop of any given material subjected to bending under similar loading conditions.

in either case. It is important, for the long life, to keep working range adequate, because the helix in a loop can be subjected to high bending moments. If short working range causes the bending moment to exceed the elastic range of the metal, there is a greatly increased likelihood of plastic deformation or failure. This is especially important where the base is in torsion; working range can be remarkably low where only a short section of wire is under torsion.

Strength. Strength, or the highest force that can be applied by the loop, is inversely proportional to the length of the arm. The helix has no effect on this value, for the maximum moment is the same in the entire helix, regardless of length; but in practice a helix may so lower the stiffness that large excursions make it impossible to apply a full load.

These various properties of loops are summarized in Fig. 18-16.

Sectional arches

A sectional arch is a short length of wire spanning two or more teeth, engaged in the bracket slots but not continuing around the dental arch from molar to molar as a full archwire does. Typical applications are limited to a single buccal or anterior segment of the arch.

Applications of sectional arches are usually at the extremes of tooth movement. A heavy rectangular arch may be engaged in the brackets of a few teeth to maintain their relationships, in which case there are no considerations of elasticity or movement. The other extreme in common application is where an individual tooth requires considerable movement.

Controlled movement of a single tooth over a long distance with the force stored in a complete arch engaged at most or all of the teeth can present many difficulties. If the archwire is flexible enough for large increments of movement, there will be significant reciprocal effects on nearby teeth; if it lacks such flexibility, it will also lack the potential for long movements without many small tedious adjustments.

Engaging an arch segment only to the teeth that must be involved in accomplishing the desired movement frees all others from unwanted reciprocal effects and greatly simplifies the evaluation of force actions. Span is often increased as well, which can provide a large increase in the elastic energy storage potential of the wire.

The simplest sectional archwire is one that connects just two teeth. All of the interactions that take place between two teeth connected by a sectional archwire will also be present with a complete archwire that continues on around the rest of the dental arch. The only differences are in effects on the other teeth that are engaged by a continuous arch and in the secondary effects that engagement of those teeth may have on the desired movement. The secondary effects of multiple tooth engagement can be negative, adding stiffness and limiting movement, or they can be positive in stabilizing one of the involved teeth.

Since the interactions between adjoining teeth united by a sectional arch are essentially the same as if the archwire extended on to other teeth, these effects are an ideal starting point for evaluating the function of a complete arch. The operation of the arch section is the basic action; added effects of other teeth in the arch can then be considered one by one to develop the complete picture. This modular approach to archwire analysis can make even the most complex archwire system understandable.

Vertical collateral effects with sectional arches. A sectional arch attached to only two teeth is just one step beyond the uprighting auxiliary described previously (Fig. 18-9). Instead of activation being derived from archwire engagement, it is derived from engagement directly on the other tooth. We can use the cuspid as an example once again, beginning with a simple straight archwire designed to inhibit cuspid eruption (or to move it apically) by the application of a light apical force (Fig. 18-17).

Engaging the arch in the cuspid bracket (Fig. 18-17, *B*) places an apical force on the cuspid and a reactionary occlusal force on the archwire. This activation has two effects on the molar (Fig. 18-17, *C*):

1. Distal tipping, with a tipping moment dependent on the force required to activate the arch at the cuspid and the distance from cuspid to molar ($M = Fd$)
2. An occlusal vector equal to the apical vector on the cuspid

These two effects can be modified by the introduction of loops into the arch. A helix just mesial to the molar (Fig. 18-17, *D*) can extend the range of movement available at a given force level, and so provide the light, continuous force required for the apical movement (intrusion) of the cuspid. This is especially important when relatively heavy rectangular wires are required to control the buccolingual tipping effects.

Buccolingual tipping as a collateral effect of vertical forces. Any vertical action applied to the buccal surface of a tooth crown will introduce a collateral buccolingual tipping effect. In the present example, the apical vector on the cuspid is directed along a line that lies buccal to the center of root support, so a buccal tipping moment will result (Fig. 18-18, *B*). The occlusal vector on the molar applies a similar lingual tipping moment (Fig. 18-18, *A*).

The tipping moments on cuspid and molar will be in opposite directions, so a rectangular archwire or other adequate control engagement of the archwire can effectively neutralize most of the effect by reciprocal action. That control can be extremely important; an apical vector applied to the cuspid without tipping control can easily tip the crown bucally.

Collateral buccolingual tipping is a common side effect of many orthodontic movements, some desirable and some undesirable. Some of the more common follow:

1. The occlusal vector of intermaxillary traction to the cuspid region will apply a lingual tipping moment. The archwire usually prevents lingual translation of the crown, causing this effect to be expressed in buccal root movement that can seriously compromise periodontal health.
2. An apical vector to lower incisors, which might be applied as part of an arch leveling procedure, will apply a very strong labial tipping vector because of the long moment arm to the center of support of the lingually inclined root.
3. An intrusive vector applied similarly to upper central incisors can have a very favorable effect on tipping control. Intrusion with a long interrupted ("utility") archwire extending freely from molars to incisors can intrude and

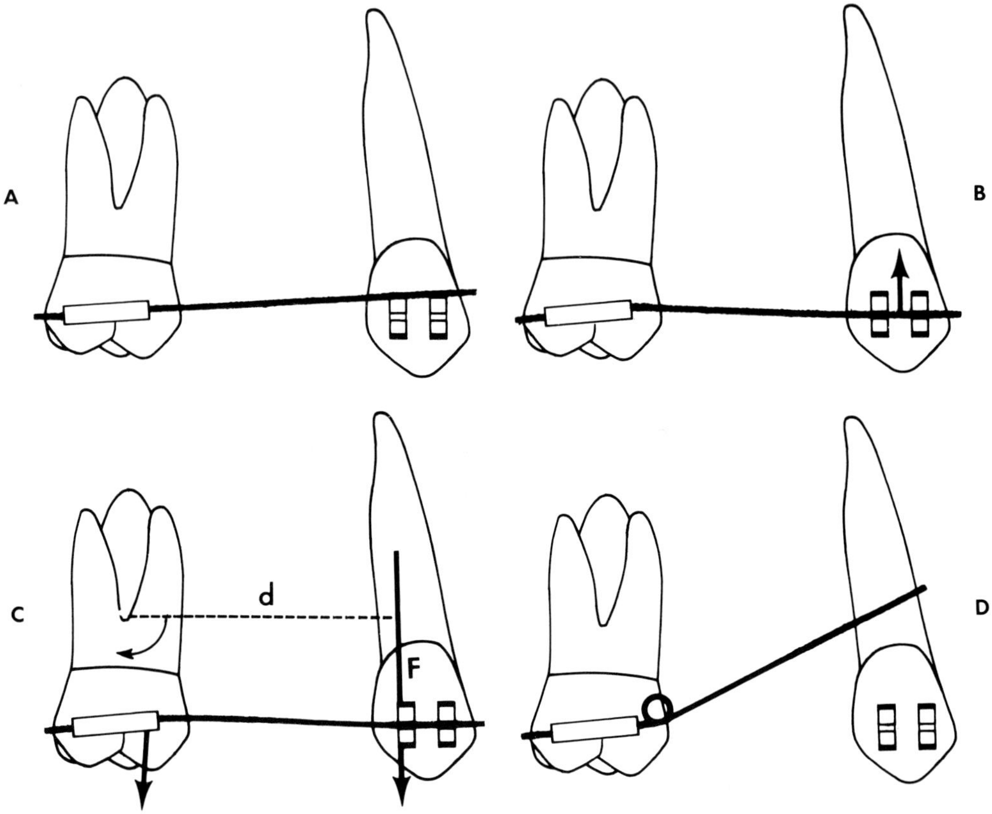

Fig. 18-17. A sectional arch designed to apply an apical vector to a cuspid. **A,** Passive. **B,** Activated, with an apical force on the cuspid. **C,** The reactionary effects on the molar are an occlusal vector equal to the apical action on the cuspid, together with a distal tipping moment applied by the activating force *F* through the moment arm *d*. **D,** A loop in the wire will extend the range and reduce the stiffness of the action, but does *not* affect the force distribution picture. Note the similarity of this configuration to the cuspid-uprighting auxiliary (Fig. 18-9).

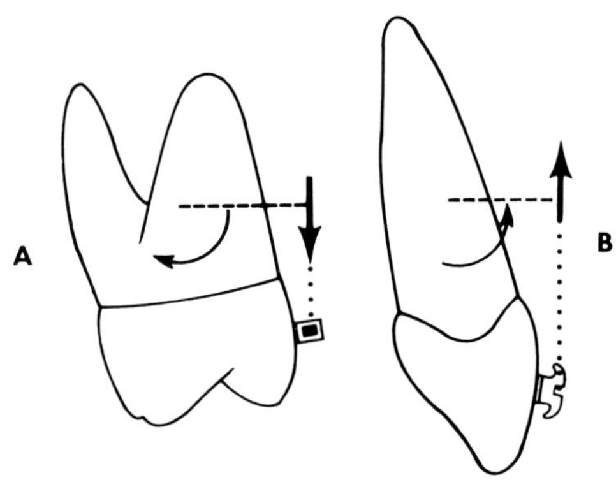

Fig. 18-18. Vertical actions applied through orthodontic attachments produce collateral buccolingual tipping effects. This illustration shows those collateral effects on the cuspid and molar shown in Fig. 18-17.

simultaneously upright lingually tipped incisors. Extraoral anchorage applied to the anterior part of an archwire can have a similar effect, making tipping control with a round wire entirely feasible as long as appropriate apical and lingual vectors are applied (Fig. 18-19).

Mesiodistal cuspid tipping. A common variation on the situation just described is the addition of an uprighting mesial tipping moment on the cuspid. This is usually applied to produce distal root movement, the same as that described previously with the tipping auxiliary. Inserting an archwire into the cuspid bracket in such a way as to provide this action results in a series of effects that are a mirror image of those just described (Fig. 18-20).

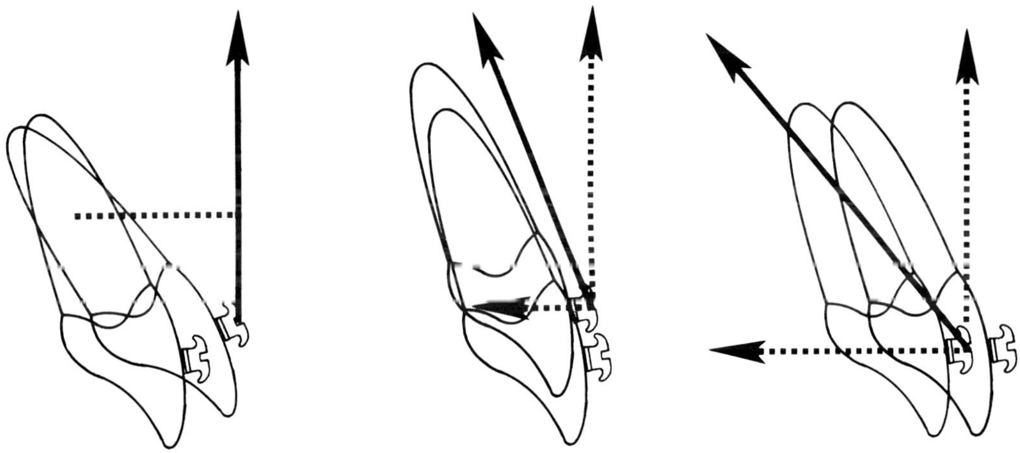

Fig. 18-19. Buccolingual tipping is an inevitable collateral effect of vertical vectors, so even round wires can provide effective tipping actions and control. An upward vector (left) will introduce a labial tipping moment. Adding a lingual vector can effectively prevent any resultant labial crown movement, with the net effect consisting of a combination of intrusion (center) and lingual root movement (right). Force levels and physiologic response will determine the relative vertical and horizontal movements.

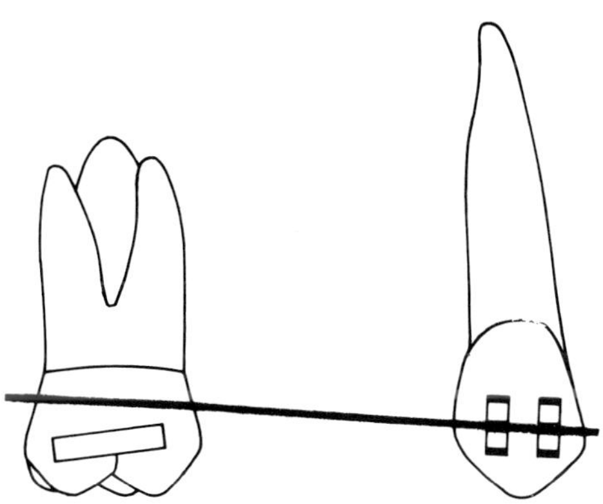

Fig. 18-20. The same auxiliary shown in Fig. 18-17, engaged at the cuspid for tipping control. Engaging it in the molar tube produces a mirror image of the actions shown in Fig. 18-17. These actions combine in the overall force picture.

These effects are best visualized by noting the passive position of the arch when it is engaged in the cuspid bracket but not in the molar, and then bringing it into position at the molar attachment. The molar in this case will receive an apical (intruding) vector, while the cuspid receives an occlusal vector and mesial tipping moment.

The collateral buccolingual tipping effects of this activation will be a buccal tipping of the molar as a resultant of the apical vector and a lingual tipping of the cuspid as a resultant of the occlusal vector, opposite effects to those shown in Fig. 18-18.

A loop immediately distal to the cuspid will increase the working range and reduce the force level for the cuspid tipping action.

Collateral horizontal effects. The mesial tipping moment on the cuspid and the distal tipping moment on the molar introduce collateral mesial and distal horizontal vectors on those teeth. If these are left uncontrolled, the two teeth will tend to separate. Mesial movement of the cuspid is especially undesirable, making such control mandatory in most cases.

Since the two teeth will tend to move in opposite directions, the reciprocal effects may be used to provide the necessary control. The two teeth may be tied together, drawn together with elastic traction, or engaged by the arch in such a way that horizontal movement will be impossible. Each of these options has unique advantages and disadvantages.

Ligating the two teeth together must be done with sufficient flexibility that the ligature does not inhibit desired movements. Typical wire ligation can effectively prevent any tipping of the involved teeth.

Elastic traction must be carefully balanced with desired effects. Too little force can prove ineffective; too much can produce undesirable tipping. The collateral tipping effects of elastic traction between two teeth are exactly opposite to the tipping action of the sectional arch under discussion.

Arch engagement is often the most predictable and reliable control method, in that it does not introduce any new actions. The major problem is doing it with precision without inhibiting desired actions.

Combined effects. The simple sectional arch just described includes many varied cuspid and molar actions. Many of the undesirable actions can be effectively neutralized by balancing them with those acting on the other tooth.

This can be done in many situations, but it should be done with full awareness of all of the actions that are involved. Many surprises can result from altering even a single variable without considering the broad range of secondary effects. Changing from rectangular to round or from conventional to superflexible wires are two examples of changes that can produce spectacular unexpected results.

Collateral effects that cannot be controlled within the archwire system require outside control. Most such control can be applied through one of the other molar attachment tubes.

A lingual arch can control many tipping and rotational effects. Extraoral anchorage can control mesiodistal tipping of the molar and buccal segment, as well as add a distal vector. Another archwire, engaging other teeth, can be inserted in another molar tube and be used to apply many different control actions.

A final option that is always available is to incorporate sectional arch functions into a full archwire. This is, of course, what is done with every full archwire. Where control needs that can be met by the full archwire outweigh any possible limitations of desired actions, this may be the method of choice.

The responsibility of the orthodontist is to look at treatment needs in light of all possible collateral effects, the controls that are required, and the potentials and limitations of each alternative, and then select and manage the appliances that will fill the needs of the individual patient.

Space closure. A somewhat different problem is space closure with a similar sectional arch. To simplify the analysis, we will apply the closing action with elastic traction. The collateral effects introduced by this action are the axial rotation induced by any mesiodistal force applied to a tooth through a buccal or lingual attachment, along with mesiodistal tipping (Fig. 18-21). Control over these effects can be accomplished by many methods, and it is important that they are either prevented or corrected in some way.

The cuspid will resist the mesial molar rotation action, but this will result in a lingual cuspid vector with a reciprocal buccal vector on the molar (Fig. 18-22).

The opposite actions resist the distal cuspid rotation: lingual vector on the molar

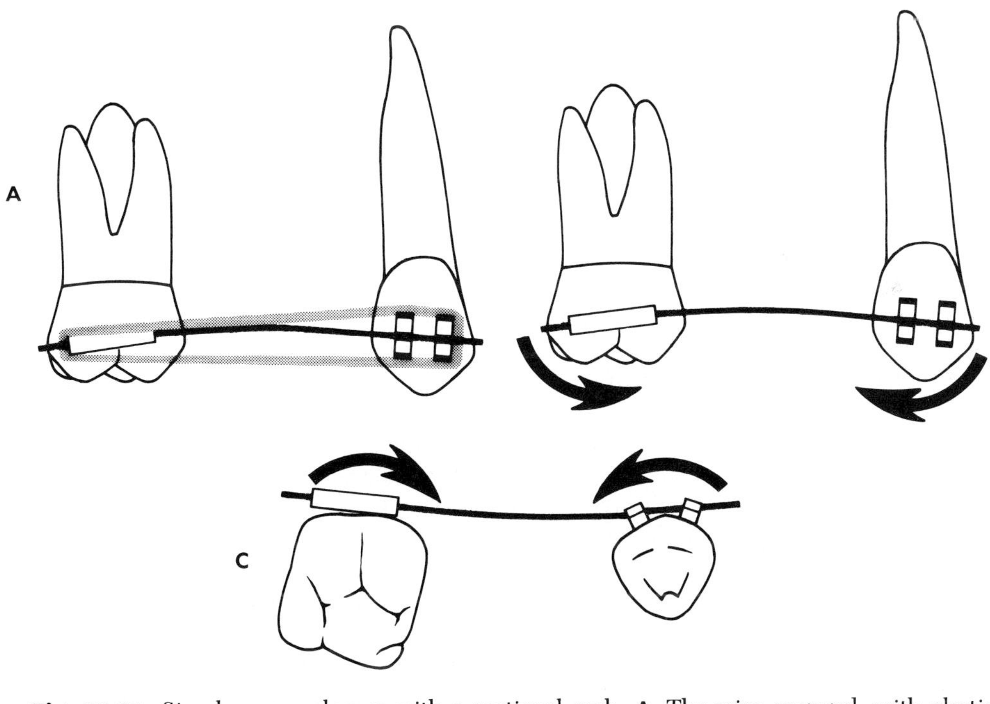

Fig. 18-21. Simple space closure with a sectional arch. **A,** The wire engaged, with elastic applied for closing action. **B,** Collateral tipping induced by the closing action. **C,** Collateral rotation. Both of these collateral effects must be controlled, either by the wire shown or by other auxiliary actions. A wire with closing loops will produce the same effects, but it loses much of its capacity to control them because of the added flexibility of the loops.

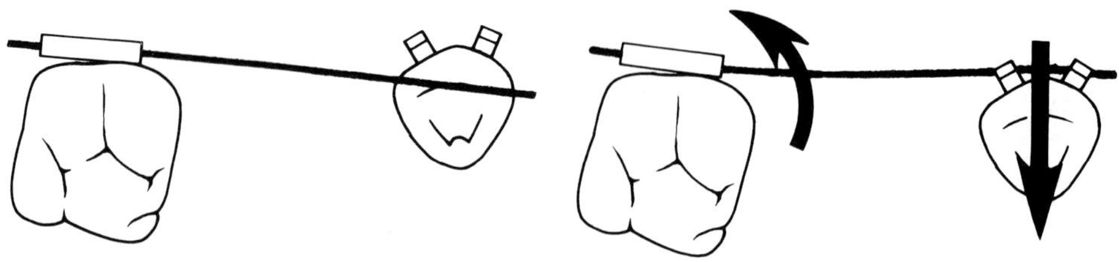

Fig. 18-22. Axial rotation control applies reactionary forces to other teeth. Here, a wire engaged to control mesial molar rotation with a distal moment will apply a lingual force to the cuspid.

and buccal on the cuspid. All of the horizontal vectors tend to balance one another, while the two strong rotating moments place a heavy bending moment on the arch.

Mesiodistal tipping effects are similar, except that they are in a vertical plane. Here the mesial tipping of the molar is resisted by apical action on the cuspid (which is usually good) and occlusal action on the molar (which is usually bad). Distal tipping of the cuspid is resisted by apical molar action and occlusal cuspid action, once again tending to balance the previous effects.

On paper, these actions appear to balance one another, but differences in teeth and in timing can disrupt that balance. The cuspid is longer than the molar, giving it a longer moment arm for the collateral tipping. This tends to favor occlusal cuspid movement, requiring a more vigorous distal tipping action on the molar to balance it. The result is that the molar may be tipped more distally at the completion of the procedure.

In the axial rotations the greater diameter of the molar results in a stronger lingual vector on the cuspid, which can result in enough imbalance to move that tooth lingually.

Balancing the vertical actions on cuspid and molar will be most effective if they are carried out simultaneously, so that opposite actions can actually cancel each other. If one takes place before the other, the fact that occlusal movements are more easily achieved than apical movements can lead to a net occlusal movement of both teeth.

For example, if the cuspid is allowed to tip as it moves distally, while the molar is held upright, both the apical cuspid action and the occlusal molar action will be operating unrestrained. Occlusal function alone may not sufficiently inhibit the occlusal movement of the molar. If the cuspid is then uprighted later, the resultant occlusal cuspid vector and apical molar vectors will also operate alone, with little restraint on occlusal cuspid movement. Assuming equal actions in each case, we can expect the occlusal movements of both teeth to exceed the apical movements.

Space closure also affects intermaxillary relationships, and the two actions may be combined to good effect. Fig. 19-2 shows elastic traction applied to close spaces in upper and lower buccal segments along with Class II correction. While this may not be the method of choice for space closure, the combination of these actions can be very effective.

Loops. All tipping and rotating actions depend on sufficient archwire stiffness to carry the required loads without excessive bending. Loops in an arch always reduce stiffness, and this reduction can seriously compromise control over these effects.

Multiple-loop sectional arches can be extremely useful in accomplishing cuspid retraction and other space closures. Loop closure is friction-free, which is a great advantage over sliding teeth along the arch, and loops that have been designed for cuspid retraction provide for delivery of effective force levels over an extended range of force movement.

The great flexibility of these units requires greatly exaggerated adjustments for tipping and rotation control; 45 degrees or more is often required, and even this may prove inadequate. Additional vertical adjustments may also be required to compensate for the vertical effects of tipping adjustments. Once again, it is important to *evaluate each activation individually*, in its final engaged position with the other end of the wire free, to evaluate side effects.

Lingual auxiliaries can be useful with sectional arches. Lingual elastics aid in rotation control, and a lingual arch can control molar rotations and safeguard against many other unfavorable effects as well. Neither of these, however, can provide mesiodistal tipping control.

A second labial arch, engaged in another molar tube, can also control many secondary effects. One or more of these aids will be useful if not essential with many active sectional arches.

Complete arches

Complete arches, extending from molar to molar, are still the primary source of control and force distribution in edgewise therapy, and their use embodies all of the principles discussed up to this point.

Force storage vs. force delivery. Archwires can serve either or both functions, and the stiffness requirements of the two are completely different. Force storage requires deflection, which places a premium on low stiffness. Force delivery places a premium on high stiffness that is essential to stable form under the loading of outside forces.

The classic force delivery archwire is the full-size rectangular edgewise arch. This wire is too stiff for effective force storage between teeth; it is useful for storage only in changing overall arch form.

The other extreme is the superflexible wire in any of several forms (p. 59). These wires are superb for storage but border on uncontrollable in delivery. It is virtually impossible to use force stored in these wires to move a single tooth without large, often undesirable movements of adjoining teeth.

The entire spectrum between these two extremes is covered by a broad range of wire sizes and materials. Further modification of stiffness with loops and long spans bypassing some teeth can be applied to all but the most flexible of those wires.

Arch fitting. Using the most effective archwire for each procedure, and using it most effectively, can make all the difference between rapid and slow progress, efficient and inefficient treatment, and gratifying or indifferent results.

Final arch form has already been discussed in detail in Chapter 14. This arch form is the final goal of treatment, and all earlier arches are aimed toward this ultimate form. The more recent innovations in orthodontic technique have done nothing to change this goal, but they have brought many changes and new options in the ways in which it can be attained.

The first arches must be formed according to the general principles of arch form laid down in Chapter 14, even though they need not be quite so exact. Only the finest details should be left for the later arches if treatment is to progress with dispatch. In some cases careful work with the first few arches can attain the goals of treatment directly, making it unnecessary to use heavier archwires to complete the correction. Every arch, *especially the first,* must be checked closely on every tooth to ensure against unwanted movements.

Where a few individual tooth movements should be accomplished first, sectional arches provide a viable alternative in the early stages.

The first arches are the lightest, and those with high flexibility are very effective for force storage as well as delivery. These are capable of the most rapid and extensive movements of any arch that will be used. For effective treatment it is essential that these capabilities be exploited to the fullest, leaving only the smallest possible corrections for the later arches. Failure to take full advantage of these light arches by adjusting them fully for all necessary corrections will result in a later situation requiring that those movements be completed with stiffer, slower-acting arches.

The first arches should correct all major discrepancies between adjacent teeth, including rotations, buccolingual displacements, overlapping, tipping, and vertical displacements. At the same time, corrections in arch form and intermaxillary relationships are begun.

The free fit and the flexibility of initial wires bring new problems of their own into the treatment picture. The tipping freedom of small diameter wires is seldom a problem with well-placed brackets, but every step in treatment must include very careful tipping adjustments. Arch form and last molar adjustments must frequently be exaggerated in flexible wires, especially where elastic traction is used. The force of rubber elastics can grossly deform these wires, and this deformation must be countered by alterations in arch form. Elastics used with these wires should usually be adjusted to exert a very light pull of not more than 50 to 100 gm (2 to 4 ounces).

Heavier archwires are required for some torque actions, but all other adjustments in tipping and tooth levels should be completed in advance of their use. The primary objective of heavy archwires is stabilization of intramaxillary relationships and arch form. These are pure force delivery wires that are of little value for storage.

Stiffness, strength, and range. All three elastic properties are important in archwires, but the one that governs most procedures and that occupies most of the orthodontist's attention is stiffness.

Stiffness requirements vary at different stages of treatment and in different parts of the arch, but most arch modifications are designed to bring about a reduction in stiffness. The reason for this is simple. We cannot increase wire stiffness, so we begin with one that will provide enough to meet maximum stiffness demands. We then modify it in the areas that require lower stiffness levels for force storage.

That is the basic principle, but practical considerations force us into many compromises, and it is the succession of these compromises through a series of arches to the final correction that constitutes an orthodontic treatment program. All of the various "techniques" represent specific series of such compromises that have proved to be workable in a sufficiently high percentage of cases to warrant their repeated use. In all of these we should never lose sight of the fact that they are compromises, that they may be applicable in many but never all cases, and that there are many other equally useful approaches.

Wire size. The most potent determinant of mechanical properties is wire size, and its selection is the first decision that must be made in arch design. Orthodontics is not a fertile field for universal rules, but the precept that we should always select the smallest wire size that will do the job comes close to fitting that description.

First, we locate our most demanding area in terms of force control requirements, and select a wire size sufficient to provide adequate strength.

Next, we consider the adequacy of the stiffness and range of that wire size. In most cases stiffness will be adequate or excessive; if it is not, we will have to select a larger size. Inadequate stiffness for molar control, where the need is usually greatest, can be compensated with a lingual arch.

Finally, we evaluate stiffness and range in other areas of the arch, where force demands are lower and greater range is often required. These will require either arch modifications with loops or the use of other force storage units such as elastic ligatures.

Wire composition. Elastic properties of conventional wires depend only on size, but the composition of the wire can also be an important factor. Composition may be altered either physically or by changes in the metallic alloy.

Physical alteration is accomplished by multistranding the wire in twisted or braided form. The fourth-power effect of diameter is immediately brought into play: three strands of .007-inch (.20-mm) wire twisted into a .017-inch (.425-mm) diameter wire have a stiffness comparable to a solid wire of about .010 inch (.25 mm), yet they will fully engage the slot of a conventional edgewise bracket.

Even more flexible than the multistrand wires are the superflexible alloys such as Nitinol (p. 59).

Exceptional flexibility introduces a whole new pattern of force storage and delivery that requires a complete reprogramming of treatment. These wires *cannot be directly substituted* for conventional wires without major and often unfavorable changes in therapeutic response. Some of the considerations in their application are:

1. Increased flexibility makes the archwire a major force storage component and drastically reduces its capacity for force distribution.
2. Wires of larger diameter are usually used. The closer fit in dental attachments greatly increases tooth movements, both desired and reciprocal, over the same force level applied with conventional wires of smaller diameter. The additive nature of these effects can compound their significance.
3. Adjustability of these wires is limited, requiring special attention to attachment position. Levels and inclinations of anterior teeth are especially susceptible to change under these conditions, and unfavorable changes can be startlingly rapid and resistant to reversal.
4. Stiffness of many of these wires is too low for effective control over arch form or curve of Spee, yet they are capable of rapid expansion of arch form.

5. Passive seating in bracket slots is especially critical for prevention of unwanted labial movements.
6. Corrective forces stored in other components should be used sparingly if at all with these wires. They can introduce collateral effects, as in space closure or elastic traction, with negligible control available from the superflexible archwire. Recovery from such unwanted effects can be prolonged.

Loops. Once wire size and composition have been selected, there is only one factor that can modify stiffness and range, and that is span. Span can be increased by bypassing some teeth, so it has valuable but limited application as an independent variable in this application. The effects are straightforward and readily determined from Fig. 4-4.

Span can also be increased by forming the wire into a loop for local modification of force delivery by the arch. All loops use combinations of the bending and torsion effects described earlier.

The objective in all cases is to attain increased deflection and movement of a tooth while keeping the bending or torsion moment at the critical section low enough to avoid excessive deformation (permanent set) of the wire. At the same time, forces are reduced to levels comparable to the normal force of the arch under smaller deflections. In other words, the loop permits large deflections without increasing either the force on the tooth or the stress on the wire. Adding helical coils, increasing length, and reducing wire diameter will help toward this end, and all three measures should be used freely wherever they will serve best.

Loop orientation. Simple U-shaped loops and all helical coils provide flexibility only in directions that lie at an angle to the arm. This fact can be used to advantage to provide more rigid control in the direction parallel to the arms, such as maintaining vertical relationships, while a loop provides horizontal flexibility for space or rotation control.

When vertical flexibility is required, a loop of this type must have at least one horizontal arm.

Rectangular loops and interrupted arches. Fig. 18-23 shows a long loop consisting of three sides of a rectangle, formed to hold space for an unerupted biscupid. This is a very useful form with many varied applications. As shown, it has a passive function, but this configuration introduces marked flexibility into the wire.

This added flexibility can be useful in many ways, but if it is not recognized and compensated for, it can also create problems.

A very useful application of this type of loop is in a complete arch interrupted by such loops extending across both buccal segments to engage only the incisors. This combines some of the effects of both sectional and complete arches. A horizontal span of this length requires a wire size of at least .016 inch (.4 mm).

This type of interrupted arch can be used for many purposes, as is reflected in the name "utility arch" applied to it by Ricketts. With the distal arms engaged against the molar tubes, as in Fig. 18-23, it will maintain total arch length.

If the distal arms are adjusted to leave a clear section of horizontal wire mesial to the molar tube, it will allow mesial molar movement or lingual incisor movement. An archwire formed in that way and then pulled back through the tubes and secured by bending the ends will provide an active arch-shortening (closing) action. This will induce active tipping and level changes that require control.

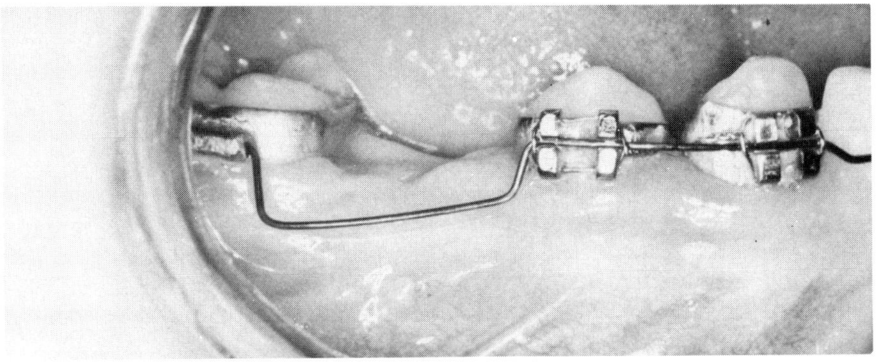

Fig. 18-23. Space-holding loop, which may be adjusted for vertical or horizontal movements.

Cuspids are free to move distally in crowded cases while total arch length is maintained by an interrupted arch extending from molars to incisors. Active cuspid movement may also be implemented with auxiliaries at this stage.

Vertical incisor action, usually apical, is possible by bending immediately ahead of the molar. The reciprocal action for these activations is molar tipping and elevation. This is a most effective means for applying the light, continuous force required for incisor intrusion, and the arch is also readily adjusted to provide the lingual vector that is needed to control collateral tipping.

Box loops. Fig. 18-24 shows a compact variation of the rectangular loop that provides flexibility in all directions. In the case shown, it is applying labial and gingival actions on the central incisor. If additional space were required, the outer vertical arms could be formed to engage the brackets of the adjacent teeth to open space simultaneously with the movement of the central incisor into that space.

Such a combined action must be checked carefully on activation, because compressing the loop by engaging the outside arms for an opening action will force the middle section either lingually or labially, with torsion in all four vertical arms. If this space opening activation is too great, it can force the displaced incisor even farther lingually with the initial adjustment, in which case the activation must be reduced and the operation carried out in smaller increments.

An *inverted box loop* can be used in an extreme form of interrupted arch to bring single teeth, usually upper incisors, out of a lingual crossbite. Fig. 18-25 shows such a loop. When formed in this way, the wire wrapping at the top of the loop secures the integrity of arch form from molar to molar so that buccolingual activations work through torsion in the main part of the arch. Vertical flexibility is provided by the long free span from molar to molar.

Vertical steps, as in Fig. 18-23, are formed to engage the molar tubes and maintain arch length to prevent lingual movement of the entire arch as the box is tied to the incisor. The combination of vertical and horizontal stiffness in such an arch formed of .018-inch (.45-mm) wire is sufficient to permit adjusting the horizontal section, which engages the bracket, to lie at its final corrected position before tying to the tooth. This type of arch should never be overadjusted or it will carry the tooth too far.

Adequate space should always be available before crossbite correction is initi-

A

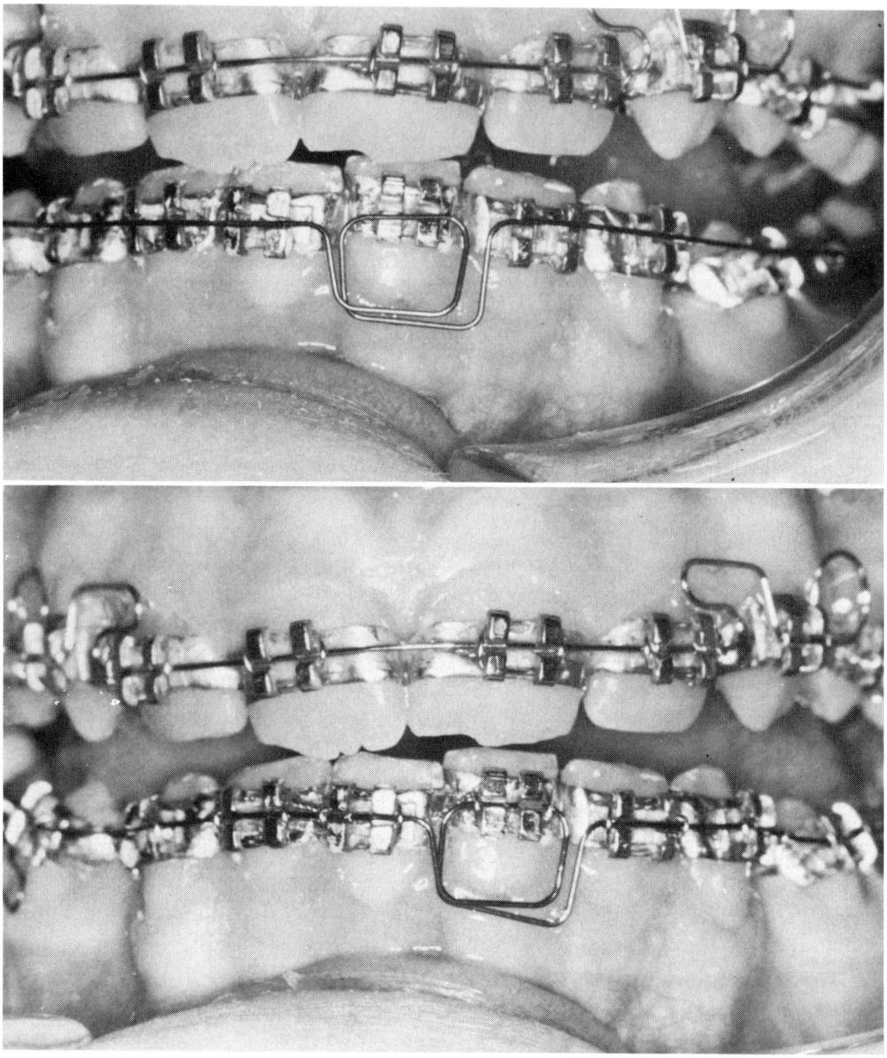

B

Fig. 18-24. A, Box loop, not engaged. **B,** Box loop, activated. Vertical arms may also be formed to engage the brackets of adjacent teeth for space opening.

ated by this or any other means, so that movement through the region of occlusal interference is accomplished as quickly as possible. Where the crossbite correction will not be impeded by slightly inadequate space, the arch may be tied to only one incisor bracket to bring that side into position first (Fig. 18-26). When this has been accomplished, a change to another arch may be indicated for space opening and rotation of the tooth into final position.

Such rotation of a crowded incisor into position is the method of choice in many situations, in preference to complete space opening before any labial movement is begun.

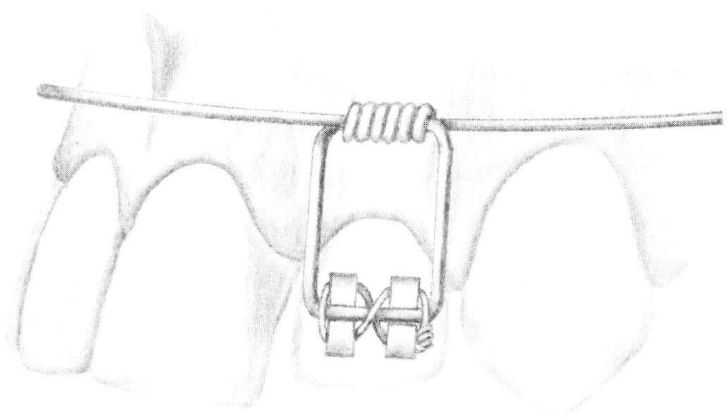

Fig. 18-25. An inverted box loop will provide light, well-controlled buccolingual force. The wire shown is .018 inch (.45 mm), with the base tightly wrapped with .020-inch (.5-mm) soft brass wire to provide stiffness for arch form control across the loop. This loop will move a single tooth out of crossbite with minimum adjustments and good vertical control.

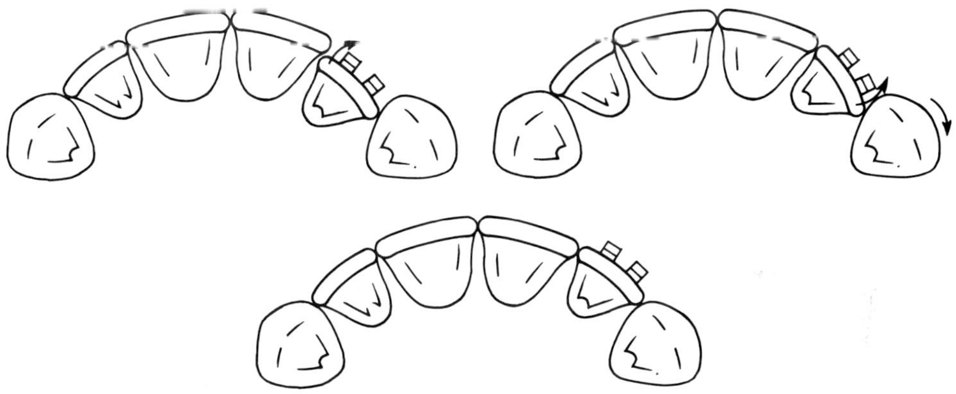

Fig. 18-26. It is sometimes more effective to rotate a tooth into alignment in successive stages, rather than attempt to force it broadside through a limited space.

Horizontal base loops. The delta-shaped loop (Fig. 18-27) functions in much the same way as a box loop, but its shape allows it to be fitted between two adjacent teeth. The key to its flexibility is the horizontal base segment, which is long enough to flex in bending for vertical action and in torsion for buccolingual movements. Full evaluation of the action of this loop requires consideration of three components as individual loops. Each arm functions with the base as a two-arm loop, while the total loop functions as two arms and a base. Angulation of the arms can introduce marked vertical effects.

The horizontal loop in Fig. 18-28 is essentially a folded version of the same loop, with similar adjustment potential.

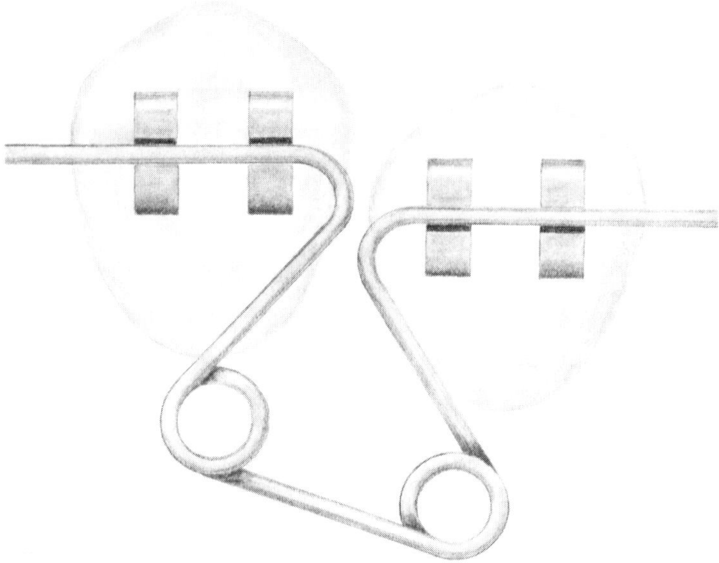

Fig. 18-27. A delta-shaped loop, with or without the helices shown here, provides good flexibility in all vertical and horizontal directions.

A

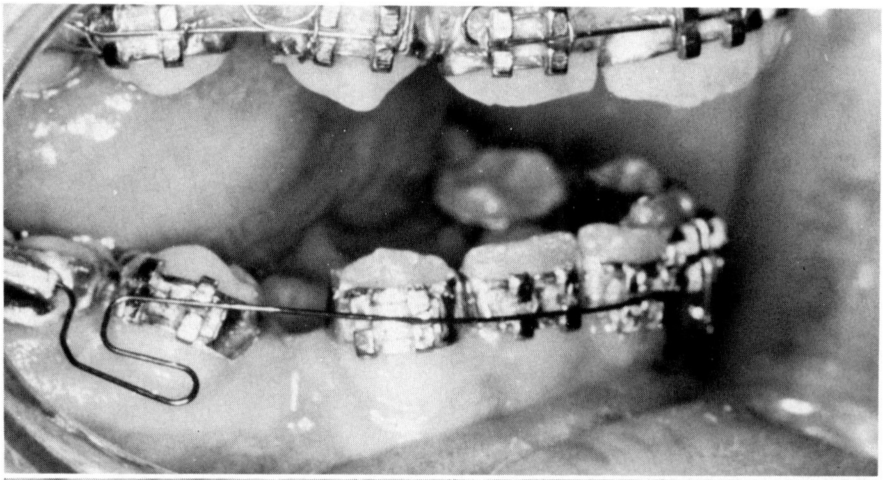

B

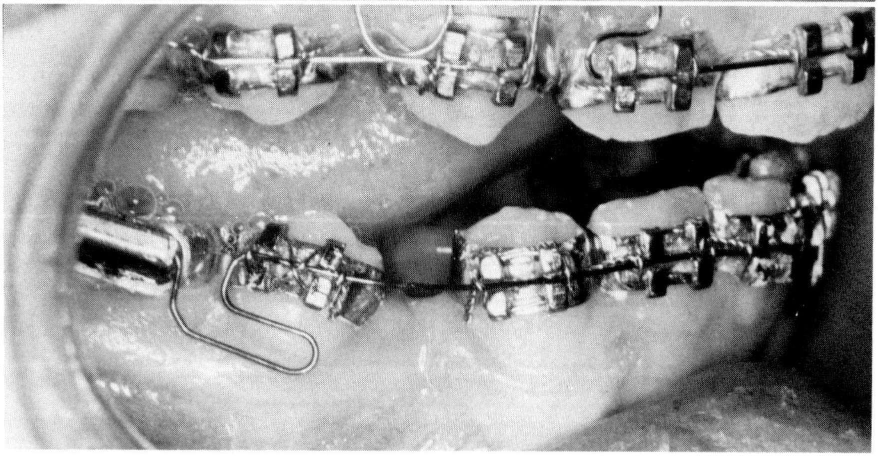

Fig. 18-28. A, Horizontal loop for vertical and buccolingual adjustment; .012-inch (.3-mm) wire, not engaged. **B,** Engaged and tied in the bracket slots.

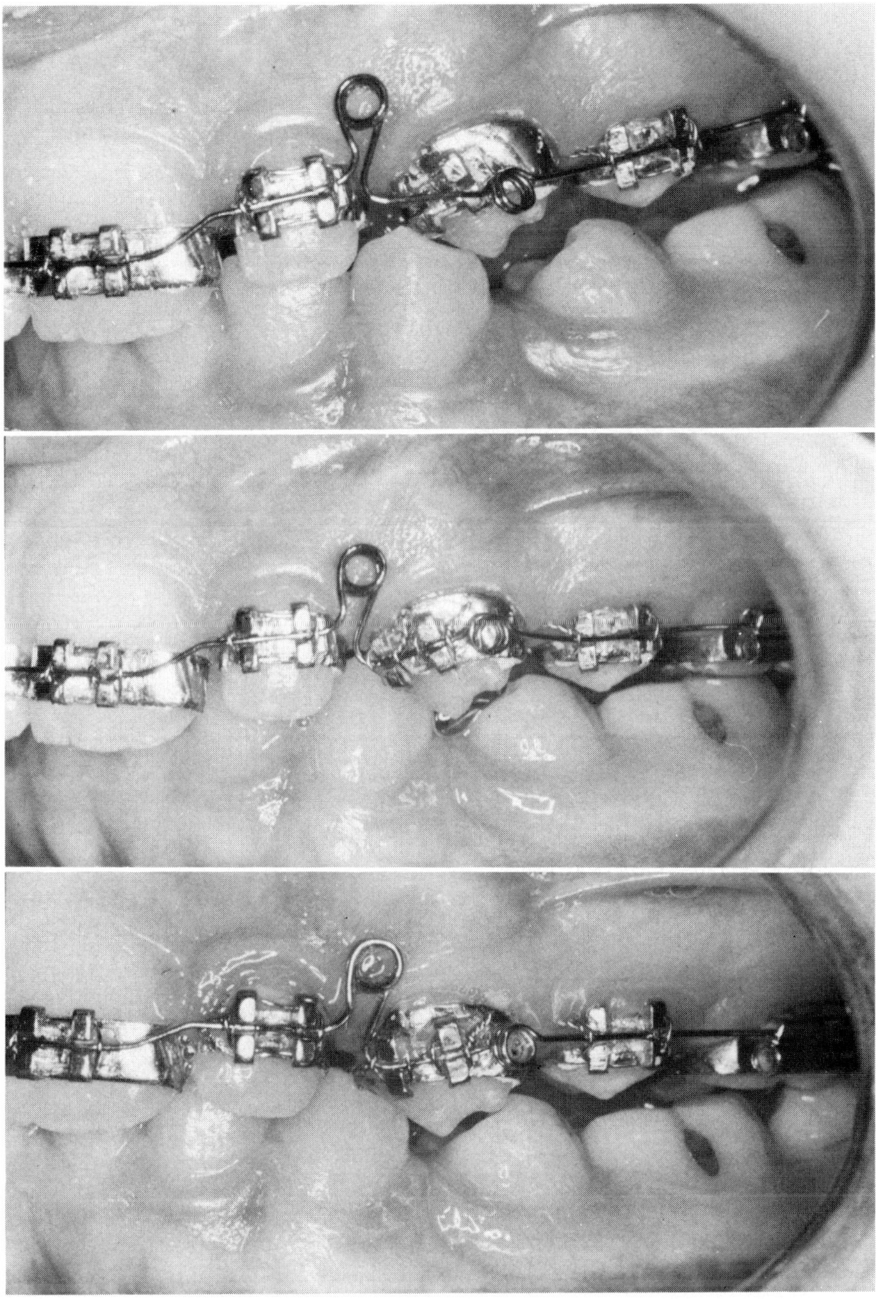

A

B

C

Fig. 18-29. A, Rotated cuspid with a .012-inch (.3-mm) arch and helical loops, before tying arch to cuspid. **B,** Activated by tying in cuspid bracket. **C,** Changes accomplished 4 weeks later.

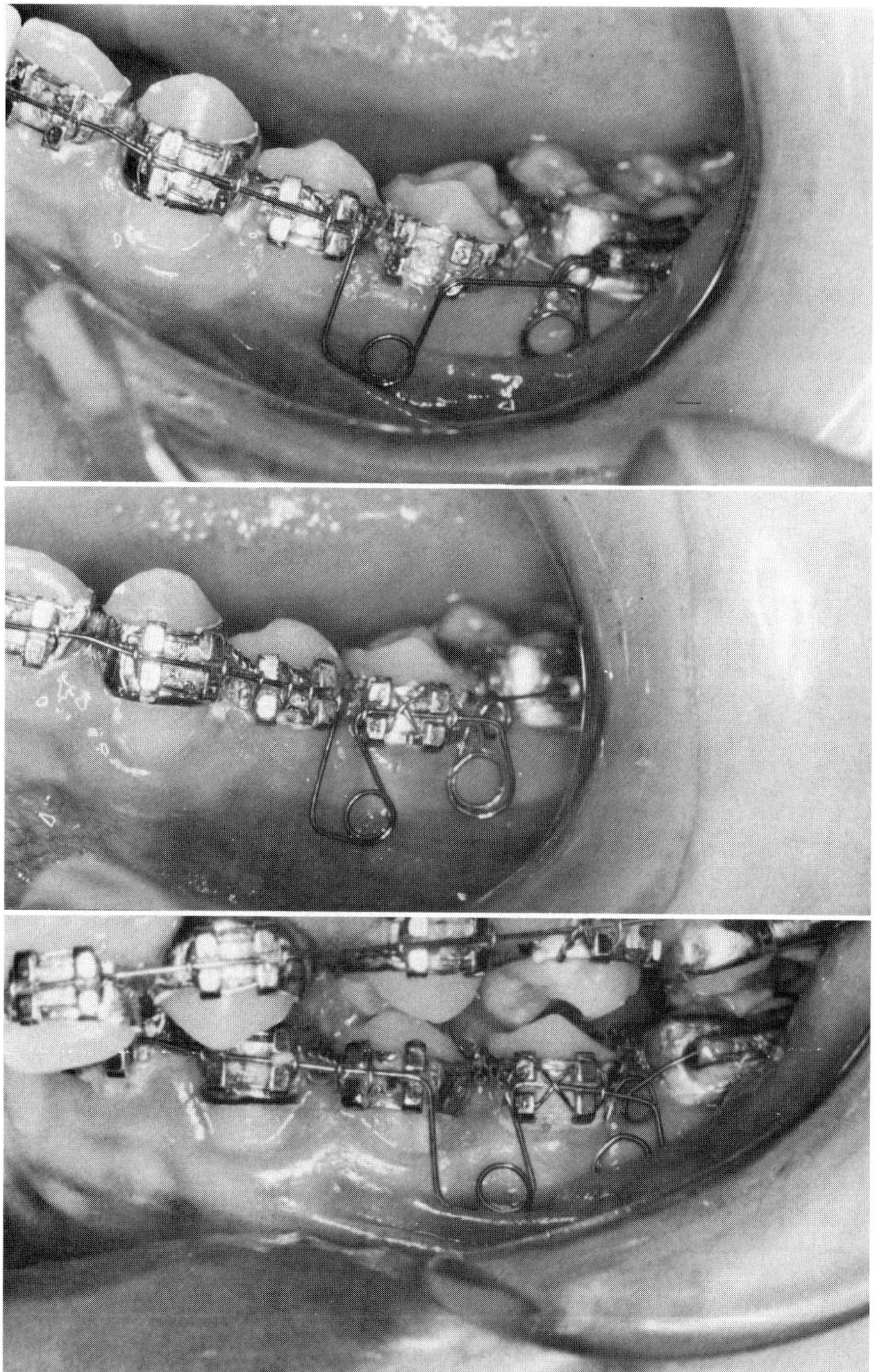

A

B

C

Fig. 18-30. A, Rotated lower second bicuspid with a .011-inch (.28-mm) arch ready for activation. **B,** The same arch after tying to the second bicuspid. This adjustment combines a rotating moment on the bicuspid with a distal action on the buccal surface. **C,** Same case 6 weeks after the initiation of movement.

Paired loops. Loops paired on opposite sides of a tooth can be used to move it in any direction, including axial rotation, without the gingival impingement that can accompany some actions with a box loop.

The most useful application of paired loops is in severe rotations, those in which both brackets cannot be engaged on the arch for rotation with elastic ligatures. Such rotations almost invariably require significant horizontal movement in addition to the rotation, and some may require tipping (uprighting) as well. Paired loops can be designed to perform all of these actions simultaneously, as is shown in Figs. 18-29 and 18-30. These are extreme deviations that are not readily controlled with elastic ligatures because of lack of bracket engagement.

The "boot hook" mesial to the upper cuspid in Fig. 18-31 shows another application of this type of loop. This loop is relatively small and stiff, intended only for small adjustments in tooth position. The same configuration can be enlarged slightly, with or without helices as shown in Fig. 18-32, to increase flexibility as required.

Loop/hook/stop combinations. Loops provide a convenient place to attach ligatures or elastics, as well as a means for preventing an arch from sliding through an attachment. A single loop can sometimes serve all three functions.

The simplest stop loop is the short vertical loop seen at the lower molar in Fig. 18-31. This may be varied as shown by the dashed line to shorten wire length, but *any* loop introduced into an archwire will reduce stiffness. In this position these changes will significantly affect molar control, especially over the collateral effects of elastic traction. This is no problem if a lingual arch is used for molar stabilization.

The upper boot hook in this same illustration is actually a triple-function loop. It provides the adjustability of a loop, a place to attach elastic traction, and also

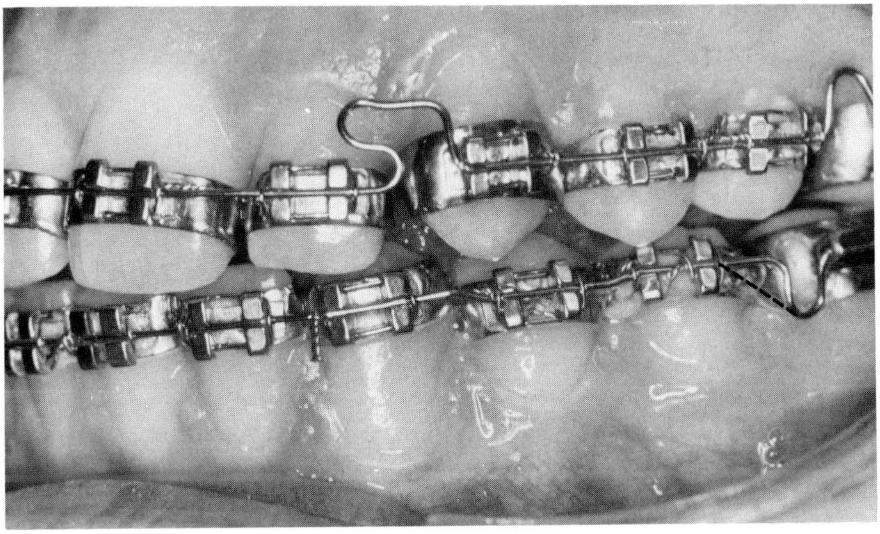

Fig. 18-31. Stop loop mesial to lower first molar tube. An alternate design is shown by the dashed line (lower right). The boot hook in the upper arch is paired with a similar loop on the other side to control intercuspid arch length.

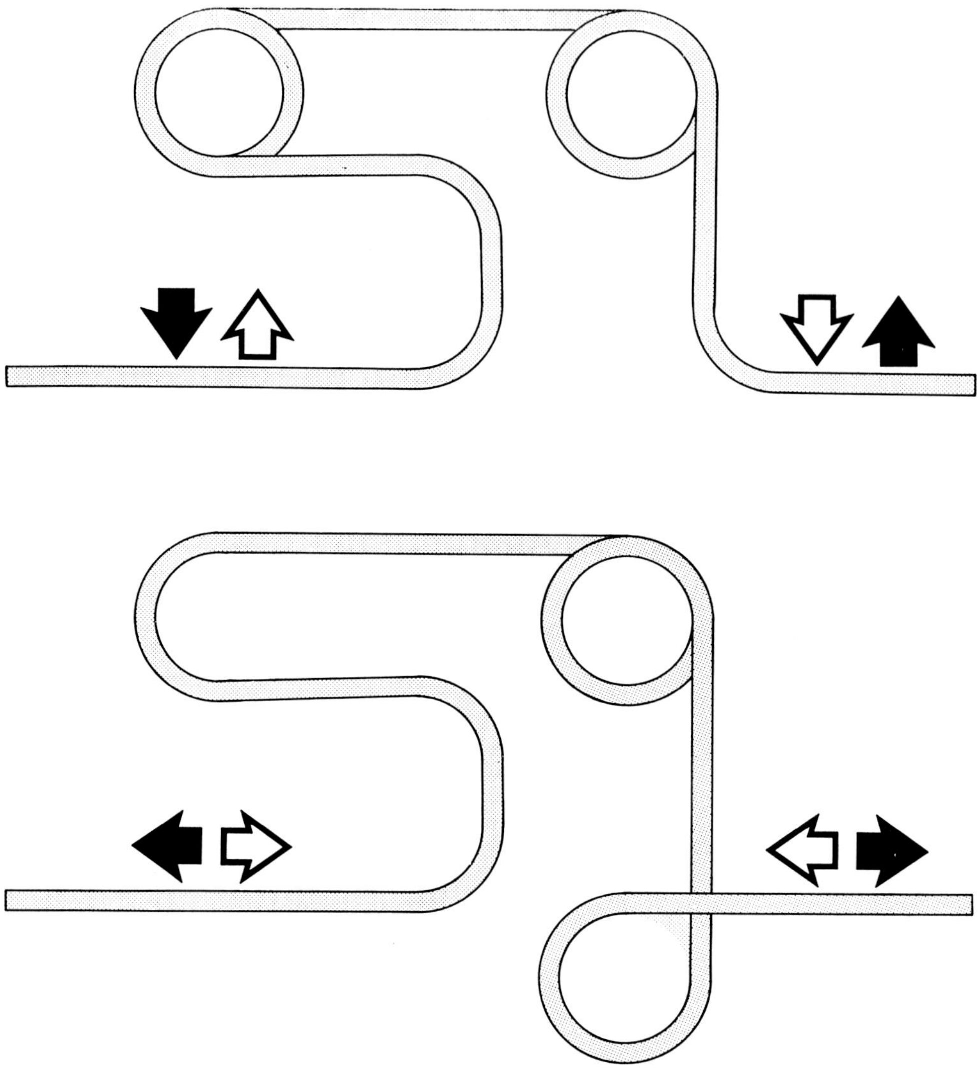

Fig. 18-32. For greater vertical flexibility, helical coils may be added at both ends of the upper horizontal section of a boot hook, and for greater mesiodistal flexibility they may be added at both ends of the distal vertical arm.

serves to keep the arch from sliding distally at the cuspid. In combination with a similar loop on the other side of the arch, it provides precision control over intercuspid arch length and ready adjustability for fine positioning of incisors. *These loops can be a useful part of almost every arch.* The torquing loops shown in Fig. 18-33, *A*, also function as arch stops.

Whenever elastic traction is attached to a loop, consideration must be given to the way in which the archwire will be distorted by that traction. For example, an elastic attached to the boot hook in Fig. 18-31 will bend the anterior segment

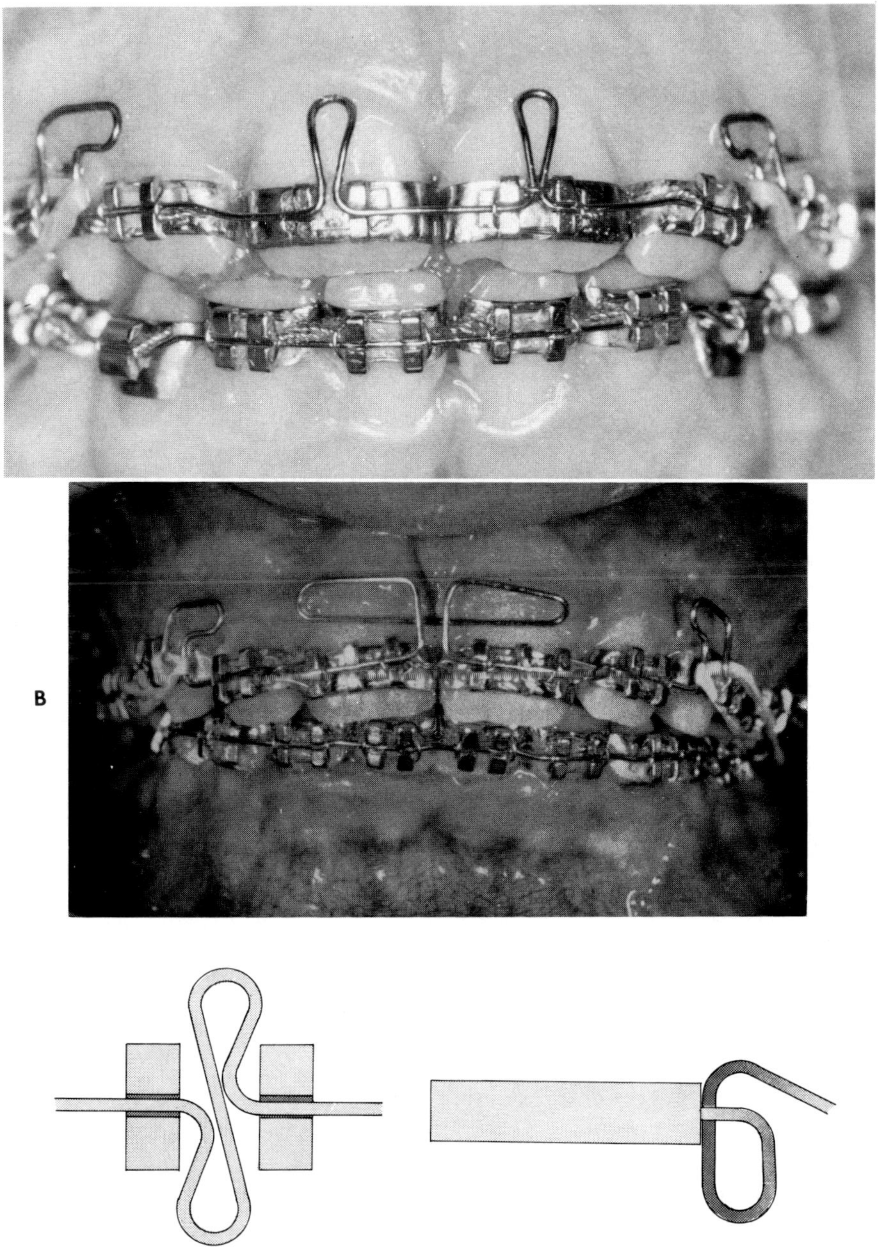

Fig. 18-33. Torque-controlling loops. **A,** Individual loops engaging the gingival region for labial tipping, with a lingual vector applied by intramaxillary elastics so that the net effect will be lingual root movement with little movement of the crown as the tooth tips. **B,** A single loop engaging both central incisors in the gingival region for a similar tipping action. This loop also provides adjustability in arch length and rotation, which may be useful in some cases, but these actions require great care in adjustment. **C,** A loop formed to fit between the brackets on an individual tooth to control rotation (rolling) of the archwire. This loop may also be used for buccolingual tipping, but a single extension in the required direction as in **A** or **B** is usually preferred for that purpose. **D,** A stabilizing/stop loop at the molar engages tooth and tube to control arch rolling in the tube as well as arch length.

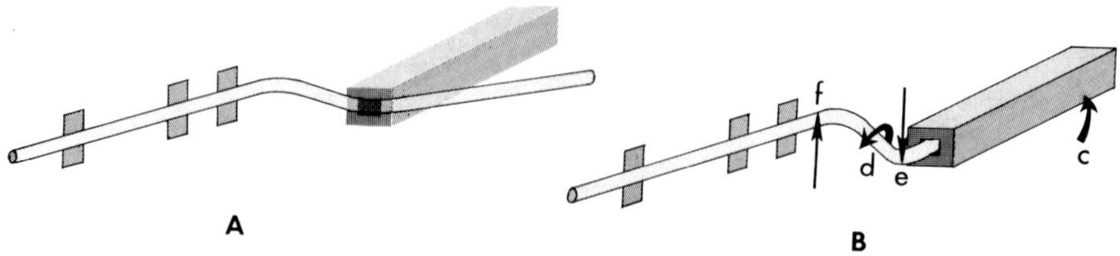

Fig. 18-34. Wires can distort and "roll" considerably when three-dimensional stresses are introduced. **A,** shows a wire with large molar offset adjusted to tip the first molar distally. **B** shows the effect of introducing this wire into the molar tube. Elevation of the distal end, *c*, introduces a torsion stress, *d*, at the offset, which in turn has a depressing effect, *e*, on the molar and an elevating effect, *f*, on the bicuspid. These changes also apply torsion to the rest of the archwire. The initial effects are almost exactly the opposite of the desired movements, and the long span that has been twisted mesial to the offset has little power to return the arch to its original form to provide the intended molar tipping. A rectangular wire undergoes the same actions, with torque effects on molar and bicuspid limiting the range of movement.

downward, requiring a compensatory adjustment at the time that the arch is placed to prevent this effect. Provision of a loop hook for the elastic in the distal arm of this same loop can reverse this particular effect of the elastic.

Torquing loops. Loops can be formed to engage individual teeth, especially incisors, in such a way that the root will be tipped in a labiolingual plane. Fig. 18-33 shows several loops of this type. All of these reduce stiffness in varying directions, which must be considered in relation to arch form as these loops are activated.

There are important mesiodistal effects related to buccolingual root movement of anterior teeth. This must always be considered in relation to intermaxillary corrections. The distal elastic traction that is visible in Fig. 18-33, *A* and *B*, is an essential compensating adjunct to these corrections.

Arch "rolling"

Adjusting any arch in more than one plane will often cause unwanted movements due to the archwire turning on its long axis or rolling in the bracket slots. This problem is most severe with small round wires, but it is present to some degree in all arches, including rectangular wires.

These effects can become very complex, but a brief description will help the operator to identify and avoid such problems.

Subtle effects occur in such situations as when a mesiodistal tipping action is combined with buccolingual adjustment, as in Fig. 18-34. Here an effort is made to tip a molar distally with an arch that has a buccal offset. Inserting this arch in the tube and bracket will place the offset section under a torsion stress. Mesial to the bend, where the arch is restrained, it will twist slightly, changing the direction of the offset. This will be expressed primarily at the molar, where the wire will roll in the tube and so change the effective direction of the bend that was intended to tip the molar distally. The net result of this action is depression and mesial tipping of the molar and reciprocal elevation of the bicuspid, essentially opposite to the intended action.

These effects can shift the actions of intended adjustments in many ways. Torque-controlling loops (Fig. 18-34, *C* and *D*) will help, but we cannot lose sight of the fact that they may also place a possibly undesirable torquing action on the tooth. Rectangular wires limit the effect both by their stiffness and by an action similar to that of the torque-controlling loops, but only if they fit closely in the attachments.

The most effective control for this problem is prevention. Placing all attachments at the same level and carefully orienting molar tubes will eliminate the need for compound compensating bends. Single bends between teeth do not have the complex reactions seen with compound bends like those in Fig. 18-34. Molar offsets can be used sparingly in combination with active light-wire adjustments. Small adjustments in critical areas will make less elastic energy available for diversion into these undesirable effects.

19

Intermaxillary and vertical actions

Intermaxillary relationships are described by the Angle classification of malocclusion as mesiodistal disharmonies between opposing first molars, and in a limited way between incisors. Buccolingual and vertical relationships can be equally important. While certain combinations of these may be more common than others, any discrepancy in one plane may occur along with any in another plane.

Horizontal problems, either lateral or anteroposterior, are usually corrected with relatively straightforward force applications from any of several sources. Choice of specific methods is often based more on collateral vertical effects than on the primary action.

Vertical relationships depend heavily on mandibular and tongue function and posture, and in turn may influence these structures. Occlusal tooth movement "raises the bite" and brings the teeth into occlusion with the mandible in a more "open" position. This rotates the chin into a more inferior and retruded position, which is usually unfavorable. One common and reasonably reliable cephalometric index of this effect is the mandibular plane angle, which increases as the mandible opens. It may also change with growth.

A mandible that has been opened in the course of treatment will return to its original balanced posture if muscle function remains unchanged. Those cases where muscle function is inadequate may retain the new position, and in some the angle may even increase farther as growth progresses. Some of the factors operating in these situations are covered in more detail in the *Atlas of Orthodontic Principles*,[34] but in the present context of treatment mechanics we will merely consider such changes in the level of occlusion as an effect to be considered and usually minimized.

CROSSBITE

Buccal crossbite corrections can be accomplished with buccolingual (crisscross) elastic traction (Fig. 19-1), buccal arch, or lingual arch. The elastics are effective with a cooperative patient where single pairs of teeth are involved, but more extensive problems are usually better corrected with more positive control.

Buccal arches in sizes .018 inch (.45 mm) or larger are at their best where expansion is required. A *straight* .018-inch (.45-mm) arch in that size range that

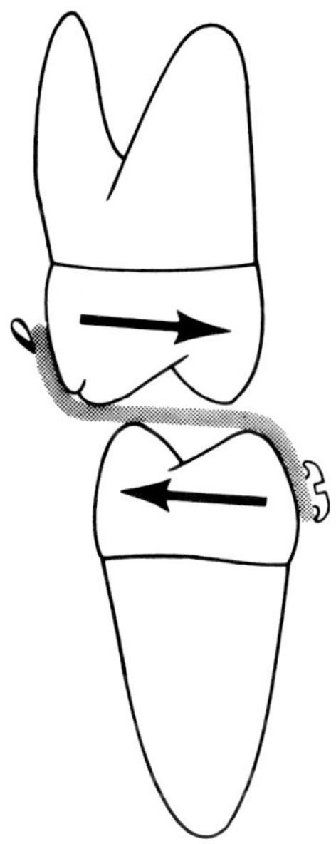

Fig. 19-1. A small elastic attached buccally and lingually to opposing brackets or hooks will correct many buccolingual crossbites involving only two opposing teeth. Major limiting factors are patient cooperation and interferences from occlusion or space deficiencies.

engages only molars or buccal teeth will exert a light but effective expansion action with no tipping control. Of course, effects on individual teeth must be considered carefully with such an arch. Rectangular wires can be used where it is necessary to control tipping, including unilateral tipping to accelerate or retard movement on opposite sides.

Lingual arches are the method of choice where maximum molar control is called for. These arches in .036-inch (.9-mm) stainless steel with horizontal tubes will provide precise control over intermolar width and buccolingual tipping of each molar. When teeth other than the molars are involved, buccal arches can be added to control their relationships to the molars, which are in turn controlled by the lingual arches.

Control in both dental arches is often required in crossbite cases, sometimes because both arches need adjustment and at other times to prevent change in an opposing arch due to occlusal contacts.

ANTEROPOSTERIOR RELATIONSHIPS

Rubber elastics

Relationships between arches are frequently adjusted with rubber elastics extending from the cuspid region in one arch to the molar region of the opposing arch. This is a reciprocal action that will influence both arches with equal force (Figs. 12-3 and 19-2).

Movement in response to these equal forces can be influenced to a limited

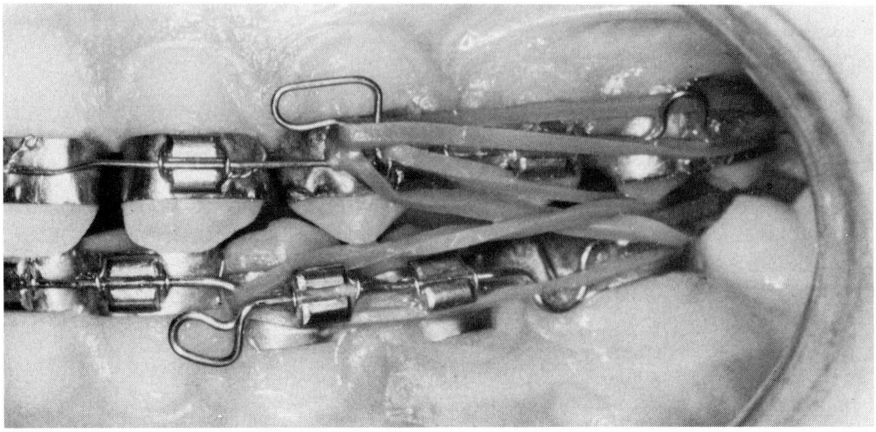

Fig. 19-2. Elastics simultaneously closing spaces and correcting Class II relationship.

extent by applying concurrent tipping actions to the teeth with the individual arches. For example, lower teeth may be tipped distally to help resist anterior forces, and upper teeth may be tipped distally to encourage distal movement. Care must be taken not to carry such tipping to excessive lengths, or the normal occlusal and contact relationships may be disrupted. Bringing such teeth back to normal axial inclination can nullify the original gain.

Intermaxillary traction introduces collateral tipping of the entire occlusal plane, due to the occlusal vectors imposed at both upper and lower attachment points. This in turn causes opening of the mandible. Light elastic traction over an extended period offers the best possibility for occlusal function to resist this side effect.

Extraoral traction

Extraoral traction offers the only available means for moving teeth without reciprocal forces acting on other teeth. These appliances direct reciprocal forces to the cranium or neck, where no undesirable effects have been observed. The improvement and reintroduction of extraoral anchorage by Kloehn[35] has added immeasurably to the potential range of orthodontic intermaxillary adjustment.

Extraoral traction devices are available in many variations, designed to exert force in various combinations of distal and vertical directions to effect changes in the maxilla. This in turn alters intermaxillary relationships.

Fig. 19-3 shows a cervical elastic and facebow, which is one of the most commonly used of the extraoral appliances. This device exerts a distal action on the upper first molar to which it is attached. In addition to the distal force, there are tipping and elongating actions that can be controlled in varying degrees by adjustment of the wire bow.

This appliance is attached to the dentition by means of bands cemented to the upper first molars, or occasionally to other teeth. The bands are equipped with round tubes, usually .045 or .050 inch (1.15 or 1.25 mm) attached to their buccal surfaces. The remainder of the appliance consists of removable inner and outer

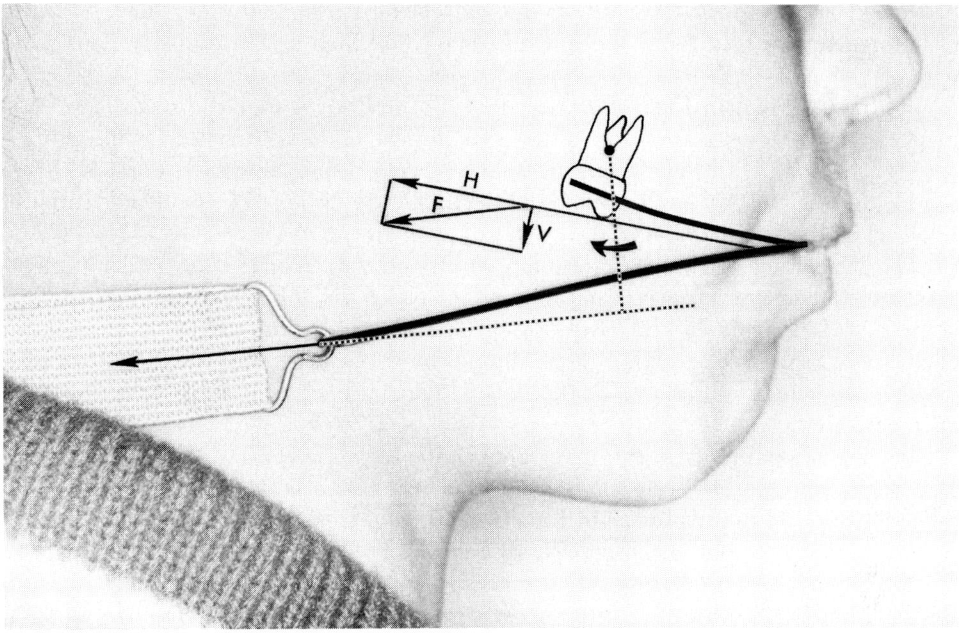

Fig. 19-3. Cervical appliance in place. Dotted extension of force arrow shows direction of pull. Dotted line from the center of root to line of force is the moment arm acting to tip the molar as shown by the curved arrow. Rectangular vector diagram shows linear forces acting on the molar. The diagonal arrow, *F*, is parallel to the direction of the elastic force. The long horizontal arrow, *H*, is drawn parallel to the occlusal plane, with the vertical arrow, *V*, drawn at right angles to it. Lengths of these three arrows are proportional to the respective forces, indicating the relative horizontal and vertical components acting on the tooth.

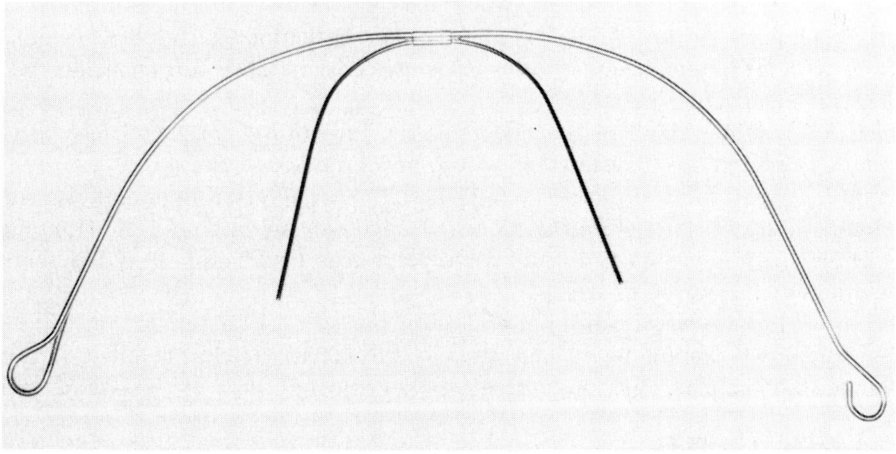

Fig. 19-4. Cervical bow assembly with hooks formed for elastic strap. This is the preferred flexible type, with a small anterior attachment between arch and bow. Large rigid reinforcements in this area limit the potential for adjusting intermolar width and rotations.

bows, fixed together at the center, and the elastic strap. The inner bow is formed of wire to fit the tube, and the outer bow of .059 inch (1.5 mm) or similar heavy wire.

A bow is shown in Fig. 19-4 with hooks formed for the elastic strap. The right hook is closed to keep that end of the elastic permanently attached, while the left serves as a hook with light snapping action to retain the removable end. All hooks are formed inside-out so that they will neither impinge on the cheek nor catch on bedding as the patient sleeps.

The inner bow (or arch) is normally equipped with stops at the molar tubes to prevent contact with the incisors and direct all of the force to the molars. These stops may be bends in the wire, small sleeves welded in place, or snug-fitting closed-coil springs of suitable length slipped over the wire.

The inner bow is adjusted to the normal parting level of the lips with the appliance activated.

Vertical adjustments in the outer bow control tipping actions on the teeth. Figs. 19-3 and 19-5, *A*, show one configuration in which the molar crown is tipped distally. Raising the outer bow as in Fig. 19-5, *B*, reverses the tipping moment on the molar, so that the root is tipped distally.

Other extraoral appliances. The cervical appliance is only one of many extraoral devices, but it is very effective for most situations. When the problem requires an upward force, as in cases requiring apical movement of upper anterior teeth, a high-pull appliance may be used. These may be attached to the molars in the same way as the cervical appliance or to a heavy labial arch in the anterior region. With the latter appliance, forces are exerted almost directly along the axes of the upper incisor roots, so that the action is mostly apical, with comparatively little distal effect.

Horizontal-pull appliances eliminate the downward component of the cervical appliance. These are very useful where this result must be accomplished, but neither the horizontal-pull nor the high-pull appliance is as comfortable or convenient for most patients as the cervical appliance. The orthodontist should consider the possibility of this factor reducing the patient's cooperation when choosing the appliance for a particular patient.

Fig. 19-5 shows some of the effects of the direction of extraoral force on the resultant molar actions. These all show the bow attached at the molar.

When an extraoral appliance is attached in the anterior region, it is usually through a nonrigid connection that does not introduce an external tipping moment. The effect in these cases is that of a simple linear force applied at the point of attachment to the intraoral arch.

The junction between the inner and outer bows in the incisor region will move up or down as the appliance is activated by the elastic traction to effect a tipping action on the molars. This movement is a reliable indicator of the actual tipping effect.

Rising of the junction on activation is an indication of counterclockwise (as viewed from the right) rotation, with mesial tipping of the molar. This will place a distal vector on the molar root and a mesial vector on the crown, helping to keep the molar upright as it moves distally. A strong tipping action in this direction can actually cause the crown to move mesially in spite of the distal traction of the

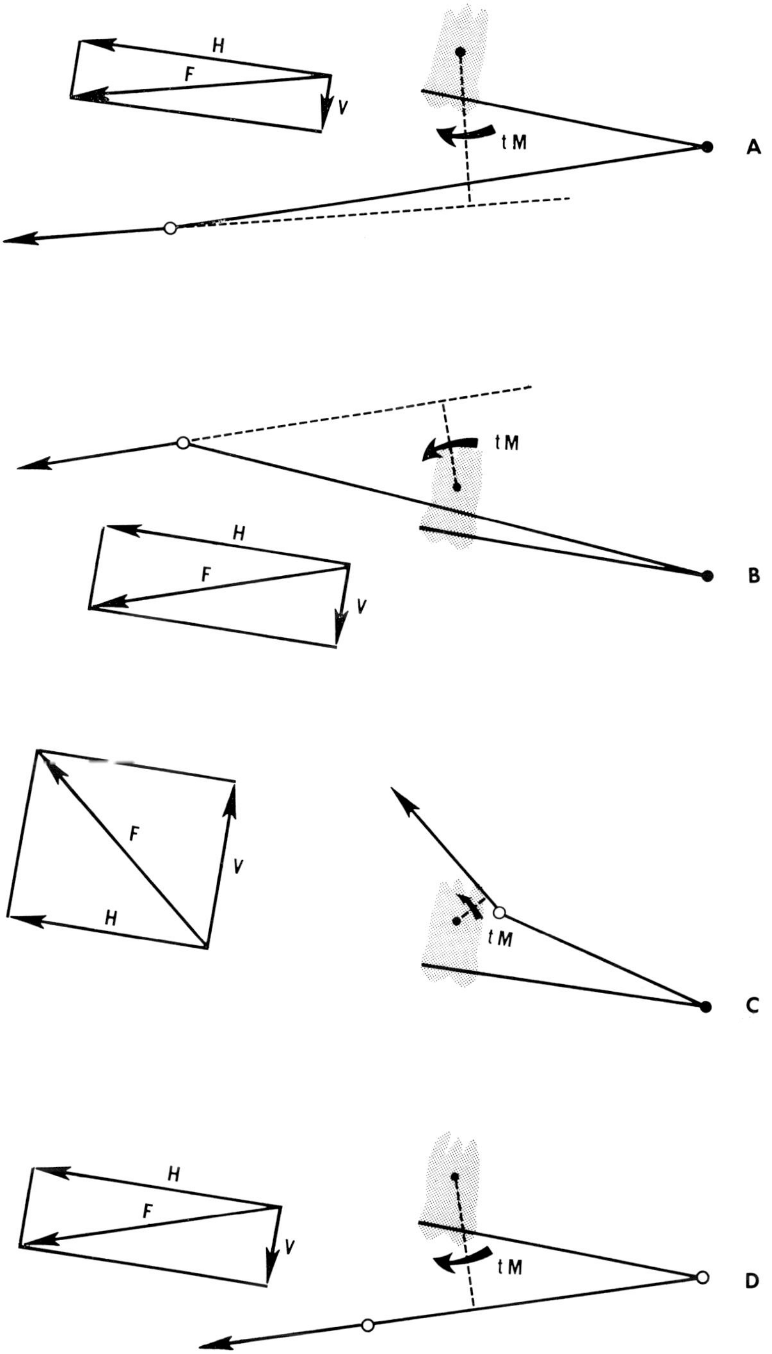

Fig. 19-5. Variations in extraoral forces on the first molar. Force diagrams are the same as in Fig. 19-3. Curved arrows, *tM*, represent the tipping moment on the molar (and maxilla). **A,** Rigid inner and outer bow, with outer bow low, will tip the molar crown distally. **B,** Raising the outer bow will apply a mesial tipping moment that combines with the distal vector to tip the molar roots distally. **C,** High pull headgear with shorter outer bow increases apical action with a reduction in distal action. Length of bow and exact direction of pull can alter the effect on the tooth from that shown here. **D,** Hinged outer bow, free to swivel where it is attached to the inner arch, gives no control over tipping except through changes in elastic position. "Stress-reducing" loops in the outer bow function in a similar way as limited hinges, reducing stress on the bow only insofar as they depreciate control over tipping. An exact force analysis can be made in any individual case by drawing diagrams as above on a tracing from a cephalometric radiograph made with the appliance in place *and activated.* Relationships before activation are unimportant except as they affect activated relationships.

elastic, although such extreme effects are more common with high-pull than with cervical traction.

Downward movement of the junction indicates a clockwise rotation at the molar, with a distal crown vector and a mesial root vector. This action maximizes distal crown movement at the cost of increasing distal tipping, which may or may not be desirable.

Tipping control can be the most critical adjustment in extraoral anchorage therapy, requiring close monitoring at every patient visit. Excessive tipping in either direction should be avoided, and most cases should be kept within relatively narrow limits.

Distal tipping provides rapid crown movement, sometimes accompanied by extrusion and bite opening. Mesial tipping (distal root movement) may be inhibited by an unerupted distal molar or lead to further impaction of that tooth. Any distal movement against a developing molar should be carefully evaluated and closely monitored.

Lateral adjustment of the inner bow. Lateral adjustment of the inner bow is important to keep upper and lower arch widths coordinated as treatment progresses. Molars moved distally will move into a wider part of the arch, requiring a steady but gradual expansion as treatment progresses. Relationships to adjoining and opposing teeth provide basic references, but the relationship between root and alveolar process should also be closely monitored.

Rotation control is also essential for good occlusal relationships. Every adjustment of arch width will have an effect on the molar rotation, and rotation adjustments will affect width. These effects must be checked with even the smallest adjustment, making compensatory adjustments in both actions as required, so that all movements will progress in concert toward the desired end result.

Lateral adjustment of the outer bow. Lateral adjustment of the outer bow is primarily for the patient's comfort, but it is also possible to exercise some control over the symmetry of action by this means. Normal adjustment of the outer bows should keep them close to the face or in very light contact. Adjusting the bow laterally on one side, so that the end of the elastic is held well away from the face, will increase the distal force on that side.[36] This can be helpful in the correction of asymmetrical mesiodistal discrepancies.

The cervical appliance should be worn approximately twelve hours every day, usually during the evening and night. Progress is possible but slow if it is worn only eight or nine hours.

The elastic should be adjusted to the highest tension that the patient can wear with comfort for the full period. Patients vary widely in this regard; many prefer the secure feeling of a very tight elastic, whereas others can tolerate very little tension. Progress, of course, is related to this tension, but a tension that awakens the patient during the night and leads to removal of the appliance will be less effective than a lighter tension that can be worn all night.

Alternate attachments. Extraoral appliances may be attached directly to the arch of the edgewise appliance instead of to the molar. This is often done with the high-pull appliance.

Several different devices can be used to engage extraoral appliances to the arch.

This configuration directs the vertical action to the anterior teeth, but it should not be applied to arches that are smaller than .018 inch (0.45 mm), or where the teeth on either side of the point of attachment are unbanded, without careful precautions concerning the bending effects on the arch. Extraoral forces can distort small arches or long spans and greatly alter arch form. This places an undesirable back-and-forth action on the teeth as the arch rebounds with the daily placement and removal of the outside force.

When to use extraoral appliances. Extraoral appliances may be used before the edgewise appliance, concurrently with it, after it, and sometimes instead of it. The decision concerning the use of this force depends on overall maxillofacial relationships and the complete orthodontic diagnosis, including growth potential.

These appliances can move upper molars and the complete upper denture distally. They can inhibit anterior growth of the maxilla and so bring it into a more harmonious relationship to the mandible. They can crowd and impact upper second or third molars. They can bring anterior teeth and lips into greatly improved relationships before the face and dentition have fully matured, producing a much more normal relationship of these structures than can be achieved by later orthodontic correction alone. All of these factors and others must be considered along with the purely local occlusal relationships.

ANTERIOR OVERBITE

The functional aspects of the overbite problem and their overriding importance in treatment have been discussed on pp. 116-119. Careful diagnostic evaluation is essential in these cases because of the very different directions that therapy may take. The following are all viable courses for correction, depending on individual needs.

Apical movement of upper incisors

Apical movement of upper incisors is one possible course. This is most commonly applicable where the central incisors have erupted well beyond the buccal occlusal plane of the upper arch, although apical movement of lateral incisors or cuspids may also be desirable in some cases.

This movement must be based on a determination of optimum functional level for the occlusal plane of the upper arch. Possible movement may be limited in some cases by inadequate height of the upper alveolar process. Cephalometric radiography provides the only reliable evaluation of this factor, by direct inspection of the relationship between the apices of the incisors and the nasal floor. Inadequate apical clearance is a contraindication for the apical movement of these teeth.

The method of choice for this movement is the "utility" type of bypassing arch, .016 to .018 inch (.4 to .45 mm), engaging the molars and the incisors to be moved. Where other leveling methods have left the occlusal plane tipped downward, a high-pull headgear may be used to augment the anterior intrusion. Apical movements are best accomplished with very light, continuous forces, so wherever possible the arch should provide the primary activation to these teeth, with the extraoral appliance used to control reactive effects such as molar tipping or extrusion.

Buccolingual tipping (torque control) is essential in all apical movements. A

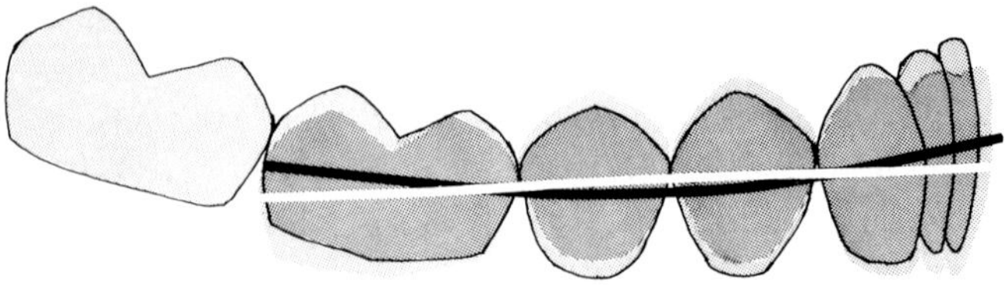

Fig. 19-6. Leveling the lower arch with archwire alone will intrude anterior teeth and molars while elevating bicuspids. When second molars are not controlled, this can seriously disrupt the contact relationship on first and second molars.

careful balance of lingual and apical vectors can accomplish this even with round wires. Where this type of control is not applied, it will be necessary to use torquing loops or rectangular wires, either in the course of the apical movement or as a separate finishing procedure.

Apical movement of lower anterior teeth

Apical movement of lower anterior teeth is required in a high percentage of cases, because these teeth frequently overerupt when their upper antagonists are displaced anteriorly.

This movement is accomplished in the same manner as that described for the upper teeth.

The major contraindications are uncommon but important. One is deficient total symphysis height, and the other is deficient alveolar height. The important consideration in alveolar height is the area of attached gingivae between the gingival margins and the muscle attachments at the reflection of the vestibule. Apical movement of teeth will reduce the height of the attached gingivae, so it should be limited to a range that leaves a sufficient area for protection of the gingival margins from negative periodontal effects of muscle action (Fig. 21-5). Where the problem is high muscle attachment rather than inadequate alveolar height, surgical gingivoplasty may be indicated.

Occlusal movement of buccal teeth

Occlusal movement of buccal teeth with a complete arch as shown in Fig. 19-6 is a common approach to overbite correction. The inevitable resultant mandibular opening is a major diagnostic consideration.

In deep bites, especially those with buccal tongue interference, molars may move apically with little anterior improvement. This will require banding of second molars or their occlusal control from a lingual arch or buccal auxiliary to add their vertical anchorage. Vertical vectors from intermaxillary elastics may help to maintain molar levels, but reciprocal occlusal vectors on upper anterior teeth often negate any desirable effects in deep overbite cases.

20

Orthodontic treatment is an exercise in ongoing diagnosis.

Coordination of intensive treatment

Orthodontic treatment is far more than a simple episode in the life of the ever-changing dentofacial complex. It is an intricate ballet, with infinite possibilities for choreographic variation.

In fixed appliance therapy, such as edgewise, the major occlusal corrections are accomplished in a coordinated intensive stage that brings the entire dentition into balance and harmony. Sequence and balance of the induced actions have far greater significance than merely determining when a certain effect will be elicited. They actually play a major role in determining *what* the treatment effects and ultimate results will be.

DENTAL ATTACHMENT UTILIZATION

Dental attachments provide direct mechanical control of individual teeth, but they are far from an unmixed blessing. They do not just introduce a *means* for control; they actually create a *need* for active therapeutic control.

Every engagement of an archwire in an attachment *requires* adjustment for all potential movements, *even if the only reason for the adjustments is to prevent the movements.*

Teeth will move wherever they are pushed, so the most dependable and physiologic way to prevent unwanted movements is to leave teeth free of attachments and consequent archwire influences whenever there is no clinical need for those influences. Crude systems that dictate immediate placement of attachments on all teeth impose constraints on tooth movements that can seriously compromise potential for some favorable movements as well as induce some undesirable side effects.

Most archwires should engage all teeth that are fitted with attachments. Bypassing individual attachments can be difficult, and it also introduces added flexibility into the archwire that can limit force distribution capabilities. Merely not ligating certain attachments that may be partially engaged by an archwire opens a risk of the wire slipping out of the slot and engaging other parts of the attachment, producing large unexpected tooth movements.

Auto-expansion

All appliances that use buccal attachments are prone to expansion. Even the most minute buccolingual clearance between a passive archwire and its seated po-

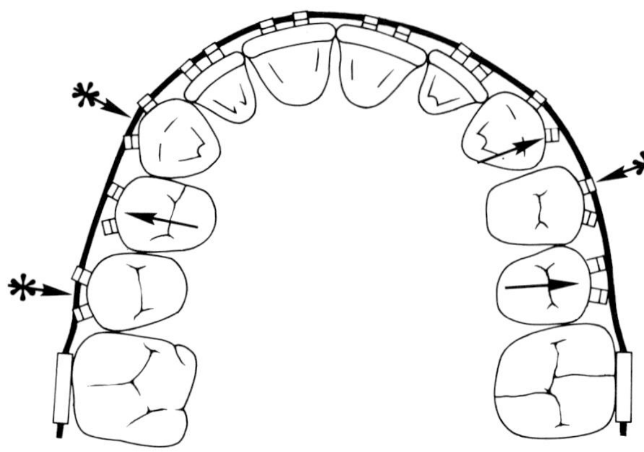

Fig. 20-1. All labial arches are expansion prone. Every minor discrepancy that leaves an arch short of seating in a bracket will induce labial movement on ligation. The arch above is seated in the brackets marked by the lingual arrows with asterisks. Even though the objective may be to move these teeth lingually, the ultimate effect of ligation will be to move the adjoining teeth labially.

sition will cause buccal movement of the affected tooth when it is fully seated. Anything short of unattainable absolute passivity will have such local expansion effects, and attempts to overcompensate will simply shift the effect to adjoining teeth (Fig. 20-1).

The cumulative effect of successive archwires, along with ligations and adjustments, is an insidious buccal and labial expansion of the arch. These small increments can add up to a major effect that may be desirable in some cases, unimportant in others, and disastrous in still others.

Such expansion is difficult if not impossible to reverse with a buccal arch. A moderately stiff full buccal arch is incapable of delivering force in a lingual direction in most situations. Most such efforts deliver equal or greater buccal vectors to other teeth. Arch constriction is practical only with lingual anchorage, which may be combined with a flexible buccal arch-shortening wire or ligation, or with a sectional arch for local action.

The advantage of prevention by assiduous attention to archwire fitting and adjustment is obvious. Prevention can be further enhanced by elimination of unneeded attachments; a tooth that is not attached to the archwire cannot be drawn buccally. Additional control derived from lingual arches and restriction of increases in arch length rounds out the preventive armamentarium.

Auto-extrusion

A similar effect also occurs in the vertical plane as archwires are engaged. Discrepancies between adjoining teeth tend toward resolution by extrusive movements rather than intrusive because of the ease with which teeth move in that direction. The net result is a raising of the bite and hinging open of the mandible.

Superflexible wires can produce great vertical effects in this way because of the vertical waves that are introduced into the archwire when it is engaged into the brackets of tipped teeth. Uprighting by this means is almost entirely the result of extrusion to a common level. Since these effects depend on archwire engagement in adjoining slots, they are most pronounced with large wires, which fit closely in the bracket slots.

Recovery from extrusion can be even more difficult than from expansion. Occlusal function will gradually return the mandible to its normal posture for those with good function, but patients with mouth breathing or inadequate musculature will tend to retain the altered mandibular posture.

Posttreatment functional recovery from therapeutic extrusion has a collateral bite-closing effect that should be closely watched in patients whose original malocclusion included a deep overbite.

Careful arch fitting and attention to *all* vertical adjustments from the start will also provide the best control in the vertical plane.

TREATMENT STAGES

Treatment progresses in a succession of stages. Initiation phases the various procedures into action, consolidation carries them through the major changes, and resolution wraps up the final details.

These stages merge together almost imperceptibly as the overall correction progresses to its consummation. The following outline covers the highlights of the many factors that must be considered in the management of that progress.

Initiation

The initial phase of treatment has two unique functions. One is initiating tooth movement, and the other is initiating the patient to tooth movement. Both of these require *gentle* forces.

The first aims of treatment will naturally govern the actual mechanism that is used. Some may not require immediate placement of fixed attachments. The following tabulation lists conditions requiring early attention, together with therapeutic possibilities:

A. Unfavorable trends, which could aggravate the orthodontic problem if not arrested
   1. *Space closure.* Space closure may occur in transitional dentitions where some permanent teeth are not fully erupted, or in extraction cases where space may be lost through mesial drift of posterior teeth.
      a. Removable space maintainer
      b. Lingual arch
      c. Bypassing arch, usually attached to molars and incisors; incisor alignment may be initiated with this arch
      d. Complete arch, if spaces are few and eruptions imminent
   2. *Trauma.* Trauma may result from teeth in a deep overbite occluding on soft tissue.
      a. Bypassing arch, molars to incisors (may include only offending anterior teeth in the beginning, to move those teeth apically)
      b. Acrylic bite plate (usually a temporary measure)

3. *Unfavorable growth patterns*
   a. Extraoral anchorage
   b. Functional appliance

B. Problems that may require an exceptionally long treatment time and so might prolong treatment if not begun early
   1. *Severe anteroposterior intermaxillary discrepancies*
      a. Extraoral anchorage
      b. Intermaxillary elastic traction

      Preliminary alignment and progression to sufficiently heavy arches may be required first
   2. *Growth problems*
      a. May need control throughout remaining growth period; early intervention enables optimum improvement
   3. *Severely tipped teeth* (especially lower molars)
      a. Usually require special auxiliaries, with much of the remainder of the arch serving as anchorage

C. Corrections requiring long retention; early completion of these corrections will initiate the tissue adaptations of the retention phase while the balance of the treatment is being completed
   1. *Severe rotations.* Method and timing of these corrections often depends on requirements of other aspects of the problem.
      a. Space opening is often the first requirement
      b. Loops, usually paired
      c. Coil springs or elastic traction
      d. Elastic ligatures, where arch engagement is possible
   2. *Large spaces*
      a. A sectional arch may be used, especially when only incisors are involved; a sectional arch that is not perfectly straight requires some provision to prevent rolling in this application
      b. Loops used on a sectional arch are best positioned distal to the teeth to avoid tipping effects (Fig. 20-2); these can also provide antirolling action
      c. Elastic ligatures. Great care is required to achieve a free-sliding fit in combination with adequate control over rolling
   3. *Overbite.* This is usually related to function, so the earliest possible correction gives the best assurance of stability. There is no one certain approach to correction, but there are several possibilities. Some of these have been discussed on pp. 285 and 286.
      a. Complete arch; reducing an overbite by leveling the curve of Spee of the entire arch, as in Fig. 19-6, will elevate the bicuspid area at the same time that molars and incisors are moved apically; the occlusal movements can be expected to greatly exceed the apical, with resultant opening of the mandible
      b. A bypassing ("utility") type arch, using a distal tipping moment on the molars to produce an apical vector on the incisors, can move teeth

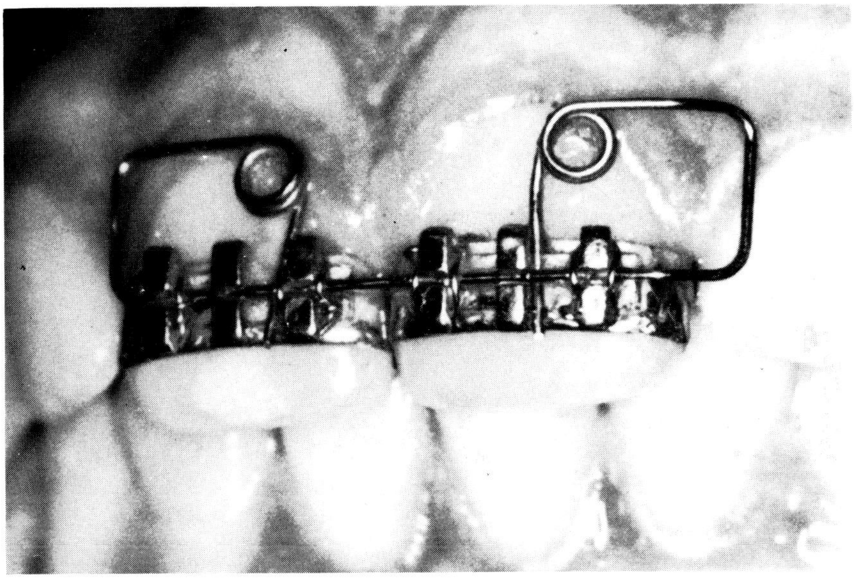

Fig. 20-2. A sectional arch that has been used to close space between two teeth. The working arms also serve to prevent rolling of the archwire. This is especially well suited for triple brackets because it can often be reactivated for a large space by merely shifting one working arm from the mesial to the middle bracket as the teeth move, as has been done in this case.

apically with varying degrees of actual molar tipping as a reciprocal effect

c. Bite plates are heavily dependent on functional and cooperation considerations for success, making case selection an important factor; these are most useful in the developing occlusion
d. A partial plastic positioner, engaging only the offending teeth with an apical action, can have an effect similar to a bite plate, with the added advantage of a lingual flange that keeps the tongue clear of the buccal occlusal surface; the major disadvantage is that it cannot be worn full-time

4. *Elimination of arch loops.* Arch loops can reduce stiffness in critical areas, and elastic traction and other forces can place collateral loads on teeth that will distort archwires without sufficient arch stiffness to maintain arch form, curve of Spee, and individual tooth position. Rotations or other movements requiring loops in these areas must be completed before such traction is applied. The same is true with highly flexible wires.
5. *Tipping and rotation adjustments* for anchorage control. For example, Class II elastic traction will subject lower molars to strong mesial tipping and rotation moments. Teeth tipped or rotated in these directions should be corrected, and some distal tipping may be desirable in advance of elastic traction.

6. *Crossbite correction* may be a part of some of the earlier considerations, but in any event it should be accomplished early. Many other tooth and arch relationships are affected by crossbite and by its correction so correction should often be accomplished before final assessment and correction of related irregularities.
7. *Removal of interferences* before movements are undertaken. Deep overbites, whether of the entire anterior segment or only between two teeth on one side, can block a Class II or other corrective effort so that only the "anchor" teeth move.

   Opposing teeth or their attachments may also block individual tooth movements such as space closure or rotation, so sometimes all that may be required will be temporary removal of an offending band.

Coordinating the initiation. The previous outline covers a broad range of possible procedures. The object is to accomplish those that may be pertinent to an individual patient as quickly as possible, with simultaneous action as a desirable objective.

The end of this phase should find all crowding eliminated, rotations corrected, continuous arches in place, and remaining corrections underway.

The first full arch is usually the most flexible arch that will be used during the course of treatment. It should be the smallest in diameter, and ordinarily it includes any required loops. This arch brings all teeth well on their way to proper alignment, level, and rotation. It should be kept in place and adjusted as necessary until gross corrections within the arch are completed.

If the first arch has many loops, the next arch may be of the same wire size but with many or all of the loops eliminated.

It is especially important to combine actions that aid one another. A simple example is rotating a tooth with an elastic ligature so as to close a space simultaneously.

A more complex example is the combination of a cuspid retracting section with an interrupted arch for apical movement of incisors as soon as adequate incisor space is available.

Fig. 20-3 shows the major actions in this combination, with each of the simultaneous elements shown separately for clarity.

The primary gain is the balancing of the mesial tipping moment of the cuspid retraction on the molar by the distal tipping moment incurred by the incisor action. The anterior apical vector from both of these actions will be divided between cuspids and incisors, as determined by the adjustments of the various segments. The occlusal vector on the molar will be the sum of the effects of all of the arches, so it will be higher than if the two actions were carried out separately; the significance of this effect must be established for each case.

Where overbite is a severe problem, it may be desirable to move the incisors apically and then maintain them there as cuspids are moved apically.

Lingual arches are especially useful in the first phase to normalize molar orientations and to guard against asymmetrical reactive forces from the many local corrections. The cuspid-incisor corrections just discussed are a case in point, with large countermoments required on the molars. Lingual arches are no protection against

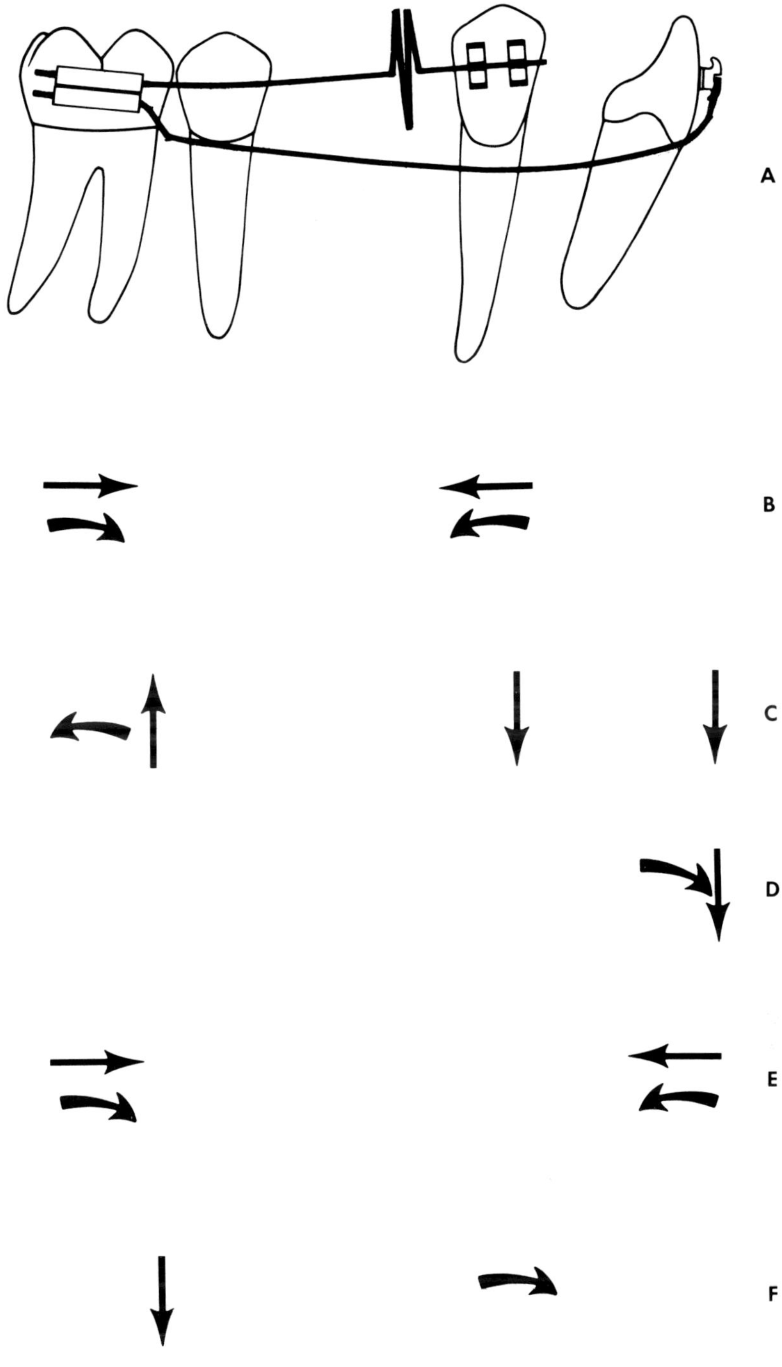

Fig. 20-3. Primary effect operating with a combination of cuspid-retracting section and interrupted arch intruding lower incisors. **A,** Schematic view of the working components of the appliance. The loops between cuspid and molar indicate a closing action, not an appliance component. **B,** The cuspid retractor applies a distal vector to the cuspid and a reciprocal mesial vector to the molar, with collateral tipping moments on each. **C,** Apical actions on cuspid and incisor place both an occlusal vector and a distal tipping moment on the molar. **D,** The apical incisor vector, applied to the labial bracket, also applies a labial tipping moment to that tooth. This is a buccal tipping moment in the case of the cuspid. **E,** A lingual vector applied to the incisor by elastic or archwire traction will provide a lingual tipping moment to counter the action in **D.** This will apply an opposite vector and moment to the molar. **F,** A mesial tipping (uprighting) moment applied to the cuspid will apply an apical vector to the molar. The timing and balance of these various actions will determine the ultimate net movement of the individual teeth.

mismanagement, but they will equalize the mesiodistal tipping effects and facilitate balancing anterior vertical relationships between the two sides.

Space closure in extraction cases is usually initiated early in this stage, but *only* to the extent required to relieve crowding or to begin intermaxillary corrections. *Space closure should not be regarded as an objective of treatment until all related corrections are complete.* The reason for therapeutic extractions is to gain space, and care must be taken to distribute the gained space to areas of need as soon as possible.

Consolidation

The consolidation phase is a relatively quiet period, where treatment settles down to a steady progression as the long-term aspects of the problem are corrected. Individual arches are already aligned, with space closure and intermaxillary corrections possibly incomplete.

This is a time for taking stock, monitoring progress, and evaluating changes in relation to the original plan. Changes with extraoral traction, intermaxillary corrections, overbite, and mandibular posture all require regular evaluation not only for their therapeutic effects but also for possible mechanical or functional interferences with those actions.

The final phase checklist should be reviewed periodically as treatment progresses through this stage to identify any problems that may need special attention.

Arch succession. Steps in size between succeeding arches will vary, but ordinarily each arch should be at least .002 inch (.05 mm) larger than the previous one. Greater increases in size may be made at one time, but care must be taken not to try to advance in size too rapidly. If an arch must be adjusted considerably to make it fit discrepancies between teeth, it may be more efficient to use an intermediate wire of a smaller size.

With rare exceptions, each successive arch should be fully engaged in all brackets. If discrepancies between teeth make this difficult, the archwire is probably too heavy and will require too many adjustments to bring the teeth into line.

Remaining intermaxillary corrections and detailed correction of torque are completed with the final arches. This point may be reached with any size arch, but the case that "needs everything," including torque adjustments, will usually require rectangular wires for the final finishing. Spaces should be essentially closed before rectangular arches are placed.

Some cases may require a long succession of arches, but most will not. Many cases can be completed with round archwires, and others can be advanced to larger sizes in big steps. Each case must be advanced according to its own requirements, and no arch should be placed merely because it appears in some arbitrary treatment schedule.

Anterior torque should be watched carefully in all phases. There should be few severe problems of this type if vertical forces, with their buccolingual collateral effects, are carefully controlled. Many torque control problems can result from inattention in the course of other movements.

Rectangular arches. If earlier round arches have been used effectively, the rectangular arches that give the edgewise appliance its name will be the simplest of all. By this time all teeth should be in essentially correct alignment with adjacent teeth. Little should remain to be done in correcting levels, mesiodistal tipping, axial rotations, or spaces, all of which can usually be more effectively accomplished with round wires.

The diameter of the round archwire immediately preceding a rectangular arch should be within .002 inch (.05 mm) of the bracket slot width, so that fitting the rectangular wire to the bracket slots should present no great problem or excessive force.

Heavy archwires may be used to adjust arch form and torque (buccolingual inclinations) of groups of teeth, usually entire segments. They may also be used to stabilize an arch while mesiodistal arch relations are corrected by elastics or other means.

Arch formation with any of these wires follows the principles outlined in Chapter 14. *First,* the wire is formed to the desired arch form. *Second,* levels are adjusted to match bracket levels where necessary. *Third,* torque is adjusted until the wire can be placed in the mouth in an essentially passive state. *Fourth,* active adjustments are introduced where required for tooth movement. For torquing movements this can be gauged by the change in relationship of the torquing instruments as the bend is made and then further verified by insertion in the tube or bracket in question.

There will always be some freedom of fit between a wire and the bracket or tube, requiring some overadjustment for torquing action. This is easily judged by a trial insertion in the individual attachment, noting the resultant tipping effect on the position of the remainder of the arch.

These wires should go to place easily with finger pressure or a light twisting with a small torquing key to align torqued surfaces with the slot. Large changes in tooth inclination require repeated adjustments.

Hooks. Hooks for intermaxillary elastics may be soldered to the archwires, or slip-on, crimp-on hooks may be added. Free-sliding hooks will place the entire elastic force on the tooth distal to the hook. Crimping hooks to the wire to prevent sliding will place the elastic force on the wire in the same way as soldered hooks. Ligature wires may also be used to tie teeth together or to the hooks to control the distribution of force.

Space closure. Space closure is best completed before placing a rectangular wire, but it is still possible at this stage. Small spaces may be closed with elastic ligatures or with the arch tiebacks described in the next paragraph. Larger spaces can be closed with loops bent into the wire.

Spurs may be soldered to the arch slightly mesial to the molar tubes. Wire or elastic ligatures tying them to the molar tube will have an arch-contracting effect for minor space closure and to hold spaces closed throughout the arch. These same effects may be accomplished with elastic ligatures, preferably applied individually, between adjoining teeth.

Adjustment intervals. The minimum interval between orthodontic adjustments should rarely be less than three weeks. The supporting tissues require time to respond adequately to adjustments. A good normal working interval is four weeks, with a latitude of one week more or less. Deviations from this schedule are made as required for unusual situations.

Many adjustments will work for longer periods; nevertheless, the orthodontist should usually see the patient monthly to check for loose ligatures, bent wires, etc. When a light arch has been well adjusted, it can work for two months or more without major adjustments, and it should not be disturbed unnecessarily before its work has been completed. It is much more desirable to make careful and complete adjustments that will work for long intervals than to make frequent, less coordinated alterations.

Final resolution

Consolidation merges almost imperceptibly into the final resolution stage, as gross movements are accomplished and only fine details remain to be corrected. Ideally, everything should fall into place at about the same time as the treatment is completed, but there are many individual small details that must be checked as that time approaches.

Standardized preangulated and preformed appliance components do *not* reduce the need for such evaluations; they do in fact tend to *increase* that need. All of the following details should be watched closely throughout treatment, and reliance on average angulations can give a false sense of security leading to serious deficiencies in the final stages.

Average values are for statisticians, not clinicians. The statistician can be satisfied with central tendencies, but the patients treated by the clinician are the individual variants who make up those averages, and each must be treated to his or her own personal norm for each variable.

The following checklist includes the most common corrections that should be accomplished in addition to the more obvious overall relationships.

1. Rotations
    a. In the buccal segments, bicuspid and molar rotations should be adjusted for optimum interdigitation. Molars are especially critical, and they should be rotated and stabilized early in treatment whenever possible.
    b. Incisor rotations are usually obvious, but the subtle interrelationships of lateral incisor and cuspid rotations can be especially elusive as well as important. These should be coordinated so that their contact tends toward parallelism with the distal cuspid contact rather than that between the central and lateral incisor (Fig. 20-4). This relationship depends on the rotations of both teeth, but the cuspid is especially critical because of its common tendency to rotate distally. Failure to accomplish these rotations can increase the possibility of later unfavorable changes in this area.
2. Levels
    a. Cuspids should not interfere with functional movements at this stage; cuspid levels should be a reflection of function, not a restriction of function. These teeth will very easily drop into elongated positions where function permits, but they will not retract into the alveolar process after treatment

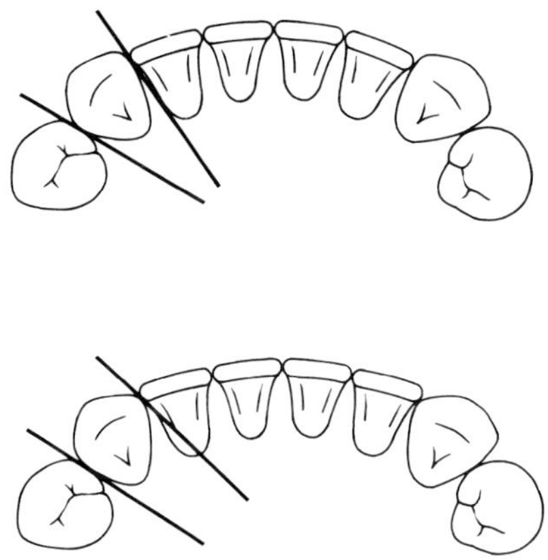

Fig. 20-4. The incisor-cuspid contact point can be especially critical in maintaining incisor alignment in both treated and untreated occlusions as intercuspid width diminishes with age. When the orientation of this contact converges with that of the distal contact as in the upper illustration, such movement will cause incisor crowding. When these contacts tend toward parallelism (below) or diverge lingually, the cuspid can slip behind the lateral with much less disruption of incisor alignment.

for the patient whose optimum functional pattern requires more freedom in lateral excursion.

b. Central incisors are easily left in elongated positions, in an exaggeration of the subtle offset between lateral and central incisors. Where required, they can be moved apically with a .018-inch (.45-mm) bypassing archwire engaging only these teeth and the molars.

c. Lateral incisors should be harmoniously upright in relation to the adjoining teeth, with no labial flare or elongation.

3. Torque, or buccolingual tipping. Central incisors are most frequently in need of this attention, and a cephalometric radiograph provides exact information for control. Careful consideration should be given to the position of the root in the alveolar process, as well as to raw angular measurements. Cuspids may also require lingual movement in some cases, especially when their initial eruption was either buccal or lingual.
4. Second and third molars. Second molar levels, as they relate to the first molars, can be an important factor in later occlusal function. It is not unusual for a lower molar to overerupt due to retarded eruption of the upper molar, and distal tipping of a lower molar can accentuate this discrepancy. Crowding and retarded eruption may also cause buccal or lingual crossbite of the terminal molars. When required, lower molars can be intruded and levels controlled by extensions from a lingual arch adjusted to engage the central fossae.
5. Arch form. This is a continuing consideration throughout treatment, so it

should require little attention at the end. Fine coordination of upper and lower arch form is essential as the active phase is finished.

6. Intermaxillary relationships
   a. Cuspid interdigitation is one of the most important criteria in establishing final intermaxillary relations, so incisor and molar occlusion cannot be judged without considering their relationships to the interdigitation of the upper cuspid with the lower cuspid-bicuspid contact.
   b. Molars must sometimes be "overcorrected," with the mesiobuccal cusp of the upper lying distal to the buccal groove of the lower in order to attain good cuspid occlusion. Molar rotations are very important in these relationships.
   c. Incisor overjet and overbite must be balanced with each other as well as with the buccal occlusion and any discrepancies between maxillary and mandibular tooth size.

21

The return to a natural environment

Finishing and "retention"

To the patient, the removal of fixed appliances marks the end of treatment, but it actually marks the beginning of the most critical phase of the orthodontic experience.

In many ways the patient is correct in regarding this point as a terminus. After an extended period tolerating a conspicuous and not always comfortable collection of foreign objects in the mouth, the teeth are unencumbered once again. After a lifetime during which the malocclusion has been the norm, *for the first time* an essentially normal dental relationship is experienced. Quite literally, this is the long-awaited day.

On the sobering side, this is also the time when the patient must be reminded of the problems and treatment that remain, with special emphasis on continuing responsibilities. The major considerations at this stage are listed below, in layman's terms that can be used as guides for patient orientation. Not all of these will apply to every case, and situations not covered here will surely arise from time to time, but at least some of these will ordinarily apply to most cases.

> Several changes must take place after appliances are removed. The first of these is the closing of the spaces between the teeth that were occupied by the bands. One set of bands on ten teeth in one arch (upper or lower) will occupy at least .088 inch (2.2 mm).
>
> Teeth will move wherever they are pushed, *at any age*. What makes them stay in one place is a balance between all of the different little pushes that go on constantly day and night.
>
> The normal forces acting on the teeth are chewing and other biting actions, plus the moving and resting pressures of the tongue and the lips. Together these forces push the teeth in many directions, but they normally balance one another.
>
> The lips and cheeks restrain the teeth from the outside and the tongue occupies the inside, working together to mold the teeth into a gentle curve from one side of the mouth to the other. If one pushes harder than the other, the teeth will move away from that strong push until it tapers off and the opposite, balancing force increases enough to equal it.
>
> Orthodontic forces are only a very temporary influence among all of the many forces in the mouth. We push the teeth with appliances for a few years at most, but you (the patient) will be pushing them all your life. This is why we must plan our work carefully to place the teeth where the normal functional forces can be in a balance that will provide stability after our appliances are removed.
>
> When the positions of the teeth before treatment have been involved in an imbalance of the supporting musculature (tongue and lips), it takes a long time for those muscles to

become accustomed to their new and more normal positions after correction. They may remain somewhat tense or too relaxed for years, making it necessary for us to give the teeth some added support in their new positions until the muscles can take over completely.

The muscles cannot adjust to orthodontic correction until after the teeth have been moved, so the end of the major tooth movement is really just the beginning of change for the musculature.

Soft tissues (gums) surrounding the teeth are very elastic, and they do not adjust to tooth movement as rapidly as bone does. When there have been great changes between adjacent teeth (as in rotations), the gums will behave much like rubber, tending to go back to their old shape and take the teeth along with them. In these circumstances the teeth must be held in the corrected positions until the tissues have had time to readjust.

Your face will continue to grow for some time yet, and that growth can make new changes in the way that the teeth fit together. That kind of change is a part of living, and it goes on with everyone.

FINAL PHASES OF ORTHODONTIC CHANGE

The changes and problems that arise after the most active (usually multiple attachment) phase of orthodontic treatment fall roughly into three groups.

Phase one changes are those occurring in the first few weeks, largely as a result of band and archwire removal. These are the favorable changes of band space closure and "settling" of the occlusion as the teeth respond to normal function unencumbered by the fixed orthodontic appliances.

Phase two changes are the succeeding changes, possibly unfavorable, in response to residual tissue tensions and unbalanced functional relationships. Although these tendencies are strongest in the first few months following treatment, they may persist for a year or two and may even continue into phase three. These are usually controlled with judicious use of finishing appliances.

Phase three changes are those due to posttreatment growth or to persistent habits or dysfunctions with lifetime effects. These are the problems that are unrelated to prior orthodontic treatment, and some may not be amenable to correction.

MECHANICAL INTERVENTION

The need for mechanical intervention following active treatment varies through all conceivable possibilities.

It has sometimes been said that a well-treated orthodontic case needs no retention, but this is only half true. There is no denying that good orthodontic treatment is a prime requisite for stability without retention, but *this alone is not enough.* An excellent anatomic relationship between maxilla and mandible, a favorable growth pattern, and a normal functional environment (good function with no undesirable oral habits) are equally important to the success of such a laissez-faire program; and to this we must add that treatment must have accomplished all substantial changes between adjacent teeth sufficiently early and in such a manner that the relapsing influence of the gingival tissues is no longer a serious factor after treatment.

In other words, only the case in which *all present and future orthodontic problems* have been solved by the initial treatment will be stable without additional help, and not all of our problems are of such a simple nature.

A more typical case requires from a few weeks to a few years of supplemental therapy to guide and maintain tooth positions, while exceptional cases at the opposite extreme require either indefinite continuation of control or acceptance of some degree of later irregularity.

Specific finishing procedures will be discussed in detail under the earliest phase of treatment in which they will ordinarily be applied.

FIRST PHASE (IMMEDIATE POSTTREATMENT ADJUSTMENT)

The most immediate problem after appliance removal is the closure of band spaces and "settling" of the occlusion. This is a short period requiring a careful balance between freedom and control over the spontaneous changes that can result in a marked improvement of occlusion.

Records

The occlusion at or near the time of appliance removal should be recorded in plaster casts regardless of the finishing procedures that are used. This point marks the beginning of a new orthodontic problem and treatment, and adequate records are just as essential as at the start of original treatment.

If phase one is expected to proceed favorably without intervention, these impressions may be postponed about a month so that the casts will represent a more stable relationship.

Cephalometric records should also be made at or near this time. If the last progress films were made near the end of active treatment, they need not be repeated at appliance removal.

No appliance

Band spaces will normally close spontaneously within a few days, and most cases are well served by a period of 1 to 2 weeks without rigid appliances. Flexible positioners may be placed immediately at the time of appliance removal.

If extraction space closure was not achieved until shortly before appliance removal, there will be a strong tendency for these spaces to reopen as other band spaces close; the teeth literally migrate together by moving away from the extraction site. Extreme rotations and other unusual conditions may also benefit from early control.

Progressive band removal

One means of controlling the closing of band spaces is the progressive removal of bands. Bands are removed from some of the teeth, and the arch may be tied back or retracted with elastics to close spaces. Only a few days are required to effect such space closure, and care must be taken not to constrict the arch excessively or permit relapse of unbanded teeth.

Bands should be retained during this stage on teeth that have been extremely rotated or otherwise grossly displaced. Sectional arches may be used to maintain control over incisor rotations or inclination of individual teeth.

If maintaining extraction space closure is expected to present a problem, all bands except those adjacent to the spaces may be removed first. These teeth may then be tied together, using a passive sectional arch on just the two teeth on either side of the space. Unless this sectional arch can be perfectly straight, it is essential to prevent it from rotating in the bracket slots, to avoid unfavorable tipping. This control may be attained by using a carefully fitted rectangular wire.

Elastic positioner

The elastic positioner is a very useful type of finishing appliance. It can be inserted during phase one or later and continued for all or part of the remainder of treatment.

Setup. The positioner is processed over a setup made by cutting the teeth from a set of plaster casts and repositioning them in wax to optimum relationships.

The entire success of the positioner hinges on the setup. The following points merit special attention:

1. A positioner is not a substitute for good primary correction. Any attempt to make large corrections with a positioner will prevent it from seating properly and lead to almost certain failure.
2. Incisor angulations cannot be altered greatly in most cases, but significant changes are possible under optimum conditions. These teeth are best set up with only subtle changes to refine positions already achieved.
3. Cuspid levels and intercuspid widths are extremely important in establishing the final stabilized occlusion. Special care should be taken to avoid elongating cuspids or expanding widths.
4. All molars should be included in the positioner whenever possible. It is especially important to include molars to control eruption when the opposing tooth is still unerupted.

Occlusal plane and overbite. Most cases will respond very favorably with a positioner made to an average bite opening and occlusal plane relationship. Problem cases with exceptional overbite problems, unusual occlusal plane angles, or temporomandibular joint symptoms require special handling in establishing jaw relationships.

Casts mounted on an articulator can be opened the required amount to establish the desired relationship in the positioner. Orientation in the articulator may be established with a facebow or by the following cephalometric technique that I developed.

In the range of jaw opening between centric and rest, the movement is normally a hinge action at the condyle. The condyle center can be assumed to be the center of rotation of the mandible, or a hinge axis may be established by other means.

The axis is marked as a dot on a cephalometric tracing, and a line drawn from that point to the incisal edge of the upper central incisor. The upper occlusal plane is drawn as determined by first molar cusps and central incisor edge (Fig. 21-1).

Only two figures are needed to use this diagram to orient the upper cast in an articulator: (1) the axis-incisor line length and (2) the angle between the axis-incisor line and the occlusal plane.

This orientation reproduces the natural relationships of the teeth to the joint and to the closing stroke of the mandible, so opening the articulator on that hinge will maintain proper relationship in the resulting positioner.

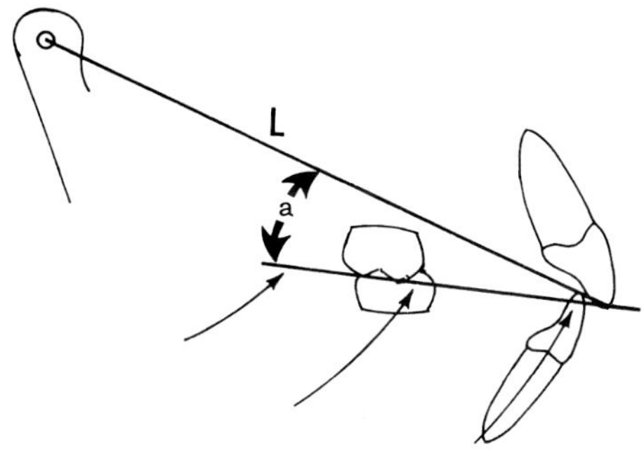

Fig. 21-1. Working dental relationships as they appear on a cephalometric tracing. Hinge axis has been arbitrarily selected at the center of the condoyle, which is essentially correct for the final closure. Orienting an upper cast on an articulator with the incisor the same distance, *L*, from the axis and with the same angle, *a*, of occlusal plane, will reproduce this relationship. Lower teeth all move in an arc centered at the axis, so the curved arrows represent actual direction of movement in closure. Note the large mesial component in movement of buccal teeth, which will place mesial forces on upper teeth and distal forces on lower teeth as they occlude.

The desired amount of opening at the incisors in the finished positioner completes the specifications. This should normally not exceed the freeway space.

For maximum accuracy the axis-incisor length can be corrected for cephalometric enlargement. With a 12-cm subject-to-film distance at a 5-foot target distance, this enlargement is 7.9%, which means that the measurement from the film must be reduced by about 7 mm in the usual case.

The line drawn from hinge axis to the incisor or *to any other functioning occlusal contact* lies perpendicular to the direction of the occlusal stroke at closure. This can also be a valuable diagnostic guide in considering the relationships between function and tooth inclinations, although it is not included in the popular cephalometric analyses.

Cooperation. The key to success with a positioner, as with other removable appliances, is patient cooperation. The problem of obtaining adequate cooperation should not be underestimated, but it is not significantly greater with positioners than with other removable auxiliaries. Careful preparation of the patient can help considerably in gaining understanding and cooperation.

Before positioner therapy is planned, the patient's ability to breathe through the nose must be verified. Those with an inadequate airway must be treated with a single-arch positioner or none at all. Habitual mouth breathers with an adequate nasal airway can benefit greatly from this appliance, but cooperation problems are much greater with this group.

Questioning the patient about breathing leads into an early explanation of the positioner and the reasons for its use. Emphasis is placed on the positive points such as possible earlier band removal, the fact that no appliances are worn away from home, and the relatively short period of use (when this is anticipated). Comparison to the athletic mouth guard, emphasizing the difference in function and precision, is also helpful in preparing the patient.

Demonstration positioners are not suggested at this time because the experience of wearing one is usually less of a problem for the patient than might be anticipated from a preview without actual insertion.

Bands are not removed until after this preliminary discussion. If contraindications to positioner finishing are discovered at this time, there is still an opportunity for changes in treatment before appliances are removed.

Appliance removal. All attachments are normally removed at one time and two sets of plaster casts made immediately, one for the setup and one for reference. A cephalometric record may also be made at this time in cases in which a recent film is not already available.

Casts from an earlier date may also be used for the setup, with the positioner prepared for insertion immediately at the time of appliance removal.

Initiating positioner therapy. The positioner is placed any time from the day of appliance removal to about two weeks later. Only cases in which unusual stability problems are anticipated require rapid placement.

Proper placement of the positioner can be checked visually by asking the patient to bite firmly while the buccal flanges are retracted with a blunt instrument such as the plugger used for band seating. Clear plastic positioners greatly facilitate this inspection.

If the teeth do not seat properly in the positioner by simply closing on it, effective placement can usually be accomplished by firmly seating it on the upper molars with the thumbs while the anterior flange barely engages the incisors. Thumbs are then rolled to the buccal flanges, holding the positioner firmly in place while the teeth are closed into it. This will stretch it evenly around the arch with each tooth in its proper recess.

When the positioner is inserted, the patient is instructed to wear it a minimum of two hours daily but as near to four hours as possible—plus sleeping hours. Total time can be three or four times longer if it is worn for only sleeping hours.

The patient is also advised that it may not stay in during the night at first but that the most important time in the beginning is the period during waking hours, when active exercise by biting firmly into the positioner can keep it in place. This is required to stretch the material into its best working position. Passive wearing during early stages will have comparatively little effect. As the teeth move to their corrected positions, they will fit the positioner more easily and nighttime retention will improve. At this stage the daytime schedule can be reduced or eliminated.

The patient should expect to feel pressure on the teeth quite similar to that experienced with earlier appliances. This is pointed out at the trial placement in the office. Care should be taken to insert it in such a way that this same sensation is felt each time the positioner is worn.

The positioner is tightest at this first wearing, and the tightness should diminish rapidly as the teeth approach the desired positions. The patient is advised that this reduction in tightness is the best indication of progress, and failure to notice a change almost on a day-to-day basis is an indication that it must be worn longer and more actively each day.

Tapering off. As the positioner achieves a loose fit and the teeth show good relationships, the schedule is reduced to sleeping hours only (or to one or two waking hours if it does not stay in at night).

The next step in reduction, a few weeks or months later, is to three nights weekly. This schedule is easier to maintain than alternate nights because the appliance is always worn on the same days of the week. Under this schedule, there will be a two-day lapse once each week, and patients are instructed to note any changes in sensation following this longer interval.

Final stages are based on the same considerations that govern all finishing appliances. These will be discussed under the third phase.

Partial positioner. The maintenance of overbite reduction and anterior alignment present two major retention problems, and these do not require a complete positioner. Anterior engagement alone will provide active control in the critical segments. A lingual flange in the buccal segments adds control over buccal tongue position, keeps it out of the interocclusal space, and helps keep the appliance oriented in the mouth.

After the first phase adjustments, buccal flanges and posterior occlusal areas of the positioner can be removed, leaving only the anterior section and posterior lingual flanges.

Premolded units of this type may also be used, with appropriate adjustments for central and lateral incisor levels and gingival clearance. In selecting such a unit, size should be based strictly on arch curvature. It is important that this radius not be larger than that of the dental arch. Excessive anterior radius will tend to widen the upper arch more than the lower, with attendant incisor and cuspid overjet problems.

Many cases can be controlled with this stock premolded miniature positioner from the beginning, with the added advantage of immediate availability for insertion at the time of band removal. With the lack of buccal occlusal engagement, these are ordinarily worn with the jaws relaxed, without the active biting usually prescribed with a full positioner. It is otherwise used in the same way.

Occlusal adjustment (equilibration)

Occlusal interferences may be removed by judicious shaping of the teeth at any stage of treatment, but the first and second phases of posttreatment adjustment are especially opportune times.

Occlusal adjustment for an orthodontic patient is not the same as for a person whose occlusion has been stable for some time. The following considerations are especially important:

1. Occlusal adjustment is not a substitute for orthodontic treatment. Careful correction can minimize the need for removal of tooth structure.
2. Moving teeth creates a need for adjustment to compensate for the natural wear that did not occur due to the original malocclusion. Teeth heavily "worn in" in one relationship can be expected to present interferences when rearranged.
3. Esthetic shaping of anterior teeth can be a valuable supplementary service, along with purely functional equilibration.
4. Do not rush into equilibration. Adjust slowly, in easy stages, correcting only the most severe interferences at first. Normal phase two adjustments can substantially reduce the need for equilibration.

SECOND PHASE (SHORT-TERM CHANGES)

After band spaces are closed and the teeth have reached a more settled occlusion, several problems may still remain. Phase three problems may also appear at this stage, but the discussion here will be limited to those peculiar to this period.

Rotations were discussed in Chapter 11. This phase of posttreatment adjustment finds some gingival fibers still under tension, tending to return the teeth toward their original positions. This tendency has been shown to persist for longer than a year, and clinical experience indicates that it can continue for a much longer time.

Evaluation of these posttreatment rotation responses requires careful differentiation from the effects of arch form and crowding changes that may induce rotations as a secondary effect.

Spaces may also tend to reopen after treatment under the influence of soft tissue, in this case the compression of intervening tissues. Extraction sites present a unique situation in that two interdental papillae must merge into one before a normal condition is attained.

A space originally occupied by a large labial frenum presents a retention problem for a different reason. Regardless of whether the redundant frenum tissue is surgically removed, transseptal periodontal fibers will be absent in these cases. It follows that these teeth are deprived of a normal aid to the maintenance of a tight contact, so these cases always require prolonged retention with close attention to the maintenance of contacts of adjacent teeth. Unclosed spaces distal to the affected teeth show a strong tendency to close at the expense of reopening of the sagittal space.

Crowding as an early retention problem is often closely related to changes in arch form during treatment, and these in turn depend largely on the original diagnosis and treatment plan.

Individual patients cannot be fitted to average norms, but numerous posttreatment studies have shown a remarkable tendency for lower cuspids to return to their original intercuspid width.[20,21] This is the case in both extraction and nonextraction treatment. Extraction is an effective means for reducing the need for cuspid expansion, but it offers no protection from the penalties of expansion. On the other hand, some cases demand the calculated risk of cuspid expansion, especially those with large discrepancies between maxillary and mandibular widths. Ultimate success in these cases depends on adaptation of the musculature to the alterations, which in turn depends highly on age.

Mechanical retention of expanded intercuspid width is almost always indicated, but it must be recognized that later relapse will still be a significant possibility. Extreme care is required to avoid holding cuspids in a position that compromises alveolar support.

Buccal crossbites inevitably require some change or arch form for correction. Some will be stable as soon as normal relationships are established. Others, such as dentitions with well-worn cusps, severe asymmetries, bilateral problems with large differences in maxillary and mandibular widths, and abnormal tongue or respiratory function, may become serious long-term problems.

Mouth breathing is a common cause of crossbite and crossbite relapse. Mouth breathing after early childhood may be a mere continuation of a past habit, but patency of the nasopharyngeal airway should always be checked. A lateral cephalometric radiograph will show tonsils and adenoids and resulting displacements of tongue and soft palate.

The best prognosis for crossbite correction lies with early treatment to restore normal function and tongue space. Crossbites should be corrected and normal mandibular function established before any attempt is made to evaluate concurrent space or intermaxillary problems.

Patients coming in too late for this optimum two-stage approach must of necessity be limited to a single course of treatment, with due regard for the greater incidence of posttreatment difficulties. Those who have completed all growth with a severe bilateral crossbite and the tongue held low in the mandible are a *poor risk* for long-term stability of crossbite correction, requiring long retention of maxillary width.

Anterior crossbites are usually self-retaining with a normal overbite. The only notable exception is phase three mandibular growth.

An *overbite,* specifically incisor overbite, can be a complex and difficult problem both in treatment and in retention. (See Chapters 12 and 19.) The basic cause of the overbite is the most important factor in all stages of treatment, and ease of correction is usually a fair guide to the gravity of the retention problem.

An overbite originating as a secondary effect of a Class II relation, with no accompanying tongue habits, will usually present few problems in retention. It is the severe overbite that accompanies lateral tongue thrust or other muscular dysfunctions that will require intensive effort in treatment and retention, with sometimes disappointing results.

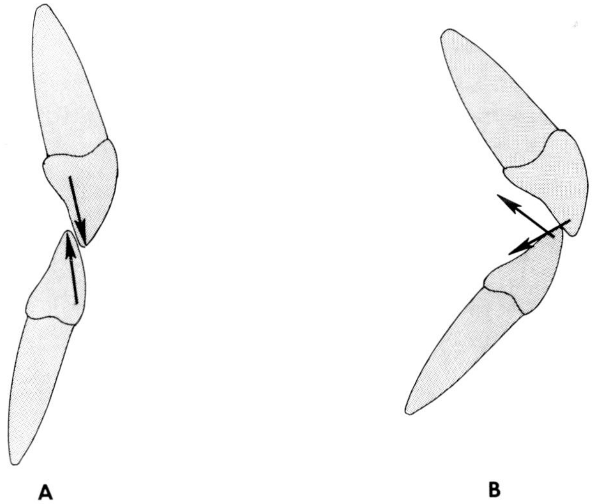

Fig. 21-2. A, Incisors with vertical inclination may tend to erupt past the normal overbite relationship. **B,** Excessive labial inclination may lead to later lingual tipping with accompanying overbite increase as shown by arrows.

All overbites must be treated to obtain as nearly normal incisor angulation as possible, often requiring torque control of both upper and lower incisors. Excessively vertical incisors will tend to bypass into a deeper overbite. Incisors tipped too far forward will tend to relapse with lingual movement of lower incisors, accompanied by increased overbite (Fig. 21-2).

Class II malocclusions are seldom an exclusively phase two retention problem. Favorable cases will remain essentially as corrected, with no problem in phase two. Patients showing a relapse tendency in phase two are usually suffering from abnormal growth or function, and long-term problems can be expected.

Second phase treatment

Hawley retainer. The classical Hawley appliance with its many variations is the most common appliace for this stage. Because it is constructed of rigid acrylic and wires, this appliance is best initiated after initial settling and space closure.

The Hawley device is made of acrylic adapted to the palate or to the lingual surfaces of the lower teeth and adjacent tissues, with an auxiliary wire to apply control on the labial surfaces of the incisors.

As a passive retainer, the labial wire can lie across the labial surfaces of the incisors, passing through the embrasure between lateral incisors and cuspids to be embedded in the acrylic. Other variations may be made as required by the demands of the case (Fig. 21-3).

A very useful variation is shown in Fig. 21-3, *C*. This appliance uses hooks lying over the lateral incisors with extensions over the cuspids. They can be adjusted as required for each of these teeth, and a light elastic can be attached between the two hooks to provide a lingual force on the central incisors.

Clasps are generally unnecessary on palatal appliances. Retention of these nearly passive appliances is adequate without them, and the elimination of clasps also eliminates the orthodontic pressures that they can exert on the attachment teeth.

Lower appliances are usually made with a lingual reinforcing wire that ends in lingual molar rests for added strength and stability (Fig. 13-11).

Bite planes (Fig. 21-4) may also be incorporated into the Hawley type of appliance as a control for overbite. Maintaining an overbite in this way is not enough to ensure stability later; unless other dental or functional relationships are normalized, overbite will inevitably increase following removal of such an appliance.

The most useful application of the bite plane is after a deep overbite correction that was accomplished initially with some degree of elevation of the buccal teeth (bite opening). A mandible thus opened will tend to gradually return to its original posture, once again "closing the bite," so incisor overbite must be controlled during this stage if overbite relapse is to be avoided.

Applications. The Hawley appliance is used primarily to maintain individual tooth alignment or to make small changes in that alignment. It can be used alone as a supplement to the rubber positioner or other appliances. An upper Hawley retainer may also be used in combination with different lower appliances such as the cemented lingual wire.

This appliance will not selectively stabilize only desirable relationships, so care is required that it does not hold minor discrepancies that might overwise settle toward improved positions. Changes in arch width in particular will be restricted by the dental margins of the acrylic, so occlusal relations with opposing teeth should be watched carefully during this period and the appliance relieved or replaced as required.

Small tendencies toward incisor procumbency may be controlled with the Hawley appliance, but it is not effective where growth or muscle habits introduce a

A

B

C

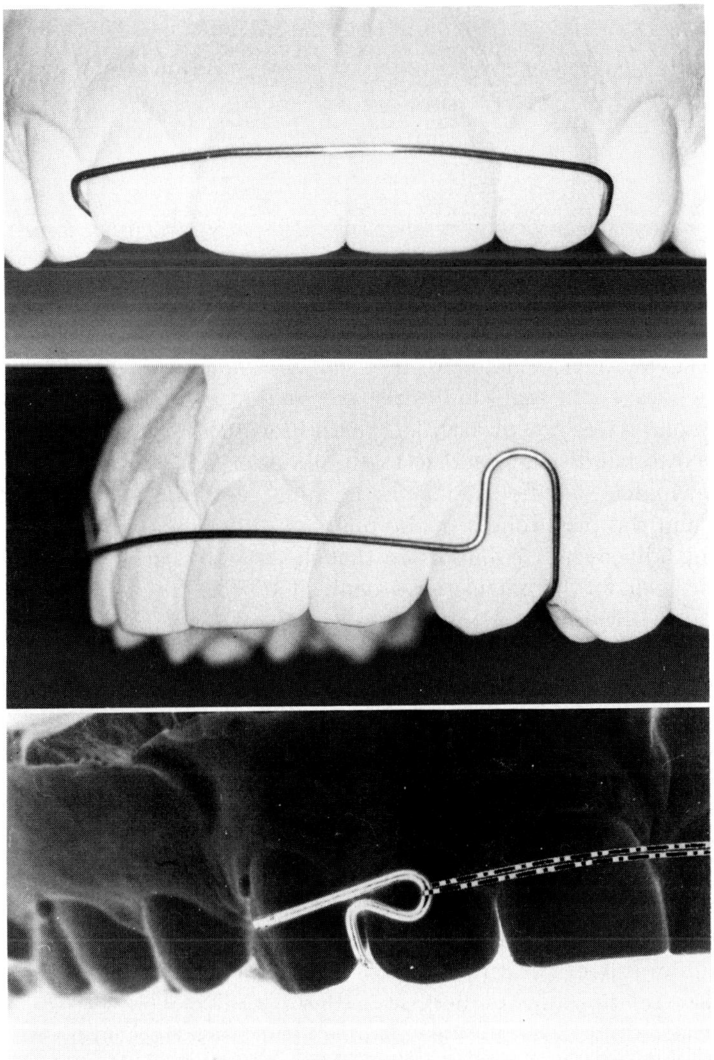

Fig. 21-3. Popular forms of labial wire for Hawley type of retainer. **A,** Conventional wire. **B,** Modified form with adjustable loop. **C,** Hooks for attachment of a light labial elastic. The hook also can be adjusted for selective action on cuspid or lateral incisor.

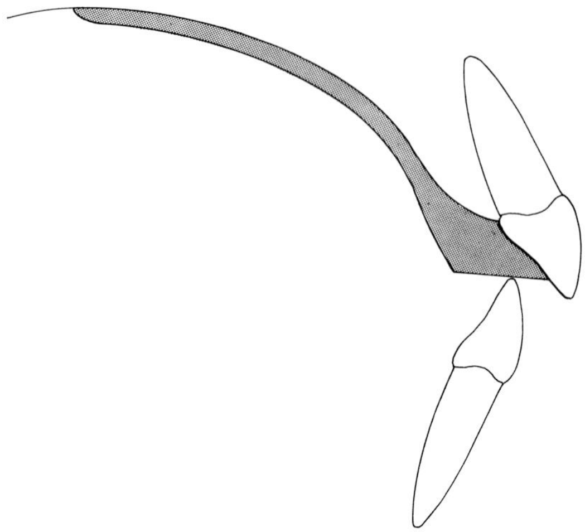

Fig. 21-4. Cross-sectional view of a bite plane. This may take many forms, with various levels and inclinations of the surface engaged by the lower anterior teeth.

strong protousive tendency. Such forces can carry the entire maxillary denture mesially, the Hawley device included; they call for much stronger action, such as the extraoral anchorage discussed under phase three.

Fixed lingual wire. Lower arch length and form can be maintained by a lingual wire soldered to bands cemented to teeth on either side. Lateral incisors, cuspids, bicuspids, or molars may be used as the terminal teeth, depending on the demands of the case and the preferences of the operator. These wires may also be attached with bonding adhesive. It is important that the wire be carefully contoured to passively touch each tooth that is to be controlled. The lingual wire is most useful where original crowding and rotations were severe, requiring retention well into phase three.

Fixed retainers have no corrective capabilities, and they inhibit favorable as well as unfavorable changes. This makes it essential that teeth controlled by fixed retainers be in precisely correct position before the appliance is placed.

Appropriate cuspid width, inclination, and rotation are all critical and variable, requiring extreme care when they are fixed in their relationships by a retainer. Cuspids that have not been adequately rotated, as described in 1b on p. 296, or that are too widely separated for muscular balance, can have a built-in relapse potential that will be expressed even after prolonged retention.

Retention of lower lateral incisors can be a most effective alternative in many cases. This is an especially attractive choice with "invisible" lingual bonding. Maintaining incisor relationships without impeding cuspid movement has important advantages. The conspicuous incisor relationship is preserved while cuspids remain free to seek their own functional balance. This provides early stability and protects the alveolar bone from excessive labial pressure.

Mucogingival surgery. Not strictly a retention procedure, such surgery may be needed before, during, or after other treatment. In the lower incisor area some

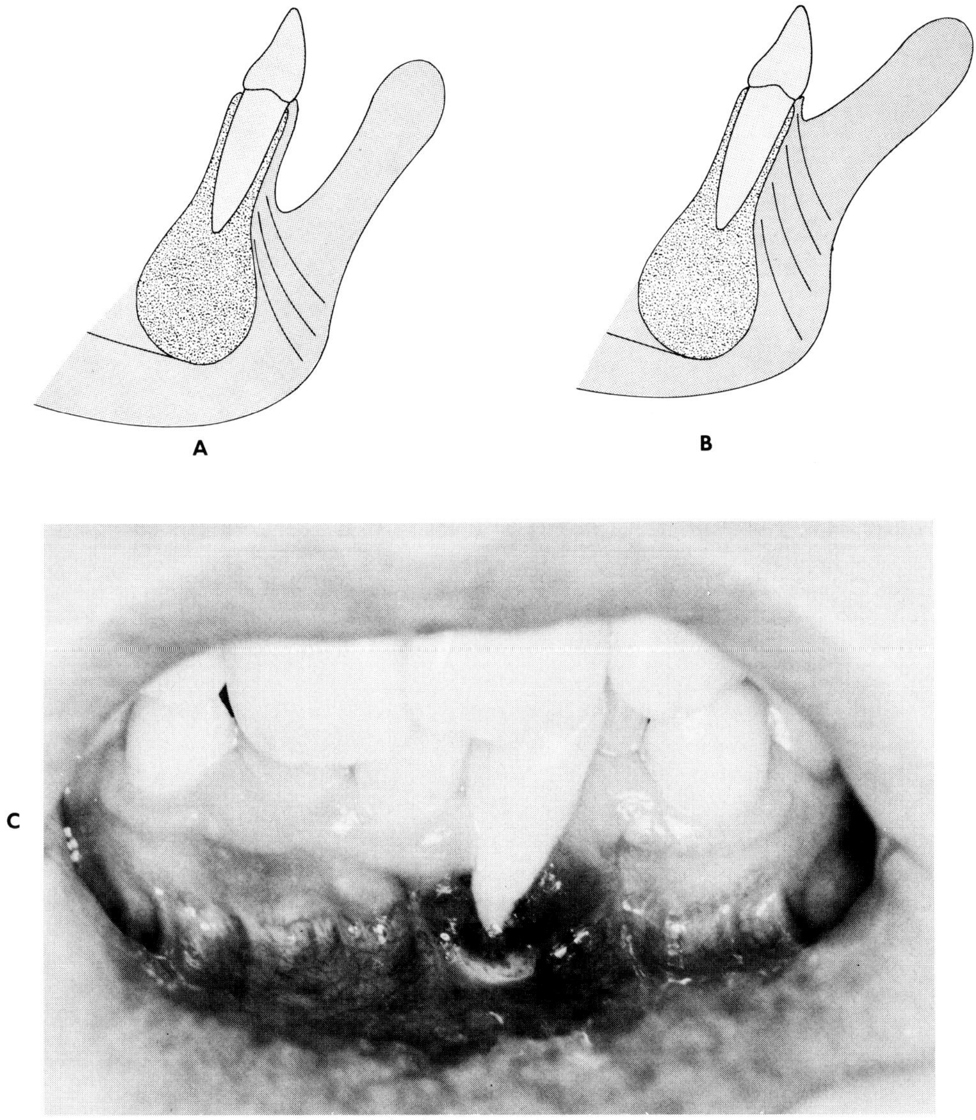

Fig. 21-5. A, Normal mentalis attachment, low on the incisor with an adequate area of attached gingivae. **B,** High mentalis attachment with little or no attached gingivae, as demonstrated by pulling lip outward. **C,** Severe gingival response to muscle action in a 9-year-old child. The lower incisor crowding and labial position of the affected tooth are the immediate precipitating causes of the aggravation of this problem, but the underlying cause is the high muscle attachment. This reaction did not occur until the gingivae had recessed to the level of the muscle attachment, thus losing the protective action of the attached gingivae. This photograph shows the lip pulled outward to demonstrate the attachment level (note tensed fibers in cuspid areas and darker color below attached gingivae). Vertical alveolar growth may advance the attached gingivae and alleviate the problem in some of these cases, but the gain is often temporary.

fibers of the mentalis muscle may extend high into the gingivae, sometimes all the way into the margin. If the soft tissue reflects directly from the gingival margin with no attached gingivae to maintain its integrity, the result will be a marked marginal recession (Fig. 21-5).

The contraction of the mentalis in this situation literally pulls the gingivae down and away from the tooth. Only surgical lowering of the vestibule and mentalis attachment, with reestablishment of an adequate area of attached gingivae, can prevent progressive gingival recession.

The diagnosis can be verified in such a case by grasping the lip and pulling it up and away from the teeth. Lack of effective attached gingivae will be immediately established by a virtual disappearance of the vestibule, as soft tissues reflect almost directly from the gingival margin. Further verification can be obtained by pulling downward on the lip and noting movement of the gingival margin.

This condition is usually accompanied by a hyperactive mentalis that is often present with a Class II malocclusion. Excessive lip pressure then combines with the muscle attachment in the overall deleterious effect on the gingival tissues. Similar problems may also arise in buccal vestibular muscle attachment areas.

THIRD PHASE (LONG-TERM CHANGES)

The third phase is the period beginning roughly one to three years after intensive therapy, when only the extreme problems remain to plague the orthodontist and the patient.

Problems at this stage are often incurable but can usually benefit from careful management. These problems generally fall into one of three classifications: (1) residual treatment problems, (2) growth, or (3) function (including habits). In all of these situations, retention through phase two is directed toward supplementing the environmental factors until they have adapted to the corrected occlusion. The normally functional case achieves this adjustment.

The more refractory case goes into phase three, and symptoms of this trend will usually arise early. The time to institute phase three measures is when the need is first established, not after some arbitrary lapse of time.

Residual treatment problems. Residual problems may be the result of an overoptimistic diagnosis, incomplete treatment, or progressive growth changes. All may entail many ramifications.

A common missed diagnosis is that which leads to excessive expansion in an effort to accommodate all of the teeth. Extraction is no cure-all, and there are some very good indications for expansion, but as a routine procedure it will incur a high rate of relapse. Treatment of borderline space conditions without extraction must recognize this calculated risk, including the prospect of some crowding in the ultimate resolution.

Indefinite retention of arch expansion is usually unwarranted, because it subjects the periodontal structures to excessive stress. Marginal problems may be improved by extraoral traction or terminal molar extractions or both, but the only alternatives in the more severe situations are either acceptance of some degree of crowding or retreatment with extraction. The crowding may well be the most physiologic alternative.

Other diagnostic problems revolve around unanticipated growth changes or habits. These problems can arise in any individual, whether orthodontic patient or not. They are actually whole new problems that must be evaluated on their own merits, but the orthodontist who has undertaken the management of an occlusion must nevertheless follow through with appropriate measures.

Incomplete treatment is of course a possibility in any type of correction, but it is most frequently seen in the incomplete correction of a Class II relationship. Failure of the patient to consistently wear elastics or extraoral appliances can effectively sabotage the best-planned therapy, and unless new motivation can be called forth later, there is little hope for further improvement during retention. The best course is usually continued extraoral traction with a second course of treatment if indicated.

Extreme habits, usually of tongue or lips or both, can become so severe that mechanical appliances cannot counter them in closing open bites or other spaces. Some of these are caused by anatomic problems that lie far beyond dentofacial orthopedic or other correction. Here again all possible measures should be taken during treatment, and if these fail the best that can usually be hoped for later is to maintain the partial correction.

Management of these problems can be summed up in the admonition to do everything possible while the appliances are still in place; correction will never be more feasible unless they are replaced later, but retention procedures can still help to maintain those gains that have been achieved.

Growth changes. The changes in growth that cause problems after treatment are mostly those that increase maxillomandibular discrepancies.

Class II problems with a skeletal imbalance are the result of the patient's individual growth pattern. Correction is a process of paddling upstream against the growth tendency, and it is folly to rest on our oars and not expect to be carried along by the stream. Growth will not carry such a case back to its original relationship; the gains of treatment can be held, but the need can continue to increase until growth ceases. This is *not* an argument against early treatment in these severe cases, because they are the ones that need it most. The point is that treatment must be continued until the total problem is expressed and corrected. A developing problem needs ongoing control.

Such extreme cases are fortunately a minority. Most Class II problems include a large functional component, and final correction is achieved near enough to the completion of growth that later changes are easily controlled.

In Class II cases with a poor growth pattern it may be necessary to continue extraoral anchorage until growth ceases. A Hawley appliance will not hold a maxillary denture in place if the entire maxillomandibular relationship is changing.

A *Class III* relationship developing or increasing after treatment presents a more unusual but also a more difficult problem. The mandible is normally the last of the facial bones to stop growing, and excessive growth in these later stages can produce a Class III relationship too severe for orthodontic correction. Placing teeth into occlusion in these cases requires such extreme tipping of anterior teeth that the esthetic and sometimes the functional result offers little improvement. Surgical osteotomy of the mandible is the only satisfactory solution.

These extreme Class III relationships may be a continuation of a pattern established early in life or they may not develop until puberty or later. In the present state of orthodontic diagnosis it is impossible to predict the course of such growth with reasonable certainty; there is no substitute for careful observation including periodic cephalometric evaluation until growth is complete.

Lower incisor crowding is a milder but much more prevalent effect of late mandibular growth. Continuing mandibular growth pushes these lower teeth forward against the lingual surfaces of the upper incisors. If the restraining musculature of the lips prevents concurrent forward migration of the upper teeth, the lower teeth will literally "pile up" behind the enveloping upper teeth.

This condition arises at about the same age that the third molars normally erupt, so circumstantial evidence obviously implicates third mold "pressure." On the other hand, similar effects are seen with the congenital absence of third molars—and of course with and without prior orthodontic treatment. Present knowledge of mandibular growth points to another source for this problem, although it is still partially related to the third molars.

As the mandible grows forward, the mandibular denture migrates upward and distally (Fig. 12-7). This has been observed cephalometrically for years, but until Björk's implant studies[23] there was some question whether this was actual distal migration or merely growth at the chin. The prodigious mandibular growth at this stage requires comparable distal migration of the denture on the mandible, and impacted third molars need only impede that distal migration (even without actual mesial force) to contribute to anterior crowding.

Molar eruption lies in a twilight zone between treatment and growth problems. Treatment is usually completed before all molars have erupted. Crowding and other factors can retard eruption, and if normal timing is disturbed, there is a strong likelihood that some of these teeth will erupt past the occlusal plane for want of an antagonist. A removable appliance can usually be used to prevent such excessive eruption and maintain the correct occlusal level until the opposing tooth erupts.

Functional aberrations. Irregularities in function include a multitude of situations, such as bruxism, tongue thrust, and lip biting. Identification of these deleterious activities is usually much easier than their cure. These largely unconscious habits are seldom amenable to dental measures alone, and most retraining efforts meet with limited success at best.

The patient should by all means be advised of the nature of such a problem and assisted as much as possible in mastering it. Dental measures can be of great help in relieving the deleterious effects in most cases if the habits themselves cannot be eliminated.

Third phase treatment

Therapeutic emphasis during this often extended period tends to shift from cure to control of the effects of aberrant growth or deleterious oral habits. These are the same services that may be required for any adult with the same problems, regardless of prior orthodontic therapy.

As a general rule, indefinite "retention" is not a satisfactory procedure. Long-term holding with appliances is not a reasonable substitute for adequate diagnosis or treatment, and the perpetuation of an unbalanced relationship can place excessive stress on supporting tissues. Whenever possible these cases should either be retreated in light of the new situation or otherwise guided into the optimum attainable *functionally stable* relationship, even if it entails some dental irregularity.

Extraoral anchorage is the appliance of choice to control continuing Class II tendencies. This type of therapy is discussed in Chapter 19, and nothing need be added here except to note that it is also possible to combine it with an elastic positioner by embedding the facebow in the positioner or embedding it in a similar fashion in rigid acrylic.[37]

During this period the primary purpose of extraoral anchorage is to counter any continuing growth discrepancies until the time that growth is completed.

A *bruxism guard* is the same as a single-arch positioner except that it is made to fit the unaltered cast instead of a setup. Worn at night, it protects the teeth from the excessive wear of nocturnal bruxism. It can be made for either upper or lower arch, and it will need periodic replacement due to wear.

A *vestibular shield,* made to fit in the vestibule around both arches, is occasionally of value to curb mouth breathing or lower lip habits. Fitting rather loosely in the vestibule, the flexible material effectively seals off the oral airway and deflects lower lip pressure from the lower anterior teeth. It can be constructed to fit loosely or closely over the dental casts, which may be modified as in a setup if indicated.

Exact conformation depends on the specific problem, bearing in mind that the teeth will be in rest position most of the time. This device is most useful in nocturnal habit control; it is definitely not a full-time appliance.

All *other* finishing appliances may be continued into this stage on a limited basis where indicated, but few cases require such an extended schedule.

Mandibular osteotomy as a treatment for extreme prognathism is accomplished in the late teens or later, after mandibular growth is complete. In some cases the excessive growth may not occur until long after intensive orthodontic therapy has been completed. Osteotomy is actually a completely new treatment, a cooperative orthodontic and surgical effort that will not be detailed here.

Molar extractions may often be indicated at this stage. Impacted lower third molars are a hazard to the second molars, and it is often the orthodontist's responsibility to recommend their removal for this reason as well as because of the possible role of these teeth in lower incisor crowding.

Impacted upper third molars usually lie extremely close to the roots of the second molars, often leading to later periodontal disease in that area. When these third molars are well developed, removal of either second or third molars may be the treatment of choice. Third molars will normally erupt rapidly after second molar extractions, with a healthy periodontium. Unless the third molar eruption is rapid, lower molar levels must be maintained as described below.

Molar level retention when eruption of opposing teeth is retarded can usually be accomplished with modified Hawley type appliances. These need not have labial wires, but they must have occlusal rests on the molars to be maintained. The distal marginal ridge or lingual fissure are usually the best locations for this rest, which can be an extension of the lingual reinforcing wire in lower appliances.

An alternate method is to place the appliance in the opposing arch, supplying an acrylic occlusal surface at the site of the unerupted tooth. This must be relieved as the new tooth erupts, so it is usually best suited for the early stages of retention where it can be incorporated into another appliance.

FINALE

As a group these phase three problems can generally be characterized as the small minority of cases that cause the majority of vexations to patients and orthodontists alike. They have often been described as orthodontic failures, but this should rarely be the actual case with adequate diagnosis and treatment.

The distinction lies in the real cause of the individual problems. Overoptimistic orthodontic efforts undertaken without adequate information and planning can result in a high percentage of diagnostic and treatment problems in this phase, but in competent hands most phase three problems will be the result of uncontrollable growth and functional aberrations unrelated to the orthodontic therapy.

As noted earlier, it is essential that these problems receive proper orthodontic care in spite of their discouraging aspects, even when they arise after the correction of the original malocclusion for which the patient first sought orthodontic help. The final decision for any treatment remains with the patient, but the orthodontist should be alert to recognize, diagnose, and advise in adult conditions as well as early developmental problems.

No one appreciates the complexities of the development of occlusion more than the practicing orthodontist, and this appreciation continues to grow with experience. Orthodontic service should not begin and end with a "one-shot" installation and management of some mechanical device. Its real value lies in the comprehensive integration of diagnosis and treatment for effective management of the occlusion through the *entire* period of development—and later, if necessary.

It is unfortunate that not everyone can have a perfect occlusion, but it is fortunate that almost everyone can have a *better* occlusion. Perfection for all is unattainable in *any* part of the body, but in dentistry, and in orthodontics in particular, we are working in what is probably the area most amenable of all to effective improvement.

With careful work we can bring all our patients as close as possible to their own individual potential for the attainment of optimum oral health, whether they be in the fortunate majority who require little or no posttreatment care, or one of the unfortunate few whose problems increase with time.

References

The following references provide basic background information for a well-rounded view of therapy utilizing the edgewise and other full-control mechanisms. Variations in application details based on these principles may be found in endless variety in orthodontic journals and supplier literature.

PART I

1. Jensen, A.: Applied strength of materials, New York, 1957, McGraw-Hill Book Co.
2. Davis, H.E., Troxell, G.E., and Wiskocil, C.T.: The testing and inspection of engineering materials, New York, 1955, McGraw-Hill Book Co.
3. Gillett, H.W.: The behavior of engineering metals, New York, 1951, John Wiley & Sons, Inc.
4. Godfrey, D.E.R.: Theoretical elasticity and plasticity for engineers, London, 1959, Thames & Hudson, Ltd.
5. The making, shaping, and treating of steel, Pittsburgh, 1957, United States Steel Corp.
6. Manual on fatigue testing, Philadelphia, 1949, American Society for Testing Materials.
7. Jefferson, T.B., and Brooking W.J.: Introduction to mechanical design, New York, 1951, The Ronald Press Co.
8. Holden, A.: The nature of solids, New York, 1965, Columbia University Press.

8a. Andreasen, G.F., and Morrow, R.E.: Laboratory and clinical analyses of nitinol wire, Am. J. Orthod. **73**:142-151, 1978.

8b. Burstone, C.J., and Goldberg, A.J.: Beta titanium: a new orthodontic alloy, Am. J. Orthod. **77**:121-132, 1980.

8c. Kusy, R.P. and Greenberg, A.R.: Influence of composition and configuration on the elastic properties of orthodontic wires, Angle Orthod., vol. 51, 1981.

PART II

9. Boyle, P.E.: In Kronfeld, R., editor: Histopathology of the teeth and their surrounding structures, Philadelphia, 1949, Lea & Febiger, pp. 361-365.
10. Bien, S.M.: Fluid dynamic mechanisms which regulate tooth movements, Adv. Oral Biol. **2**:173-199, 1966.
11. Thurow, R.C.: The periodontal membrane in function, Angle Orthod. **15**:18-29, 52-66, 1945.
12. Sicher, H.: The periodontal ligament. In Kraus, B.S., and Reidel, R.A., editors: Vistas in orthodontics, Philadelphia, 1962, Lea & Febiger, pp. 63-68.
13. Zwarych, P.D., and Quigley, M.B.: The intermediate plexus of the periodontal ligament, J. Dent. Res. **44**:383-391, 1965.
14. Gross, J.: Collagen, Sci. Amer. **204**:121-130, 1961.
15. Utley, R.K.: The activity of alveolar bone incident to orthodontic movement as studied by oxytetracycline-induced fluorescence, Am. J. Orthod. **54**:167-201, 1968.
16. Angle, E.H.: The latest and best in orthodontic mechanism, Dental Cosmos **71**:165, 168, 263-265, 1929.

17. Reitan, K.: Bone formation and resorption during reversed tooth movement. In Kraus, B.S., and Reidel, R.A., editors: Vistas in orthodontics, Philadelphia, 1962, Lea & Febiger, pp. 69-84.
18. Reitan, K.: Some factors determining the evaluation of forces in orthodontics, Am. J. Orthod. **43**:32-45, 1957.
19. Angle, E.H.: Malocclusion of the teeth, Philadelphia, 1907, S.S. White Dental Mfg. Co.
20. Strang, R.H.W.: The fallacy of denture expansion as a treatment procedure, Angle Orthod. **19**:12-22, 1949.
21. Steadman, S.R.: Changes of intermolar and intercuspid distances following orthodontic treatment, Angle Orthod. **31**:207-215, 1961.
22. Moorrees, C.F.A.: The dentition of the growing child, Cambridge, Mass., 1959, Harvard University Press.
23. Björk, A.: Variations in the growth pattern of the human mandible: longitudinal radiographic study by the implant method, J. Dent. Res. **42**:400-411, 1963.
24. Enlow, D.H.: The human face, New York, 1968, Harper & Row, Publishers, Inc.
25. Brader, A.C.: Differential orthodontic diagnosis and treatment planning, Am. J. Orthod. **51**:806-815, 1965.
26. Ricketts, R.M., Bench, R.W., and Hilgers, J. J.: An overview of computerized cephalometrics, Am. J. Orthod. **61**:1-28, 1972.

PART III

27. Haas, A.J.: Rapid expansion of the maxillary dental arch and nasal cavity by opening the midpalatal suture, Angle Orthod. **31**:73-90, 1961.

27a. Haas, A.J.: The treatment of maxillary deficiency by opening the midpalatal suture, Angle Orthod. **35**:200-217, 1965.

28. Angle, E.H.: The latest and best in orthodontic mechanism, Dental Cosmos **70**:1143-1158, 1928.
29. Angle, E.H.: The latest and best in orthodontic mechanism, Dental Cosmos **71**:164-174, 1929.
30. Angle, E.H.: The latest and best in orthodontic mechanism, Dental Cosmos **71**:260-270, 1929.
31. Angle, E.H.: The latest and best in orthodontic mechanism, Dental Cosmos **71**:409-421, 1929.
32. Tweed, C.H.: The application of the principles of the edgewise arch in the treatment of malocclusion, Angle Orthod. **11**:5-67, 1941.
33. Downs, W.B.: Variations in facial relationships: their significance in treatment and prognosis, Am. J. Orthod. **34**:812-840, 1948.
34. Thurow, R.C.: Atlas of orthodontic principles, ed. 2, St. Louis, 1977, The C.V. Mosby Co.
35. Kloehn, S.J.: Guiding alveolar growth and eruption of teeth to reduce treatment time and produce a more balanced denture and face, Angle Orthod. **17**:10-33, 1947.
36. Haack, D.C., and Weinstein, S.: The mechanics of centric and eccentric cervical traction, Am. J. Orthod. **44**:346-357, 1958.
37. Thurow, R.C.: Craniomaxillary orthopedic correction with en masse dental control, Am. J. Orthod. **68**:601-624, 1975.

Glossary

abscissa The horizontal axis of a graph; values are plotted by measuring in a horizontal direction from the vertical axis of ordinates.

acrylic Methyl methacrylate, an organic resin commonly used for the construction of dental appliances including orthodontic treatment and retention appliances.

alveolar bone The bone that provides the immediate support of the roots of the teeth.

anchorage The supporting base for orthodontic forces that are applied to stimulate tooth movement; the area of application of the reciprocal forces that are generated when corrective forces are applied to teeth. May be one or more teeth in either jaw, environmental musculature, the neck, or the cranium.

- **cervical anchorage** Extraoral anchorage based at the back of the neck.
- **cranial anchorage** Extraoral anchorage based at the back of the skull.
- **differential anchorage** A force distribution system in which movement of teeth providing reciprocal resistance is minimized. See *differential force.*
- **extraoral anchorage** Orthodontic anchorage based outside of the mouth. Dental attachments are typically linked to a wire bow or hooks extending between the lips and attached elastically to a cap, a strap around the neck, or other extraoral device.
- **facial anchorage** Extraoral anchorage based on the face, usually the chin and forehead.
- **intermaxillary anchorage** Anchorage based in the opposite jaw.
- **intramaxillary anchorage** Anchorage based on teeth within the same jaw.
- **intraoral anchorage** Anchorage based within the mouth (intermaxillary, intramaxillary, or muscular).
- **occipital anchorage** Cranial anchorage based in the occipital area of the head.
- **reciprocal anchorage** All anchorage is reciprocal; sometimes used to describe a force system in which movement of the resistance units is a desired response, as opposed to differential anchorage where movement of resistance units is to be minimized.
- **simple anchorage** Use of a tooth as a resistance unit without tipping control.
- **"stationary" anchorage** Use of a tooth as an anchorage unit with tipping control.

ankylosis Abnormal fixation and immobility. May occur in bony joints or in the attachment between the roots of teeth and supporting bone. In the case of teeth a part of the periodontal membrane is replaced by a direct bony union between tooth and bone; this prevents normal functional movements, eruption, and orthodontic movement.

apical movement Movement in an apical direction, opposite to the normal direction of eruption; intrusion.

appliance (orthodontic) Any device used for the purpose of influencing tooth position.

archwire A wire secured to two or more teeth through fixed attachments to cause, guide, or control orthodontic tooth movement.

- **full archwire** An archwire extending from the molar region of one side of a dental arch to the other.

sectional archwire An archwire extending to only few teeth, usually within a short arch segment.

axis (of rotation) The line about which an object rotates; does not necessarily coincide with any physical entity.

band (orthodontic) A thin metal ring, usually stainless steel, which serves to secure orthodontic attachments to a tooth. The band, with orthodontic attachments permanently fused to it, is closely adapted to fit the contours of a tooth and cemented to that tooth.

beam Any relatively slender structure subjected to lateral (bending) loads; an orthodontic archwire functions mechanically as a beam.

bending moment A measure of the bending effort at any specified point in a beam; measured in units of force times distance (ounce-inches, gram-centimeters, etc.).

bending rate The ratio between force and deflection in bending: $\frac{\text{force}}{\text{deflection}}$; spring rate; an index of stiffness in bending.

biteplane (or biteplate) A removable orthodontic appliance designed to occlude with teeth (usually anterior) in the opposing jaw.

bodily movement (translatory movement) Orthodontic movement of a tooth in a horizontal direction with no change in axial inclination; crown and root move the same distance.

bonding Adhesion of an orthodontic attachment directly to a tooth without the use of an interposed band.

direct bonding Individual placement of attachments on the teeth at the time of adhesion. This term is sometimes also used to describe all bonding, because the attachment is bonded directly to the tooth.

indirect bonding Positioning of attachments on a dental cast and transferring them to the teeth en masse by means of a molded matrix for simultaneous adhesion.

bracket An orthodontic attachment secured to a tooth for the purpose of engaging an archwire. The distinguishing feature of the edgewise appliance is bracket design.

buccal Pertaining to the cheek. Used to identify surfaces of the teeth that face toward the cheek and a direction toward the cheek. "Labial" has the same meaning in relation to the lips; "facial" encompasses both terms. In this book "buccal" also encompasses both terms, since the labial musculature is merely a decussation of the buccinator.

c The distance from neutral axis to extreme fiber in the cross-section of a loaded beam; this value is used in the determination of the stiffness, strength, and working range of the beam; in the bending formula, $c = \frac{I}{Z}$; for round wire, c is equal to the radius.

cephalometric radiograph A radiograph of the head made with precise reproducible relationships between x-ray source, subject, and film.

cervical appliance An extraoral appliance that uses the back of the neck as a base (cervical anchorage) for traction to the teeth.

closed bite Excessive vertical overlap (overbite) of the anterior teeth.

coil diameter The diameter of a coil spring, measured from the center of the wire on one side of the coil to the center of the wire on the opposite side.

collateral movement Movement of a tooth in response to an applied force, in addition to the intended movement and in a different direction or arc, due to the alignment of the force in relation to the support of the tooth.

condyle The articular surface at the superior end of the mandibular ramus that engages the articular fossa of the temporal bone.

couple Two equal forces operating on an object in parallel but opposite directions; a couple has a purely rotating effect that can be expressed as a moment, equal to the value of one of the forces multiplied by the distance between their lines of action.

critical section The section of a beam that is subjected to the highest bending moment and that will therefore be the first section to undergo plastic deformation and failure under increasing load; this may also be called the dangerous section.

crossbite An abnormal relationship of a tooth or teeth to the opposing teeth in which normal buccolingual relationships are reversed.

debanding The removal of cemented orthodontic bands.

debonding The detachment of bonded orthodontic attachments from the teeth.

deep bite Excessive overbite; closed bite.

deflection (beam) The distance that a specific point on a beam moves as the beam is bent under load; usually measured at the point where deflection is greatest (maximum deflection): maximum deflection describes the maximum deflection under a given load, *not* the maximum attainable under maximum load.

dentofacial orthopedics A more descriptive synonym for orthodontics; the adjustment of relationships between and among teeth and facial bones by the application of outside forces and/or the stimulation and redirection of functional forces within the craniofacial complex.

depression (dental); apical movement; intrusion Movement of a tooth in an apical direction, opposite to the direction of eruption.

developmental guidance See *guidance.*

die A metal block with an accurately formed hole through which material to be shaped is forced; a rod or wire may be formed by drawing the material through the die or by extrusion through the die under pressure; the opening in the die is lined with a hard material to resist wear; dies with internal threads are also used to cut screw threads on the external surfaces of rods by screwing the rods through the dies.

differential force A term sometimes used to describe the design and application of an orthodontic appliance to distribute the reciprocal forces of the appliance over significantly different root areas with the objective of eliciting a differential response from different teeth. Most orthodontic forces are applied in this way; the distinction is largely a matter of emphasis of objectives.

distal A direction oriented along the dental arch away from the dental midline; right or left in the anterior segment, posteriorly in the buccal segments.

drawing The process of pulling a metal rod or wire through a die to reduce its size and in some cases to alter its shape; the metal is literally squeezed to the shape of the die as it is pulled through; drawing is the basic wire-making process.

edgewise appliance A fixed orthodontic appliance, the last of those developed by E.H. Angle. It is characterized by attachment brackets with a rectangular slot for engagement of a round archwire in one plane or a rectangular archwire in two planes, with ligation adding engagement in another plan in either case.

elastic curve See *stress-strain diagram.*

elastic deformation Change in shape, brought about by mechanical force, within the elastic (proportional) limit of the material; the original form is recovered on removal of the deforming force; See *plastic deformation.*

elastic (or elastomeric) ligature An elastic thread or ring used to fasten an archwire to a tooth or to apply traction to a tooth.

elastic limit See *proportional limit.*

elastic modulus Modulus of elasticity.

elasticity The mechanical behavior of materials as they undergo changes in shape when subjected to force and return to their original shape on removal of the force.

equilibrate Reshaping the occlusal (functional) surfaces of teeth to alter functional relationships, redistributing and balancing functional loads.

extraoral anchorage Orthodontic force applied from a base outside the mouth. See *anchorage.*

extreme fiber The line in a bending beam or twisting bar that lies farthest from the neutral axis; usually the part subjected to the greatest distortion (strain).

extrusion (dental) Orthodontic movement of a tooth in an occlusal direction (the direction of eruption) from its position in the alveolar process.

extrusion (engineering) A method of forming metal or plastic in which the material is squeezed out through a small hole (die), much as toothpaste is squeezed from a tube; this method is used to form both solid and hollow shapes (rods, bars, tubes, etc.).

eyelet; staple An attachment placed on an orthodontic band in the original edgewise technique for attachment of a ligature.

facial Of or toward the face. Used to identify the surface of a tooth that lies toward the face, encompassing both buccal direction and labial direction.

flexibility A nonspecific term denoting ease of bending; it may indicate low stiffness, low strength, low working range, or low brittleness, either singly or in any combination.

free-body analysis Analysis of static forces by the figurative isolation of a part of a mechanism as a free body; all internal and all external forces in such a system must be in balance (add algebraically to zero), and this fact is used to determine the unknown forces.

freeway space Clearance between upper and lower teeth when the jaw is at rest (rest position).

fulcrum The point of support for a lever; the fulcrum may also be a point of rotation, but a point of rotation is *not* a fulcrum unless it also provides mechanical support; the point in the root of a tooth about which the tooth may tip is an axis of rotation, not a fulcrum.

gingiva(e) The tissue that immediately surrounds the tooth where it emerges from the alveolar process, consisting of fibrous tissue that is continuous with the periodontal ligament and a mucosal covering that is continuous with the lining of the mouth.

gingival attachment The fibrous attachment of the gingivae to the tooth.

growth Increase in size (as compared to development, which also includes changes in function).

guidance (developmental) Comprehensive dentofacial orthopedic control over the growth of the jaws and eruption of the teeth, with the objective of optimizing the achievement of the genetic potential of the individual. Requires a combination of carefully timed active appliance therapy and supervisory examinations, including radiography and other diagnostic records, at various stages of development.

Hawley retainer A removable plastic and wire appliance used to stabilize the teeth of the upper arch, developed by Charles Hawley. Often modified for special applications.

headgear Common generic term for extraoral traction.

high pull headgear An extraoral appliance designed to apply traction to the upper dental arch from a base above the level of the occlusal plane.

hinge axis The axis of mandibular rotation in the initial opening movement; usually passes approximately through the mandibular condyles.

Hooke's law The basic law of elastic response stating that stress is proportional to strain;

such response will be evidenced by a straight-line elastic curve: See *elasticity*, *stress*, and *strain*.

I Usual symbol for moment of inertia in bending: I = cZ.
impaction Inhibition or prevention of full eruption of a tooth by the blocking effect of another tooth, bone, or soft tissue.
infraocclusion A tooth or teeth below the normal level of occlusion.
ingot The metal casting that is the raw material for such fabrication processes as rolling and drawing of rod or wire.
intermaxillary Between upper and lower jaws.
elastic traction Use of rubber elastics to apply traction between upper and lower arches.
interocclusal clearance Clearance between upper and lower teeth when the mandible is in the postural resting position (freeway space).
intramaxillary Within the upper or lower dental arch.
elastic traction The use of elastic bands to apply traction between teeth in the same arch.
intrusion; depression Apical movement of a tooth in the direction of its long axis, opposite to the normal direction of eruption.

J Usual symbol for moment of inertia in torsion: J = cZ.
jackscrew A threaded device used to apply force between teeth or groups of teeth; typically used to widen the upper arch.

Kloehn cervical appliance The classical cervical extraoral traction appliance introduced by S.J. Kloehn. Uses a relatively light and flexible (.045-inch or 1.15-mm) inner arch rigidly attached to a long outer bow.

labial Of or pertaining to the lip. Also used to identify a surface facing the lips or a direction toward the lips. See *buccal.*
ligature A tie used to secure individual teeth to an orthodontic archwire, typically wire or elastomeric material.
linear force A force acting in a straight line; measurement is in simple force units, such as pounds or grams.
lingual Of or pertaining to the tongue. Used to describe surfaces and directions facing the tongue. See *buccal.*
load Force applied to a beam (such as an archwire) or other mechanism.

mal Prefix denoting a bad or unfavorable condition.
occlusion (relationship of teeth in occlusion). A deviation in intramaxillary and/or intermaxillary relations of teeth that presents a hazard to the individual's well-being. Often associated with other dentofacial deformities.
maximum bending moment The highest bending moment in a beam under any specific loading conditions; this maximum bending moment is one limiting factor on the capacity of a beam, and its location and measurement are important considerations in design.
maximum working load The maximum load that can be sustained within the working range of deformation
mesial Toward or facing the midline, following the dental arch. Used to describe surfaces of teeth as well as direction.
mil One thousandth of an inch (.001 inch); See *Appendix B* for conversion tables.

mixed dentition The developmental stage during which both deciduous and permanent teeth are present in the mouth (approximately 6 to 12 years old).
modulus of elasticity Ratio between unit stress and unit strain, usually expressed as pounds per square inch; an index of stiffness. See p. 54.
molar sheath See *molar tube.*
molar tube (edgewise); molar sheath A rectangular tube attached to the buccal surface of the last banded molar on each side to receive and restrain the ends of the archwire.
moment A measurement of rotational effort; moments are measured by the product of the applied force multiplied by the length of the moment arm; typical units are ounce-inches, pound-feet, and gram-centimeters.
moment arm The distance from the fulcrum to the line of a force associated with a rotation; measured over the shortest distance from the fulcrum to the line of the force, which is along a line lying perpendicular to the line of the force.
moment of inertia (of beams) A property of the cross-section of a beam that is proportional to the effect of the cross-section on resistance to bending or twisting (stiffness); the usual symbol for moment of inertia in bending is I; in torsion the usual symbol is J; I = cZ; J = cZ. See *Appendix A* for additional formulas and figures.

negative pressure In tooth movement, the local condition in which a tooth is moved in such a way that the volume of the periodontal space is increased beyond its normal resting volume; See *pressure* and *tension.*
negative tension In tooth movement, the local condition in which the periodontal fibers are subjected to less than their normal resting tension (shortened). See *tension* and *pressure.*
neutral axis The part of a beam that is neither elongated nor compressed in bending; in a symmetrical beam the neutral axis is a plane through the long axis perpendicular to the plane of bending; in torsion it is the axial center.
normal (engineering) Lying (or directed) at a right angle.

occlusal Pertaining to the chewing surfaces of the posterior teeth. May be used to identify those tooth surfaces as well as the direction toward the occlusal plane (upward in the lower arch, downward in the upper).
movement Movement of a tooth in an occlusal direction; extrusion.
plane The imaginary plane on which the teeth meet in occlusion. It is actually a compound curved surface but is commonly approximated by a plane (straight line in the lateral view) based on specific reference points within the dental arches.
occlusion The relationship of the maxillary and mandibular teeth as they are brought into functional contact.
open bite A malocclusion in which some teeth cannot be brought into functional contact with opposing teeth.
ordinate The vertical axis of a graph; values are plotted by measuring in a vertical direction from the horizontal axis or abscissa.
origin (of a graph) The intersection of the vertical and horizontal axes, at which values on both scales are zero.
ortho A prefix denoting straight or correct.
dontic related to the orthopedic correction of abnormal dental relationship, including related abnormalities in facial structures.
pedic correction of abnormal form or relationship of bone structures. May be accomplished surgically (orthopedic surgery) or by the application of appliances to stimulate changes in the bone structure by natural physiologic response (orthopedic therapy). Orthodontic therapy is orthopedic therapy applied through the teeth.

osteotomy Surgical procedure involving the cutting of bone.

overbite Vertical overlapping of upper teeth over lower teeth, usually measured perpendicular to the occlusal plane.

overjet Horizontal projection of upper teeth beyond the lower teeth, usually measured parallel to the occlusal plane. When not otherwise specified, the term is generally assumed to refer to central incisors and is measured from the labial surface of the lower to the labial surface of the upper at the level of the upper incisor edge. Unique conditions may sometimes require other measuring techniques.

periodontal fibers The connective tissue fibers in the periodontal membrane that attach tooth to bone; these are inelastic fibers, and their ends are embedded in the cementum of the root and in the supporting bone.

periodontal membrane (or ligament) The tissue that occupies the space between tooth root and alveolar bone, providing physical attachment of the tooth to the bone. It also provides nourishment to the bone and cementum surface of the root.

periodontium The investing and supporting tissues of the teeth; the periodontal membrane and alveolar bone.

plastic deformation Change in shape, brought about by outside force in excess of the elastic (proportional) limit of the material; the original form will *not* be recovered on removal of such force; plastic deformation is a permanent change in shape (permanent set).

positioner A removable elastic orthodontic finishing appliance, typically used to achieve fine adjustments and retain corrected positions in the finishing stages of treatment. Fabricated by molding to fit the teeth in a "setup" made by repositioning the teeth from a plaster cast. The material may be rubber or elastomeric plastic.

pressure A compressive stress; in tooth movement, the local condition in which a tooth is moved in such a way as to reduce the volume of the periodontal space below its normal resting volume. See *negative pressure* and *negative tension.*

progressive appliance placement Placing orthodontic attachments on the teeth successively over a period of time as dictated by treatment needs, as opposed to placement of all attachments at the beginning of treatment.

proportional limit; elastic limit The maximum load or deformation that can be attained under Hooke's law; exceeding this limit will bring about increased deformation proportionately greater than the increase in load, with permanent plastic deformation.

protrusion Teeth and/or jaws protruding farther forward than normal.

radiograph A permanent image, typically on film, of an image produced by ionizing radiation. Sometimes incorrectly called an "X ray" after the most common source of image-producing radiation.

range; working range The maximum deformation that can be sustained without exceeding arbitrary limits of plastic deformation; range is inversely proportional to "c"; in this book, range is generally shown as a relative value, comparing different materials or forms of wire with one another.

reciprocal forces The typical method of applying corrective orthodontic forces; each applied force is balanced by a reciprocal force elsewhere in the definition or surrounding structures.

reciprocal movement Movement of teeth or groups of teeth in response to reciprocally applied forces. Variously used to emphasize the movement of teeth at opposite ends of the force distribution mechanism.

resiliency The capacity of a material for the elastic storage of energy; depends on the *combined* effects of stiffness and working range; resiliency is a property of the material itself and is unrelated to size or form.

resorption Physiologic or pathologic removal of hard tissue (bone or root) by the activity of multinucleated giant cells (osteoclasts).

rest position The normal resting position of the mandible, with teeth apart and muscles relaxed.

retainer Any orthodontic appliance, fixed or removable, used to maintain teeth in corrected positions during the period of functional adaptation following corrective treatment.

retention The passive treatment period following active orthodontic correction during which retaining appliances may be used. May also include fine adjustments of individual tooth positions.

retraction Orthodontic movement of teeth in a posterior (distal) direction.

retrusion Teeth and/or jaws posterior to their normal positions.

ribbon arch appliance An appliance developed by E.H. Angle prior to the edgewise appliance, using a rectangular wire in a vertical rather than horizontal (edgewise) slot to gain multidirectional control.

rolling A process for shaping metal bars or sheets by passing them through successive pairs of rollers; rolling may be carried out at high or low (room) temperatures.

root movement Orthodontic movement in which the root of a tooth is moved without moving the crown, or with minimal crown movement, as in uprighting.

rotation, axial Rotation of a tooth around the long axis of the root; direction of such rotation is defined by the relative change in position of the buccal or labial surface in relation to the axis (unrelated to other movements that may simultaneously shift the axis in the same or opposite direction).

rotation, tipping The rotation of a tooth around a horizontal axis. See *tipping*.

section modulus A value of the cross-section of a beam proportional to maximum load-carrying capacity (strength); the usual symbol is Z in both bending and torsion, although values are different in each case: $Z = \frac{I}{c}$. See *Appendix A* for additional formulas and specific values.

separation An orthodontic procedure for slightly separating teeth in order to place bands on them for orthodontic attachments.

setup A laboratory procedure in which teeth are removed from a plaster cast and repositioned in wax. May be used as a diagnostic tool to evaluate alternatives, as when some teeth are missing; also used to produce the mold to make a positioner appliance.

shear modulus A value comparable to the modulus of elasticity based on a shear stress instead of a tension stress: an index of stiffness in shear (including torsion).

sheath a synonym for a tube used as an orthodontic attachment.

simple tipping See *tipping, simple.*

sliding (in tooth movement) The local situation in orthodontic tooth movement in which the surface of the root moves essentially parallel to the surface of the adjacent bone; may occur alone or in combination with pressure or tension.

slope (of a curve) The ratio between increases in ordinate and abscissa at any point on the curve; steepness of the curve; determined by the slope of the tangent to the curve at the point in question.

space maintainer A prosthetic replacement for prematurely lost deciduous teeth, intended to prevent closure of the space before eruption of the permanent successors.

Spee, curve of The anteroposterior curvature of the mandibular occlusal "plane" from cuspids to terminal molars. Normally concave upward.

split palate A removable palatal orthodontic appliance that is divided in the sagittal plane with the two halves connected only by a jackscrew that is progressively lengthened to widen the palate and upper dental arch.

spring rate; spring constant; bending rate The ratio between force and deflection: $\frac{\text{force}}{\text{deflection}}$; an index of stiffness.

staple See *eyelet.*

static analysis Analysis of static forces, both within and outside a mechanism; see free-body analysis.

statics The field of engineering concerned with static forces and their effects (forces without associated motion).

stiffness Resistance to elastic deformation; in bending or torsion, stiffness in a measure of the amount of force required to produce a specified deformation; the stiffness of a wire is proportional to the moment of inertia of its cross section; there is no consistent relationship between stiffness and strength or range.

stop A bend or auxiliary attachment placed on a wire to limit its sliding into a tube or other orthodontic attachment.

strain Change of shape (deformation) of a structure such as an orthodontic wire or the periodontal fibers when a force (stress) is applied.

strength Capacity to resist a deforming load without exceeding arbitrary limits of plastic deformation; depends on both stiffness and range but bears no consistent relation to either one alone; used here to describe properties of materials, wire sizes, and beam configurations; strength is proportional to the resiliency of materials and to the section modulus of beams.

stress Force applied to a mechanical structure; application of stress produces deformation (strain) within the structure; stress may be from an outside source or from forces within the material (such as those produced in heating, cooling, or work hardening).

stress-strain diagram A graph showing the relationship of stress and strain as a material is subjected to increasing loads; usually plotted with stress as the ordinate and strain as the abscissa; the curve produced in this diagram may also be called the elastic curve.

tensile curve The elastic curve (Stress-strain diagram) for a material subjected to a tensile force.

tension An extending stress; in tooth movement, the local condition in which a tooth is moved in such a way as to extend the periodontal fibers beyond their normal resting length; See *negative tension* and *negative pressure.*

tipping; mesial, distal, buccal, or lingual Tipping movement in which the position of the crown is shifted in the direction specified in relation to the apex of the root; this may involve *any* combination of crown or root movement; the *only* change defined by these terms is in the relationship of crown to root.

tipping, simple Moving a tooth by applying force to the crown without control over tipping; the tooth tips, with rotation around a horizontal axis usually lying in the mid-root area.

torque (engineering) A force (stress) causing twist in a structure; the resulting twist of the mechanical part is called torsion; torque and torsion therefore occur together; for this application, the word *torsion* is used instead of *torque* in this book wherever possible to avoid confusion with *torque* as it is used in the orthodontic sense; torque is measured as a moment, in pound-feet, ounce-inches, gram-centimeters, etc.

torque (orthodontic) Buccolingual root tipping in which movement of the crown is minimized and movement of the root apex is maximized. Usually accomplished orthodontically through the application of force by means of mechanical torsion in the archwire.

torsion A twisting strain in a material; torsion is the result of a twisting force (torque); torsion is measured in degrees of twist; since torque and torsion exist together, this situation is described in this book as torsion whenever possible to help differentiate from torque as it is used in the orthodontic sense.

traction The act of pulling, usually by an elastic force.

transitional dentition The final phase of the transition from deciduous to permanent teeth in which most deciduous teeth have been lost or are in the process of shedding and the permanent successors are not yet in function.

transseptal fibers Gingival fibers traversing the septum between teeth, providing a fibrous connection between the teeth.

translation Horizontal (in relation to the alveolar process) tooth movement in which the axial inclination of the root is unchanged.

tube See *molar tube.*

tuberosity The posterior end of the maxillary alveolar process.

uprighting Tipping a tooth into a more vertical position, usually by moving the apex of the root instead of the crown.

vector A translatory action that may be defined by force magnitude and direction, unrelated to point of application; a vector is a purely linear effect; in most orthodontic applications it will exist in combination with a moment of rotation.

work hardening Change in the internal structure of metal, brought about by plastic deformation; in work hardening, the crystalline structure becomes more rigid and the elastic limit is increased.

working range See *range.*

Young's modulus Modulus of elasticity.

Z Symbol for section modulus: $Z = \frac{I}{c}$.

APPENDIX **A**

Tables of properties of wire sections in bending and torsion

The elastic behavior of wires when they are bent or twisted depends on the size and shape of their cross-section.

Tables 1 to 3 present the values for physical constants that determine this behavior. Absolute values are shown, but these can usually be applied in practice by simply comparing the appropriate values for different wires as a ratio.

These values are absolute physical constants of the cross-sections. They are completely independent of the physical properties of the structural material and the form of the mechanism in which they are used. Such other factors affect stiffness, strength, and range in their own right, *in addition to* these properties of the cross-section.

Descriptions of these individual properties follow:

Wire size refers to the diameter of round wires and to the width and thickness of rectangular wires. This is shown in mils (thousandths of an inch).

c is the distance from the neutral axis to the extreme fiber in bending and from the center to the extreme fiber in torsion. For round wires, *c* is equal to the radius for both bending and torsion. For rectangular wires, *c* is one-half the thickness in the plane of bending and one-half the diagonal in torsion.

c is inversely proportional to working range, the amount that a wire may be bent or twisted without taking a permanent set.

In terms of the two following values:

$$c = \frac{I}{Z}$$

Values of c in Tables 1 to 3 are shown in mils.

Moment of inertia (I for bending, J for torsion) is proportional to stiffness, the force that is required to produce a bend or a twist.

For round wires:

$$I = \frac{\pi d^4}{64}$$

$$J = \frac{\pi d^4}{32}$$

where d = diameter of the wire.

For rectangular wires:

$$I = \frac{wt^3}{12}$$

$$J = \frac{\pi\, t^2\, w\, \sqrt{t^2 + w^2}}{32}$$

where w = width and t = thickness in the plane of bending. In torsion, t must be less than w.

In terms of the other two characteristics:

$$I = cZ$$

$$J = cZ$$

Values in Tables 1 to 3 are shown in inches $\times\ 10^{-12}$, which means that true values in inches will be obtained by moving the decimal twelve places to the left. This can be ignored in making relative comparisons.

Section modulus (Z) is proportional to strength, the maximum force that a wire can apply or support without sustaining a permanent set.

Section modulus is equal to the moment of inertia divided by the value c.

$$Z = \frac{I}{c}$$

Values in Tables 1 to 3 on the following pages are shown in inches $\times\ 10^{-9}$.

Table 1. Properties of round wire sections

		Bending		Torsion	
Diameter (mils)	c (mils)	Section modulus (Z) (inches × 10^{-9})	Moment of inertia (I) (inches × 10^{-12})	Polar section modulus (Z) (inches × 10^{-9})	Polar moment of inertia (J) (inches × 10^{-12})
5	2.5	12.272	30.680	24.544	61.36
6	3.0	21.256	63.617	42.412	127.24
7	3.5	33.674	117.86	67.348	235.72
8	4.0	50.265	201.06	100.53	402.12
9	4.5	71.569	322.06	143.14	644.13
10	5.0	98.175	490.88	196.35	981.75
11	5.5	130.67	718.69	261.34	1,437.4
12	6.0	169.65	1,017.9	339.29	2,035.8
13	6.5	215.69	1,402.0	431.38	2,804.0
14	7.0	269.39	1,885.8	538.78	3,771.5
15	7.5	331.34	2,485.1	662.68	4,970.1
16	8.0	402.12	3,217.0	804.25	6,434.0
17	8.5	482.33	4,099.8	964.67	8,199.7
18	9.0	572.56	5,153.0	1,145.1	10,306
19	9.5	673.38	6,397.1	1,346.8	12,794
20	10.0	785.40	7,854.0	1,570.8	15,708
21	10.5	909.20	9,546.6	1,818.4	19,093
22	11.0	1,045.4	11,500	2,090.7	22,998
24	12.0	1,357.2	16,286	2,714.3	32,572
26	13.0	1,725.5	22,432	3,451.1	44,870
28	14.0	2,155.1	30,172	4,310.3	60,344
30	15.0	2,650.7	39,761	5,301.5	79,522
32	16.0	3,217.0	51,472	6,434.0	102,940
36	18.0	4,580.5	82,448	9,160.9	164,900
40	20.0	6,283.2	125,660	12,566	251,330
45	22.5	8,946.2	201,290	17,892	402,580
50	25.0	12,272	306,800	24,544	613,600
55	27.5	16,334	449,180	32,668	898,360
60	30.0	21,206	636,180	42,412	1,272,300
70	35.0	33,674	1,178,600	67,348	2,357,200
80	40.0	50,266	2,010,600	100,530	4,021,200

Table 2. Properties of rectangular wire sections in bending

Wire size (mils)	Direction of bending	c (mils)	Section modulus (Z) (inches × 10^{-9})	Moment of inertia (I) (inches × 10^{-12})
8 × 20	Edgewise	10.0	533.3	5,333.3
	Flat	4.0	213.3	853.3
8 × 25	Edgewise	12.5	833.3	10,416.6
	Flat	4.0	266.7	1,066.7
8 × 28	Edgewise	14.0	1,045.3	14,634.7
	Flat	4.0	298.7	1,194.7
8 × 32	Edgewise	16.0	1,365.3	21,845.3
	Flat	4.0	341.3	1,365.3
10 × 20	Edgewise	10.0	666.7	6,666.7
	Flat	5.0	333.3	1,666.7
10 × 25	Edgewise	12.5	1,041.7	13,020.8
	Flat	5.0	416.7	2,083.3
10 × 28	Edgewise	14.0	1,306.7	18,293.3
	Flat	5.0	466.7	2,333.3
11 × 22	Edgewise	11.0	887.3	9,760.7
	Flat	5.5	443.7	2,440.2
11 × 25	Edgewise	12.5	1,145.8	14,322.9
	Flat	5.5	504.2	2,772.9
11 × 28	Edgewise	14.0	1,437.3	20,122.7
	Flat	5.5	564.7	3,105.7
16 × 16	Either	8.0	682.7	5,461.3
16 × 22	Edgewise	11.0	1,290.7	14,197.3
	Flat	8.0	938.7	7,509.3
16 × 25	Edgewise	12.5	1,666.7	20,833.3
	Flat	8.0	1,066.7	8,533.3
16 × 28	Edgewise	14.0	2,090.7	29,269.3
	Flat	8.0	1,194.7	9,557.3
17 × 17	Either	8.5	818.8	6,960.1
17 × 22	Edgewise	11.0	1,371.4	15,084.7
	Flat	8.5	1.059.6	9,007.2
17 × 25	Edgewise	12.5	1,770.8	22,135.4
	Flat	8.5	1,204.1	10,235.4
17 × 28	Edgewise	14.0	2,221.4	31,098.7
	Flat	8.5	1,348.7	11,463.7
18 × 18	Either	9.0	972.0	8,748.0
18 × 22	Edgewise	11.0	1,452.0	15,972.0
	Flat	9.0	1,188.0	10,692.0
18 × 25	Edgewise	12.5	1,875.0	23,438.0
	Flat	9.0	1,350.0	12,150.0
18 × 28	Edgewise	14.0	2,352.0	32,928.0
	Flat	9.0	1,512.0	13,608.0

Table 2. Properties of rectangular wire sections in bending—cont'd

Wire size (mils)	Direction of bending	c (mils)	Section modulus (Z) (inches × 10^{-9})	Moment of inertia (I) (inches × 10^{-12})
21 × 21	Either	10.5	1,543.5	16,207
21 × 25	Edgewise	12.5	2,187.5	27,344
	Flat	10.5	1,837.5	19,294
21 × 28	Edgewise	14.0	2,744.0	38,416
	Flat	10.5	2,058.0	21,609
22 × 22	Either	11.0	1,774.6	19,521
22 × 25	Edgewise	12.5	2,291.7	28,646
	Flat	11.0	2,016.6	22,183
22 × 28	Edgewise	14.0	2,874.6	40,245
	Flat	11.0	2,258.6	24,845

Table 3. Properties of rectangular wire sections in torsion

Wire size (mils)	c (mils)	Polar section modulus (Z) (inches × 10^{-9})	Polar moment of inertia (J) (inches × 10^{-12})
8 × 20	10.78	251.33	2,709.3
8 × 25	13.12	314.16	4,121.7
8 × 28	14.56	351.86	5,123.1
8 × 32	16.49	402.12	6,631.0
10 × 20	11.18	392.70	4,390.4
10 × 25	13.46	490.88	6,607.2
10 × 28	14.87	549.78	8,175.2
11 × 22	12.30	522.68	6,429.0
11 × 25	13.66	593.96	8,113.5
11 × 28	15.04	665.23	10,005.1
16 × 16	11.31	804.25	9,096.1
16 × 22	13.60	1,105.84	15,039.4
16 × 25	14.84	1,256.64	18,648.5
16 × 28	16.12	1,407.44	22,687.9
17 × 17	12.02	964.67	11,595.3
17 × 22	13.90	1,248.39	17,352.6
17 × 25	15.11	1,418.63	21,435.5
17 × 28	16.38	1,588.86	26,022.3
18 × 18	12.73	1,145.11	14,577.3
18 × 22	14.21	1,399.58	19,888.0
18 × 25	15.40	1,590.43	24,492.6
18 × 28	16.64	1,781.28	29,640.5
21 × 21	14.85	1,818.39	27,003.1
21 × 25	16.33	2,164.76	35,366.9
21 × 28	17.50	2,424.53	42,429.3
22 × 22	15.56	2,090.73	32,531.8
22 × 25	16.65	2,375.83	39,557.6
22 × 28	17.81	2,660.94	47,391.3

APPENDIX **B**

Metric-English conversion tables

Table 4 shows two columns for metric equivalents. The one labeled "exact" shows the precise value, and the one labeled "nominal" shows the rounded value that identifies an equivalent substitute for wires and similar appliance components. These are well within manufacturing tolerances for most wires. For slot or lumen sizes it is recommended that the exact value be consulted to determine tolerances and clearances.

Table 5 shows two columns for English equivalents. The one labeled "exact" shows the value rounded to the fifth decimal. The "nominal" value identifies the commercial equivalent for wires and similar appliance components. These are well within manufacturing tolerances for most wires. For slot or lumen sizes it is recommended that the exact value be consulted to determine tolerances and clearances.

Table 4. English to metric conversion (inches to millimeters)

English inches	Exact millimeters	Nominal millimeters
0.001	0.0254	
0.005	0.1270	
0.006	0.1524	0.15
0.007	0.1778	
0.008	0.2032	0.20
0.009	0.2286	
0.010	0.2540	0.25
0.011	0.2794	
0.012	0.3048	0.30
0.013	0.3302	
0.014	0.3556	0.35
0.015	0.3810	
0.016	0.4064	0.40
0.017	0.4318	
0.018	0.4572	0.45
0.019	0.4826	
0.020	0.5080	0.50
0.021	0.5334	
0.022	0.5588	0.55
0.023	0.5842	
0.024	0.6096	0.60
0.025	0.6350	
0.026	0.6604	0.65
0.027	0.6858	
0.028	0.7172	0.70
0.029	0.7366	
0.030	0.7620	0.75
0.031	0.7874	
0.032	0.8128	0.80
0.034	0.8636	0.85
0.035	0.8890	0.90
0.036	0.9144	
0.037	0.9398	
0.038	0.9652	0.95
0.039	0.9906	
0.040	1.0160	1.00
0.043	1.0922	
0.044	1.1176	1.10
0.045	1.1430	
0.046	1.1684	1.15
0.049	1.2446	
0.059	1.4986	
0.060	1.5240	1.50
0.065	1.6510	1.65
0.069	1.7526	1.75

Table 4. English to metric conversion (inches to millimeters)

English inches	Exact millimeters	Nominal millimeters
0.070	1.7780	
0.075	1.9050	1.90
0.079	2.0066	2.00
0.080	2.0320	
0.100	2.5400	
0.200	5.0800	
0.250	6.3500	
0.300	7.6200	
0.400	10.1600	
0.500	10.7000	
1.000	25.4000	

Table 5. Metric to English conversion (millimeters to inches)

Millimeters	Exact inches	Nominal inches
0.10	0.00397	0.004
0.15	0.00591	0.006
0.20	0.00787	0.008
0.25	0.00984	0.010
0.30	0.01181	0.012
0.35	0.01378	0.014
0.40	0.01575	0.016
0.45	0.01772	0.018
0.50	0.01969	0.020
0.55	0.02165	0.022
0.60	0.02362	0.024
0.65	0.02559	0.026
0.70	0.02756	0.028
0.75	0.02953	0.030
0.80	0.03150	0.031
0.85	0.03346	0.033
0.90	0.03543	0.035
0.95	0.03740	0.037
1.00	0.03937	0.039
1.05	0.04134	0.041
1.10	0.04331	0.043
1.15	0.04528	0.045
1.20	0.04724	0.047
1.25	0.04921	0.049
1.30	0.05118	0.051
1.35	0.05315	0.053
1.40	0.05512	0.055
1.45	0.05709	0.057
1.50	0.05906	0.059
1.55	0.06102	0.061
1.60	0.06299	0.063
1.65	0.06496	0.065
1.70	0.06693	0.067
1.75	0.06890	0.069
1.80	0.07087	0.071
1.85	0.07283	0.073
1.90	0.07480	0.075
1.95	0.07677	0.077
2.00	0.07874	0.079

Index

Page numbers in italics refer to main discussion.

D